BIRTH, DEVELOPMENT AND GROWTH

The Birth of a Baby

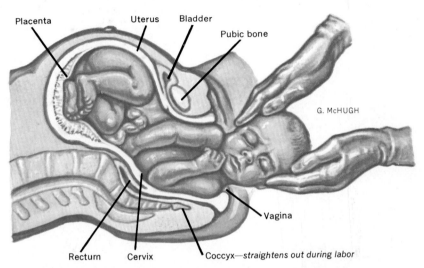

Delivery of the Baby is practically complete after the head—the largest presenting part—and the shoulders are out of the mother's pelvis. In this illustration the mother's abdomen is in contraction with a labor pain that is expelling the baby.

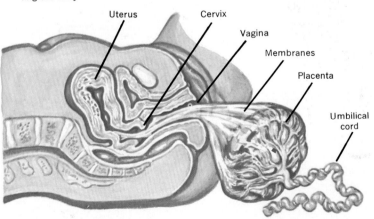

Delivery of the Placenta or Afterbirth occurs within 5 to 20 minutes after the baby's delivery. Here the membranes that enclosed the bag of waters are peeling away from the uterus. Note the dramatic contraction of the uterus after delivery. This seals off the blood vessels that had nourished the baby.

The Growth of the Fetus and the

Fetus is the term used for the developing child in the mother's womb. Pregnancy is calculated in lunar months of four weeks each and the period of gestation—from the time of conception to the time of birth—at forty weeks or ten lunar months. Births may occur two to four weeks earlier—the average time being thirty-eight weeks.

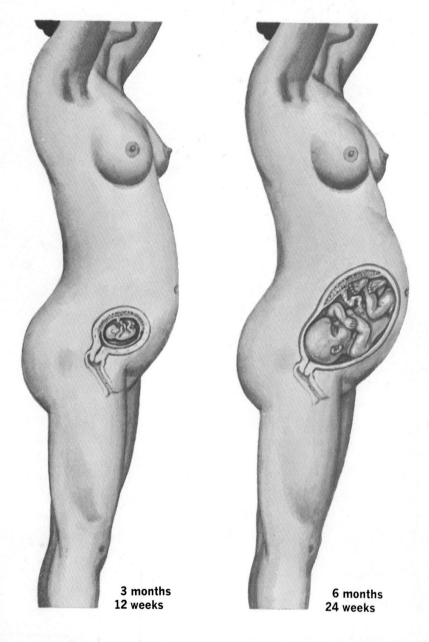

**3 months
12 weeks**

**6 months
24 weeks**

Changing Contours of Pregnancy

During the last two weeks of pregnancy the baby's head drops down into the mother's pelvis (lightening) and the contour of her abdomen suddenly changes, taking on a lower bulge as shown in the last figure. The average weight of the full term fetus is from seven to seven and one-half pounds with boys weighing slightly more than girls at birth.

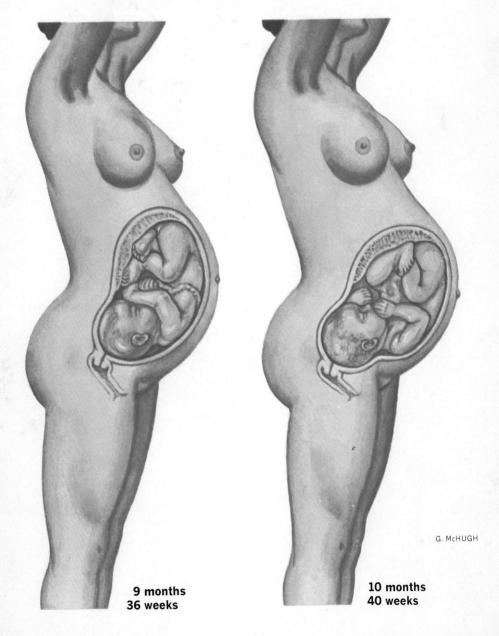

G. McHUGH

**9 months
36 weeks**

**10 months
40 weeks**

Growth and Development

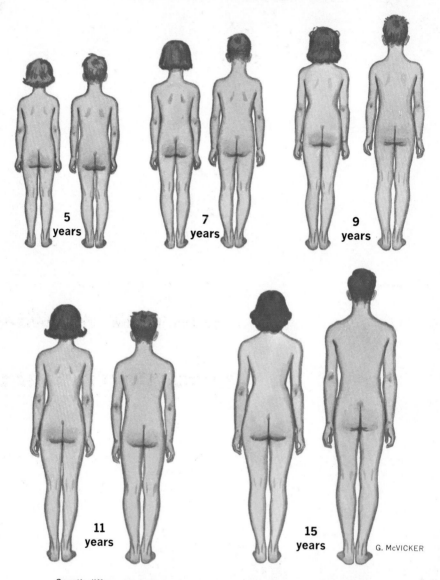

Growth differences between boys and girls are shown in this series of figures. During childhood the boy grows faster than the girl, but around age eleven the girl overtakes the boy and is temporarily taller. Girls mature earlier than boys, a state most apparent at junior high school age, and their growth is complete by age thirteen to fifteen. Boys continue to grow, reaching their maximum height at about seventeen. Growth rate slows after fifteen. When all the bones of the skeleton are completely ossified growth stops, but there may be many changes in body form after that. G. McH.

The figures and information on this page are based on studies made by Dr. Nancy Bayley at the University of California Institute of Child Welfare.

THE *New*

ILLUSTRATED

MEDICAL

and # HEALTH

ENCYCLOPEDIA

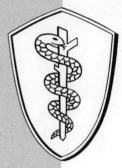

Home Library Edition

COMPLETE IN 4
VOLUMES

This 4 volume edition contains new
entries, illustrations, anatomical
charts and MEDIGRAPHS not
included in previous editions as
well as revised and up-dated entries
from the previous editions.

VOLUME

2

CHILD CARE
• • • • • • • • • • • •
HARELIP

THE *N*EW ILLUSTRATED MEDICAL and HEALTH ENCYCLOPEDIA

EDITED BY

MORRIS FISHBEIN, M.D.

EDITOR, Medical Progress
EDITOR, Modern Home Medical Advisor
EDITOR, Excerpta Medica
CONTRIBUTING EDITOR, Postgraduate Medicine
MEDICAL EDITOR, Encyclopedia Book of the Year
FORMERLY EDITOR, Journal of the American Medical Association

**With the Collaboration
of 27 Leading Specialists in
Medicine and Surgery**

H. S. STUTTMAN CO., Inc. *Publishers*
New York, N.Y. 10016

CHILD CARE. Many parents are bewildered by the responsibilities implied in the arrival of a new baby. They feel that they have before them a highly scientific task with which they, in their ignorance, will be unable to cope. This attitude is erroneous and should be discarded. There are facts about child care that should be known, but if parents use common sense and are really fond of their child they will not make serious mistakes.

At one time, pediatricians had their information neatly packeted in concise crisp form and parents were told exactly what to do for their babies in each situation. More recently, however, pediatricians have discovered that babies cannot be treated in this rigid fashion. Just as babies are different from one another in size, color, and other characteristics, so are they different from one another in their likes and dislikes, in their feelings and sleep habits, in their ways of growing, in their dispositions.

Babies should be treated as individuals; no one else can understand the idiosyncrasies of a baby as well as the parents. The parents should not expect the doctor to tell them what to do in every conceivable situation. He will guide and instruct the parents from his wealth of experience with babies in general, but they will have to adapt what he tells them to their own baby. Parents must learn to rely on their own judgment not only because of the child's individuality but also because it is only through this hard schooling that they really acquire the art of parenthood. Theoretical knowledge and expert advice cannot take the place of practical experience.

Modern pediatrics has returned to a "naturalistic" attitude toward child care. The natural attitudes which adults have assumed toward babies since the earliest days actually are the most desirable ones. It is good for the baby to be picked up from time to time, to be hugged and patted and rocked and sung to.

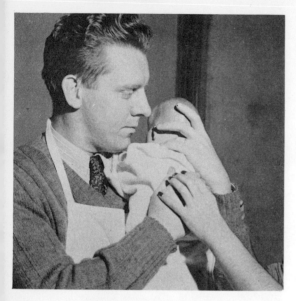

Child Care—Prospective fathers are interested in learning the correct ways of handling and caring for babies. In special classes for such gentlemen, instructions are given and techniques practiced until mastered. Photograph shows the correct placement of the hands and correct position of the baby for burping after feeding. Dolls are used for demonstration purposes.

Indeed, some pediatricians look to the time when the cradle will again have a place in the nursery.

Bringing up a baby should be a pleasure. If it is not, something is wrong with the situation. Parents will not enjoy their baby if they are worried because he is not getting enough vitamins or minerals, or because he had not been outdoors for several days, or because someone neglected to open a window in his room one night, or because he cried when a stranger approached, or because he weighs less than a neighbor's baby. Parents should learn to take it easy. If their baby is under a physician's care, they can assume

that he is getting an adequate diet. Being indoors for a week or even longer will not hurt him; and, as for the weight of a neighbor's baby, it should be remembered that, within reasonable limits, there is no relation between health, happiness and body weight. Babies thrive best in a warm, affectionate, orderly atmosphere.

Structure and growth. The average infant weighs about seven pounds at birth, girls generally weighing about half a pound less than boys. It is not unusual or abnormal for a child to weigh eight or even ten pounds. Babies born weighing less than five and a half pounds are classified as premature, regardless of how long the pregnancy has lasted, and require special care. Most babies will double their birth

Child Care—A prospective father is learning how to bathe and dry the baby while other fathers-to-be look on. The doll is quieter than a live infant, but it provides good practice in handling tiny humans.

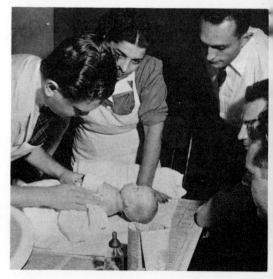

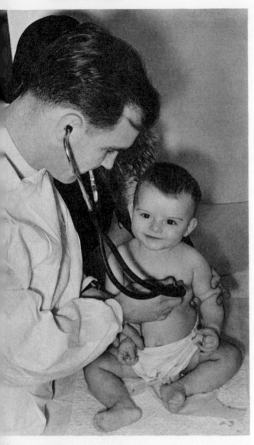

head size grows rapidly, increasing two and a half inches in circumference by the end of the first year. The bones of the skull are soft at birth and often the skull is misshapen from the effect of labor and may be molded right after delivery. An odd-shaped head should not cause alarm; within a few weeks the skull will assume a normal contour. Since the bones of the baby's skull are soft and easily molded into an incorrect shape, the infant should not lie in one position too long during the first year. He should lie on the left side after one feeding, on the right side after another, and be encouraged to sleep on both stomach and back. *Fontanelles,* the two soft spots in the skull, are places where the skull bones have not yet fused. The spot toward the back of the head usually fills in by the fourth

Cranial Measurements—The head grows rapidly during the baby's first year of life. The cranial measurements are being taken as a part of an extremely careful and thorough check-up.

Child Care—Regular physical examinations are very important in the baby's life, especially during the first year. The baby grows so quickly that changes must be carefully watched. Regular check-ups are valuable because indications of poor health or faulty nutrition are detected early. Photograph shows a healthy, happy baby undergoing a complete examination.

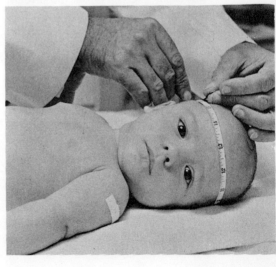

weight at six months of age and triple it at a year.

Length at birth is generally between nineteen and twenty-one inches and by the end of the first year the baby will have grown an additional ten inches. The baby's head and chest circumference should be equal at birth. Thereafter, the

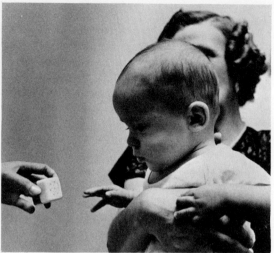

Mental Awareness—The mental alertness and awareness of the baby can be measured. Photograph shows a cube being held forward to test the prehensile and interest attitudes of the child. The baby's mental development as well as physical growth should be checked at frequent intervals.

the end of the second year. Sometimes a slippery floor or crowded play area, or ill-fitting shoes discourage the child from walking. Occasionally muscle disease, rickets, or nerve damage may be involved but this is rare. Parents should be patient with the child who is reluctant to start walking. Urging him to walk before he is ready can only make him insecure. Letting the child play with other toddlers will encourage him to imitate them and try to walk himself.

Seeing and hearing. At birth babies can distinguish between light and dark, but they are not able to

Blocks—What a child does with blocks is a good test of mental growth. Though monotonous to the adult observer, this girl's activities are everything one could desire of a child her age. Given a cup and a set of blocks, she will continue filling and emptying the cup endlessly until distracted.

month, and the spot in the front by the eighteenth month. Special care of the spots is not necessary, but they should not be disturbed.

Learning to walk. Some children will begin to creep about the seventh month, while others sometimes wait until as late as the tenth or eleventh month. By the end of the first year the child should easily be able to pull himself into the standing position and to walk holding on to something. Usually he can walk at about eleven months if someone holds his hand. Walking unaided usually starts at about twelve to sixteen months. Of course, some children progress faster than others, but about 40 per cent of children can walk at a year, and 67 per cent at fourteen months. Occasionally, if the child is fat or has been ill, he may not walk until

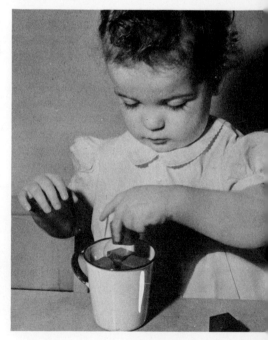

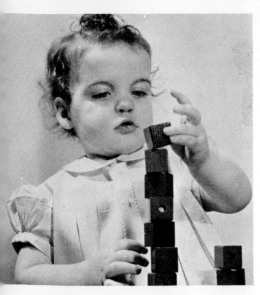

Blocks—Photograph illustrates the mental development of this child. Given a number of blocks, she will begin to pile them one on top of the other without further direction. She will not, at this age, build in two directions, but will continue piling them only in a vertical column.

fix their attention on any object until about two weeks of age when the eyes can focus on light. Usually, at four weeks, the child can look at something and at two months follow a moving object with his eyes. During the first few months, difficulty in focusing correctly the delicate eye muscles may cause the eyes to look crossed. Parents should not be alarmed since this difficulty normally disappears soon.

Babies recognize noises and voices soon after birth, but are unable to distinguish specific sounds for two or three months. An infant of two or three months enjoys listening to music and often will stop crying if the radio or phonograph is turned on softly.

Babies do not have a developed sense of taste as a rule and can usually distinguish only between sweet and sour foods.

The first six years. The most rapid growth period in a child's life is the first four months. At one month, the baby will look at a person near by, hold objects placed in his hand. His eyes can follow a moving object and he can hold his chin up when lying on his stomach. Whether or not the child really smiles, or just has a gas bubble in his stomach, is difficult to say, but at two months he definitely smiles when he sees his parents and persons who give him attention or when

Motor Development—Testing the baby's mental development. Fine motor movements permit a precise grasp of the small pellet given her, and she is able to drop it into the flask without any trouble. Given two objects such as these, most children of this age will proceed to use them in this way.

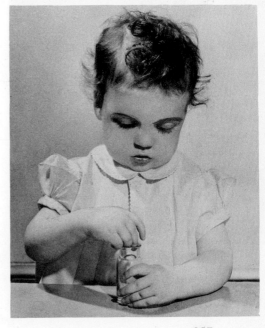

357

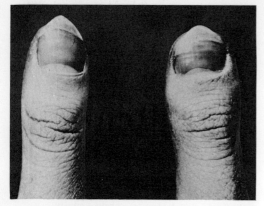

Thumb-sucking—If the bones are soft and the habit persistent, the thumb may be deformed by thumb-sucking. Photograph shows the difference in formation of thumbs in a patient who had the thumb-sucking habit during childhood.

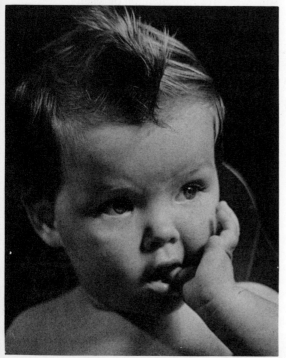

Thumb-sucking—Thumb-sucking habit in a child. Thumb or finger sucking can cause malocclusion which may result in facial disfigurement. To prevent irregular growth of teeth, this habit should be discouraged.

he feels contented. The two-month-old baby will coo, hold up his chest when prone, and turn his head away from bright lights. He turns toward a spoken voice and sometimes is frightened by loud noises.

At three months the baby can hold his head steady and may laugh. He can roll over, so it is not safe to leave him unprotected on an open bed. He gurgles and grasps objects. He may prefer his mother or whoever takes care of him to anyone else.

A four-month-old baby loves to study his hands, fingers, and objects around him. His attention is easily distracted by the world around him and feeding time may become a problem.

By five months, the child will sit propped, and recognize and be afraid of strangers. He will begin to scratch and to put toys in his mouth.

By the end of the sixth month, the child may sit briefly without support, reach for things he wants, and pound on furniture. He will probably love to watch himself in the mirror, and will stretch his arms to go to his parents or those he likes.

When he is seven to eight months, the baby will play peek-a-boo, pick up small objects, and often stand, if held. He may pull his mother's hair, and can wave good-bye.

In the last four months of the first year, the child will begin to recognize his own name and names of persons around him. He can open boxes, play with appropriate toys, walk alone or by holding on, notice other babies, and repeat simple words.

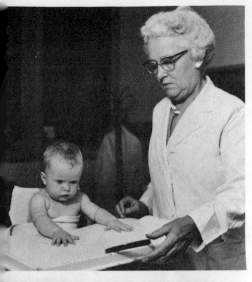
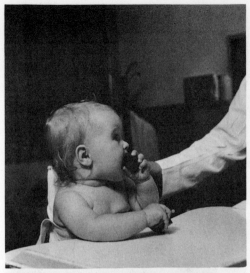
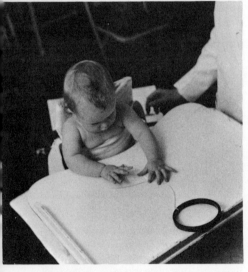
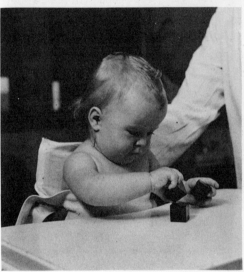

Psychometric tests of various kinds are often utilized to determine or indicate the rate and extent of mental, psychological, and psychomotor development in children. On this and the succeeding pages, photographs of the administration of such a test designed specifically for infants are shown. This and similar tests can give both the doctor and the parents a valid idea of the mental and physical progress and development of the baby. If any unusual or alarming symptoms or manifestations become evident as a consequence of the test, appropriate corrective measures can be instituted at this early stage, with considerably greater chances of success than is often the case at a later age. Conversely, any manifestations of exceptional intelligence should similarly be demonstrated by tests of this nature. On this page, the psychomotor development of a 9-month-old baby is illustrated. In the left-hand pictures, the ability to pull a ring by a string is tested. The baby here pulls at the string while looking at the ring —characteristic for her age. In the right-hand photographs the ability to grasp blocks is tested. Tests of this kind are fun for baby as well as informative.

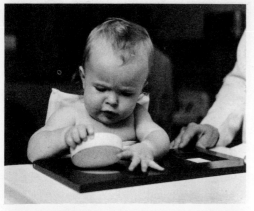
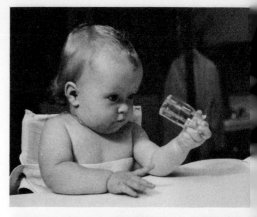

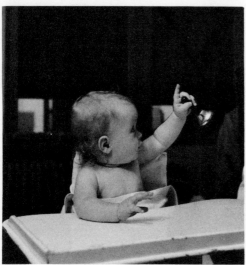
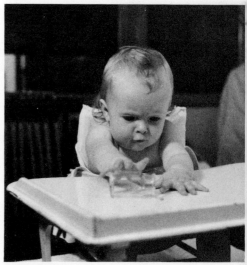

Top: Although she is unable to replace the block in hole, baby tugs until it comes out. She shows interest in pellet in bottle, characteristic behavior for her age. **Middle:** She imitates examiner who has rung bell, advanced behavior for her age. Interest in the bottle, rather than the pellet outside, is normal perceptual behavior for a 9-month-old baby. **Below:** Baby exhibits ability to handle her own bottle. Right, the ring shown on preceding page is secured by pulling the string.

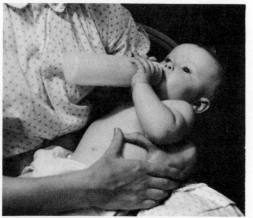
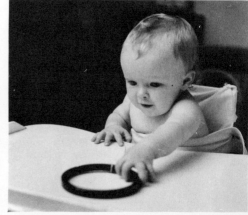

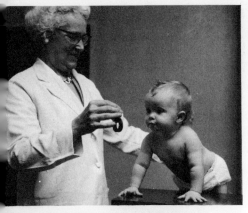

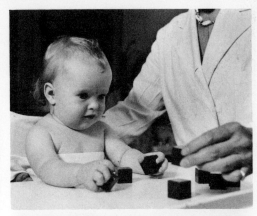

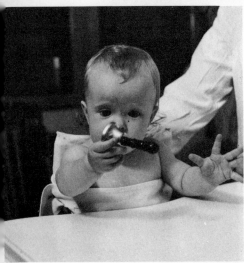

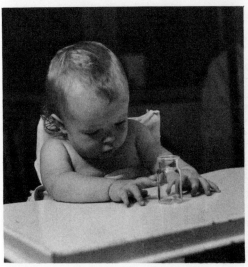

This baby's postural control is excellent. She easily achieves stance shown above. She can grasp a block in each hand, but building a tower is still beyond her. This ability is more characteristic of a one-year-old. But she watches and tries. She transfers the bell from hand to hand, displaying good manual dexterity and exploitiveness. She sees the pellet in the bottle, but has not yet learned to overturn the bottle to get it out, as she will do at a later age. Repeated efforts will eventually succeed.

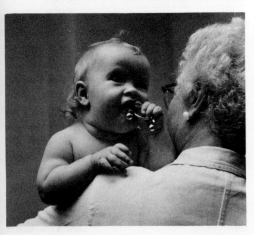

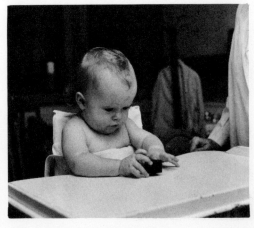

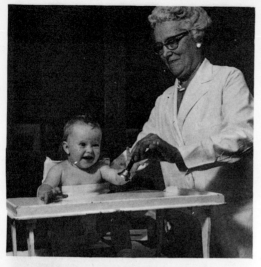
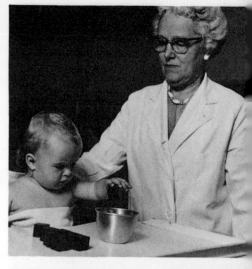

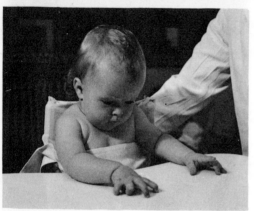
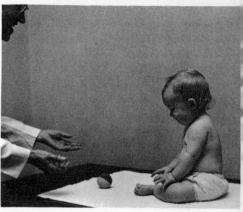

Baby shows eager responsiveness to bell. She is not yet able to release cube into cup. This is a still undeveloped adaptive function of the central nervous system. The attempt to pick up the pellet with the thumb and forefinger is unsuccessful. Baby approximates this maneuver by rolling the pellet into her palm, characteristic of a 9-month-old. She can release a ball on the table but can't throw it to examiner. This baby showed no interest in "patty cake" —unusual but not an alarming divergence.

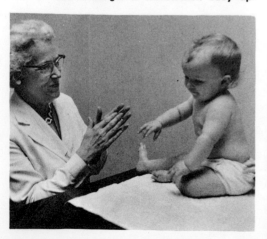
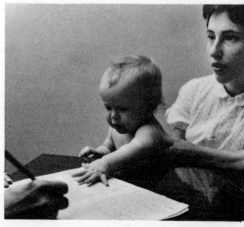

Speech is a significant means of testing development of the child. At the age of one year, a child can say a few simple words.

At two years of age the child should be able to fold paper, name familiar objects such as keys, pennies, and watches, listen to stories, look at pictures, and attempt to describe his own experiences. He will ask for things by their own names and begin to make sentences of about two to three words.

According to the Stanford-Binet tests, at three years of age the child of average intelligence will be able to point out his mouth, nose, and eyes and repeat two numbers, but not consecutively. He will look at a picture and pick out four or five objects meaningful to him such as a boy, dog, tree, or car. Most children do these things quite easily, and failure to accomplish these simple tests may necessitate special training.

At four, the child should know his sex, and be able to name three familiar objects shown to him, such as a spoon, book, and pencil, and to repeat three nonconsecutive numbers.

At six, the child should know whether it is noon or evening, and to define the use of a fork, chair, knife, or table.

Crying. Physiologists recognize the value of crying for the new baby. Crying helps ventilate the baby's lungs, forcing out old air and replacing it with fresh air. The thrashing about of arms and legs associated with crying helps develop the body musculature. Also crying is

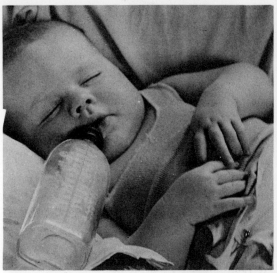

Facial Deformity—Permitting the child to sleep with the nursing bottle in the mouth may deform the face. Later in life, facial disfigurements are of great psychological import. Bad eating and sleeping habits which may cause deformity of the face or malocclusion should be interrupted as soon as possible. Good care and close supervision can prevent the development of these habits.

the only way a baby can indicate his needs, whether it be food, sleep, a change of diapers, or love, to those around him.

Most of the time a baby cries because he is uncomfortable, and parents should check for wet or soiled diapers or an open safety pin. The child may be too hot or cold. Often crying may indicate fear or anger. A new baby enjoys being in command and if he learns that he can control adults by crying he will continue to do so. Always be sure when the baby cries that he is comfortable, dry, and has had enough to eat.

Thumb sucking. Practically all babies, some more than others, suck their thumbs. In moderation, thumb

363

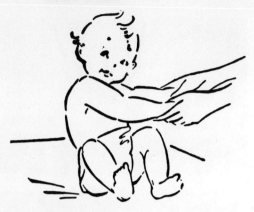

Exercise 1—The baby is laid on his back with his feet toward the mother. The mother then grasps the baby's hands and pulls him toward her. The exercise should be repeated two or three times. The baby tries to help himself up, which strengthens the arm, shoulder, neck, and abdominal muscles.

sucking does not do any harm and interference with the eruption of teeth will ordinarily not happen unless the habit continues past two years of age. Thumb sucking may indicate that the child is hungry or unhappy. It frequently occurs among babies who are weaned too soon, thus depriving them of the pleasurable satisfying practice of sucking. Artificial devices to prevent thumb sucking, such as arm splints or bitter preparations on the thumb, should not be used. It is better to try to find out the reason why the baby sucks his thumb. He may need more love and security. His hand should not be pulled out of his mouth, and the parents should avoid appearing upset about the habit. Ordinarily the child will discontinue sucking his thumb before the habit is prolonged enough to harm him.

Bed wetting (*enuresis*). Children usually learn bladder control during the daytime some time during the end of the second year. Nighttime control may not occur until the third or even fourth year, but ordinarily it is accomplished by the end of the third year. If persistent bed wetting continues beyond four years of age, consult the doctor.

Bed wetting may arise from emotional reasons, such as insecurity or jealousy of a new baby in the family. It can also occur if parents are too vigorous and rigid in insisting on early toilet training. Best results are obtained if the parents are understanding, patient, and do not push day or night toilet training and do not make a fuss about occasional accidents.

When the child is young, the bladder empties automatically, without any control from the brain. Gradually the brain becomes involved so that the child is able to control his urine when awake. Nighttime con-

Exercise 2—The baby is laid on his back with his feet toward the mother. The mother then grasps both feet and gently resists any movements that the baby may make. This resistance usually stimulates the baby to kick all the more. The exercise should be continued one or two minutes. It serves to strengthen the leg muscles.

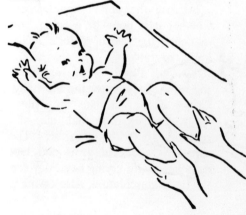

trol does not require much help from parents and if they are patient the child will eventually discipline himself.

In helping the child to keep dry at night, the following points should be remembered: (1) Water, milk, or other fluids should not be given to him after 5 P.M., unless he insists on a small drink to quench thirst. If the child complains of thirst at bedtime, or to delay going to bed, he may be given a piece of apple or orange. (2) Some parents awaken the child at ten o'clock to permit him to empty his bladder. If the child does not wake easily or has trouble going back to sleep, this practice should be avoided. (3) Protect the bed with a rubber sheet or have the child wear two diapers at night. (4) The child should be taken to the bathroom when he awakens. (5) The evening meal

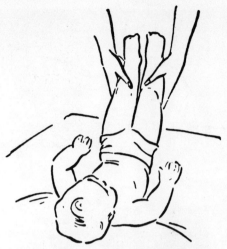

Exercise 4—The baby is laid on his back with his feet toward the mother. The legs are grasped by the mother midway between the knees and the ankles. The legs then are raised until body and legs are almost vertical, with only the baby's head and upper part of the shoulders on the table. The baby then is returned to his original position. The exercise should be repeated two or three times. It tends to strengthen the trunk and spinal muscles.

Exercise 3—The baby is laid on his back with his feet toward the mother. The baby's legs are raised and the calves grasped near the ankle. The feet are brought toward the child's nose with knees straight and thighs in contact with the abdomen. This exercise should be repeated three or four times. It tends to strengthen both leg and abdominal muscles.

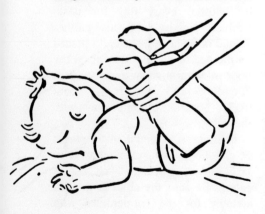

should be somewhat dry, and milk as a beverage or on cereals or puddings omitted. However, milk is, of course, to be given regularly throughout the day and used in foods when possible.

Bowel control. Bowel control is easier to teach than bladder control. The following points will help the child learn to control his bowels. (1) Do not begin bowel training until the child can sit comfortably by himself, at about the age of eight or nine months, although some authorities suggest much later. (2) The child may be placed on the toilet two or three times during the day at about the time he usually moves his bowels. This may be fol-

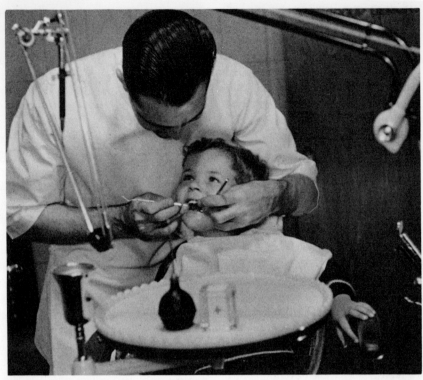

Dental Care—Regular dental examinations are essential to ensure proper development of the teeth. Scrupulous care of the teeth should be part of every child's education.

lowing meals and just before bedtime. (3) Soiled diapers should be promptly changed. (4) Do not leave the child on the toilet seat for more than a few minutes at a time, and do not permit the child to play with toys while on the seat. (5) Undue fuss should not be made over moving his bowels, or failing to do so.

Many mothers, because of excessive modesty, teach the child all sorts of tricks to indicate that he wishes to go to the toilet. Often strange gestures and queer words are used. The child should learn from the beginning the correct words used for this normal function.

Exercise. Babies need exercise as much as adults do, though often of a different kind. Kicking and moving about vigorously is really strenuous exercise for a baby and time should be allowed every day for unrestrained activity. All his clothes should be removed, the child placed on the bed or a thick blanket on the floor in a warm room and then permitted to kick and move about freely. Someone should play with the baby.

Exercise is essential in all stages of childhood, but violent play is to be avoided, especially just before eating. Be sure the child is dressed suitably for the temperature with

366

clothing that is loose and unconfining.

Care should be taken in exercising the small baby not to push him into activity for which his body is not ready. The baby will indicate when his muscles are ready to perform such actions as sitting or standing. Playpens are good places for babies to learn to stand and move about without danger when they cannot be closely watched.

Bathing the baby. Many hospitals today hold baby care classes for parents, either before or after the birth of the child, which include instructions for bathing a baby. Most babies should not have a soap-and-water bath until the umbilical cord falls off. Until then their bodies are washed with cotton balls dipped in bland baby oil. The bath is given in a warm room with a temperature about 98°F and drafts guarded against. It should only take a few minutes, and afterward the baby should be dried thoroughly, but without vigorous rubbing, with an absorbent towel. If the child's skin is exceptionally delicate, a handful of table salt to a gallon of water helps to lessen irritation. As the child grows older, a warm bath just before bedtime may help promote more restful sleep.

All the bath equipment and change of clothing should be assembled before the child is undressed. The head and neck of the baby must be supported during his bath. It is

Dental Care—This six-year-old child is proud of himself when the dentist tells him he has been doing a good job brushing his teeth. At this age, the permanent first molars erupt.

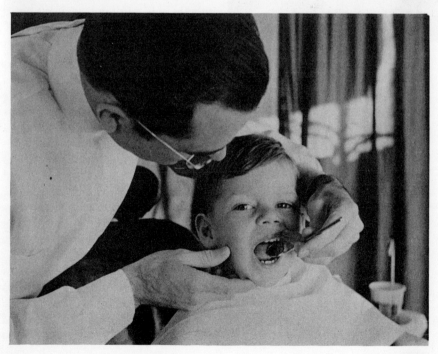

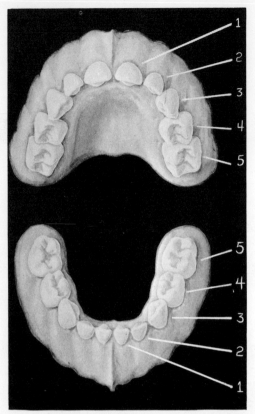

Dental Care—The teeth must not be overlooked in child care. Many dental diseases can be prevented if the child is brought to the dentist regularly even though dental attention seems unnecessary. The first set of teeth are called *deciduous*, commonly known as milk teeth or baby teeth. These teeth are twenty in number and are smaller than the second set of teeth. Photograph shows the upper and lower jaws of a set of deciduous teeth. Upper jaw: (1) *central incisor*, (2) *lateral incisor*, (3) *cuspid*, (4) *first molar*, and (5) *second molar*. Lower jaw: (5) *second molar*, (4) *first molar*, (3) *cuspid*, (2) *lateral incisor*, and (1) *central incisor*.

neither necessary nor advisable to wash the baby's mouth or clean his ears and nasal passages with a cotton-tipped stick. Any discharge from these areas should be reported to the family doctor.

If the scalp develops a slight irritation, overactivity of the sweat and fat glands may cause *caking* or *cradle cap*, a type of dermatitis. This caking is caused by a mixture of fat and secretion with layers ·of skin and dirt. Warm oil or petroleum jelly rubbed on the scalp, which helps to soften this condition, followed by a bland-soap shampoo will eradicate the difficulty.

After the bath, powder may be used but it is not essential. If used, care must be taken to keep the powder out of the child's reach, and not to spray it about since irritation in the lungs can be caused if too much powder is inhaled. The use of oil on the baby's body is also not necessary.

Breast feeding. The best possible food for the infant is its mother's milk, particularly during the earlier months of life. For unknown reasons, many women today are unsuccessful in nursing their babies, but fortunately many excellent substitutes are now commercially prepared which resemble mother's milk. The new mother should not feel disturbed or guilty if she is unable to nurse her baby.

Babies can derive benefit from breast feeding for about six months or even as long as nine months. When the baby cannot get at least half his food supply from his mother's breast, it is advisable to begin weaning. Most babies require weaning by the fourth to sixth month.

All mothers should make every effort to breast feed their babies, since breast-fed infants have a much lower incidence of infection, and seem to develop a little faster. In only rare instances does the milk of the mother fail to agree with the child. Occasionally diarrhea occurs if some element in the mother's diet disagrees with the child, but this can easily be detected and corrected in most cases.

Diet for nursing mothers. A common belief persists that a mother who wants to produce sufficient good rich milk for her baby should eat plentifully, drink excessive amounts of milk, cocoa, or even beer. This is not true; many women who have done this have become unpleasantly fat, disgusted with nursing, and inclined to discontinue. Actually the diet for a nursing mother is little different from that of any healthy adult woman, with about an extra quart of fluid, half of which is whole milk, each day. The diet should be about 2500 to 3000 calories, which usually does not lead to any increase in the mother's weight. The nursing mother should avoid taking substances such as strong laxatives which deplete her body's fluid resources, or which stimulate the kidneys, such as excessive amounts of coffee or tea.

The theory that a nursing mother should avoid gassy or sour foods such as cabbage, salads, and raw fruits is also without foundation, unless, of course, she herself is allergic to such foods. Fried foods may be eaten when a woman is nursing, but it is best to avoid chocolate. The best flow of milk results from regular nursing of the baby because the sucking action actually stimulates the formation of milk in the mother.

The diet of the nursing mother should contain about one quart of milk each day, some butter, four eggs a week, two green vegetables daily, and fresh fruit every morning, particularly oranges or tomatoes which are rich in vitamin C. Butter provides vitamins A and D; to provide a full supply of these vitamins the mother may take cod liver oil as directed by her doctor. The milk drunk daily may be whole, or nonfat dry milk if she is overweight. If she doesn't wish to drink milk, it may be used in food such as ice cream, custards, or cocoa drinks.

Mothers often worry about taking medicine, fearing that it will appear in the breast milk and harm the baby. Actually few drugs will do this, but if in doubt consult the doctor.

Secretion of milk begins a few days after the baby is born. In some cases, the breast may leak fluid during the last few weeks of pregnancy. During the first few days, the flow is usually scanty but becomes

Child Care—The following pages present information in handy capsule form about the psychological development of children from infancy to adolescence. Actually, of course, every child has his own individual idiosyncrasies and develops at his own unique pace. The observations made here should be regarded as pertinent to the average child and his representative characteristics. Any markedly unusual situations which might arise are best handled by consultation with a child psychiatrist.

what your baby needs from you in his
FIRST TWO YEARS

He needs to be carried often to develop his sense of balance and his feeling of security.

Giving the baby prompt attention when he cries develops his sense of safety and trust.

Singing, rocking, patting or holding your baby when he's wakeful helps him sleep.

A room of his own is important for baby's quiet and comfort and your own privacy.

Companionship and play with parents are important to any baby.

Needs matter-of-fact parental attitudes. Show no disgust at elimination.

With a little help a child toilet trains himself when he is ready.

Needs practice in talking and listening, to develop his ability to communicate.

Needs to be given as much freedom as is sensible, not hedged in with Don'ts.

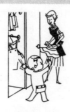

By asserting himself, he gains the sense of being an individual.

He also needs to feel that he is a member of a family group.

Among his needs are toys and materials he can master—not ones he can't manage.

Here's the first in a unique series of pictographs which depict the all-important needs of children as they grow from birth into the teens. These features are based on scientific studies and research

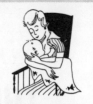

Baby needs mothering—being held and caressed—especially at feeding time.

New baby needs several hours of sucking a day.

Needs frequent, open display of affection—since he learns to love by being loved.

Let him feed himself when he shows interest—even though he makes a mess.

Be sure your baby has room and opportunity for free movement and exploration.

His first playthings should be ones that satisfy his need to handle, bang, suck, throw.

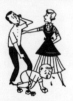

Needs to have his parents realize that he is not a little adult.

A child needs to grow at his own pace and be appreciated—not pushed.

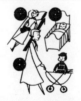

Needs a relaxed, responsive mother who plans rest and recreation for herself and her baby.

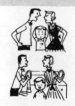

A cooperative, harmonious home atmosphere is important—tensions distress a baby.

A child needs to be able and encouraged to display love for others.

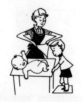

He needs to consider all parts of his body as clean and acceptable.

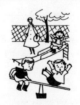

The young child needs to climb, run, pull, be physically active.

He needs to play freely and be allowed to get dirty.

Three is a delightful age. A child has greater self-control, is friendly and cooperative and learning to manage social relationships. Let's follow him through a typical day.

introducing the
THREE-YEAR-OLD

Will cooperate in clearing the table, tidying his own room— if asked.

Sometimes creates imaginary playmates, pets, or pretends that he is an animal.

Alternates between pestering brothers and sisters, and getting along with them.

Learning to ride tricycle. Likes to go marketing with mother.

Needs guidance when play gets quarrelsome. Aggressiveness expressed in words as well as actions.

Notices sex differences and sometimes worries about them. Questions should be answered simply.

May handle genitals. Can be quite matter-of-factly distracted from sex play.

Likes to have familiar stories read without change. Enjoys explaining pictures.

Likes to help prepare his bath, wash himself. Gets out unwillingly.

May try to be the center of attention if eating with family. Eats well by himself.

Outcropping fears: of the dark, dogs, other animals, fire engines. Needs reassurance.

When he knows parents are going out may say good-bye cheerfully. Or may protest until older.

Frequently whines upon awakening. May drowse off after getting mother's help in toileting.

Cheers up when fully awake. Likes to frisk around parents' room and get dressed with them.

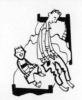

Can put on pants, socks, shoes, sweater. Able to undress easily, undo buttons —but can't button them.

Appetite usually good for breakfast. Feeds himself skillfully—not much parental help is needed.

Requests favorite foods (such as fruit, meat, milk) when meal is being prepared.

Gaining good control of elimination. Frequently has bowel movement after lunch.

Willing to rest at naptime, but frequently does not go to sleep.

Beginning to be able to play with other children, as well as beside them. Has definite choice in friends.

Affectionate toward parents. Mother is generally the favorite.

Enjoys painting, crayoning, modeling with clay. Results seldom resemble what he calls them.

Welcomes playtime with his father. Likes riddles and enjoys guessing games.

Listens to adults. Wants to please and enjoys praise. Likes to master new words.

Plays in bed for half hour or so. Usually goes to sleep without too many demands.

Begins to talk about his dreams and may occasionally be wakened in fright by nightmare.

Frequently gets up during night. May get out of bed and wander around the house.

May want to get in bed with mother. But can usually be diverted if parent stays with him awhile.

373

a pictorial guide to the
FOUR-YEAR-OLD

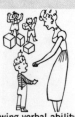

Growing verbal ability. Sometimes expressed in such ways as quarreling, tattling.

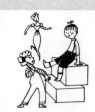

Play still needs some supervision. Quarrels may lead to too much hitting, kicking, throwing.

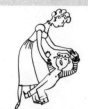

Verbally—and sometimes physically—child dissents from his mother's authority.

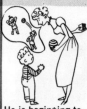

He is beginning to understand rules and restrictions such as balls for throwing— not blocks.

Vivid imagination is frequently expressed in dramatic play, imitation of adults.

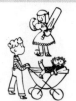

Boys may play with dolls, girls with boyish toys. All right if each enjoys his own toys, too.

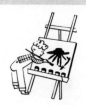

Works hard at drawing— though he may change theme in middle. Details are crude.

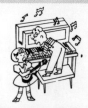

Likes to try musical instruments, play phonograph. Takes part in singing games.

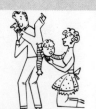

Child frequently clings affectionately to parents. Likes to be cuddled. Enjoys tumbling.

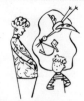

May confuse parents' answers about how babies are born with stories picked up elsewhere.

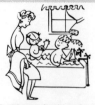

Bathing, toileting of both sexes together offer healthy ways to teach sex differences.

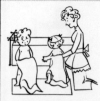

Can bathe himself if mother supervises. Can also partially dry himself.

374

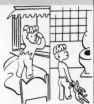

Generally wakes in morning in cheerful humor. Takes care of own immediate needs.

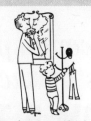

Can almost completely dress himself if clothes are ready at hand.

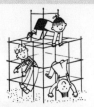

Very energetic. Adept on tricycle and climbing apparatus. Can handle some simple tools.

Enjoys nursery school or a play group, since he usually prefers play with others to solitary play.

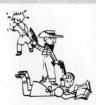

Frequently annoys older brothers and sisters, bullies younger ones.

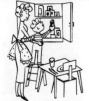

Appetite is fair but improving. Has definite likes and dislikes. Eats skillfully.

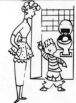

Frequently wants toilet privacy but asks for help with wiping. Controls urination.

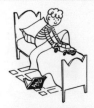

Will rest after lunch, but seldom naps. Plays quietly with books, toys.

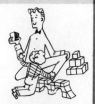

Makes intricate buildings with blocks. Admires his own work. Likes to have father help.

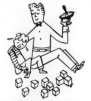

A peak age for crying and whining if bored or hurt. Needs comforting, then distraction.

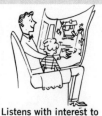

Listens with interest to verse and action stories —especially those explaining how things work.

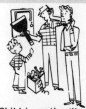

Child is continually asking questions—both to get information and to make conversation.

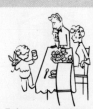

Enjoys eating with family. But interrupts progress of meal by talking, leaving table.

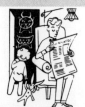

Shows fear of dark, animals, fire engines, old people. May resent mother's going out.

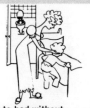

Goes to bed without serious objections— especially if he can recognize bedtime on clock.

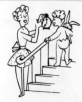

Less awakening because of nightmares now. May wake to go to toilet, needs help getting back.

375

the very special needs of the child
FROM 5 TO 7

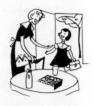

Needs a warm welcome and a chance to talk after a day at school.

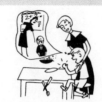

Needs understanding if he occasionally blows his top after a long day of school routine.

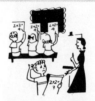

School can give him a feeling of accomplishment, even though he's slow in some things.

Needs to feel he can freely bring friends home and have parents accept them.

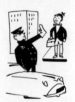

Should be able to take direction but . . .

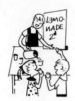

Also needs opportunities to act independently.

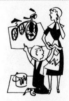

Parents should help with big projects when a child bites off more than he can chew.

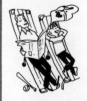

Give him time to think and dream as well as act.

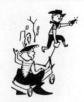

Needs to have opportunity for dressing up and dramatic play.

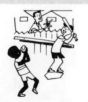

Will easily accept people from other races and groups if parents do not pass on prejudices.

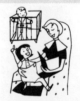

School can give him a feeling of accomplishment, even though he's slow in some things.

Boys need encouragement to develop masculine traits, girls to develop feminine ones.

What your school beginner needs at this crucial time when he is entering a big new world. A feature based on scientific studies

Make him feel that starting school is an adventure, not banishment to a disciplinary place.

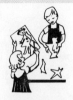

Give him opportunities for creative activity adapted to his own capacities.

Parents can help by realizing that he will learn to read when he's ready, not at a special age.

He needs simple spontaneous group play and skipping, dancing, rhythmic activity.

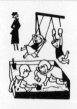

Needs space and materials for play—from which he learns much.

Needs an allowance to develop a sense of the value of money.

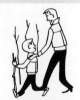

Parent of the same sex as child should make opportunities for companionship.

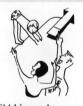

Build him up by emphasizing his strong points, rather than criticizing his weaknesses.

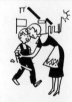

Is mature enough to spend time away from home but still needs assurance of parents' love.

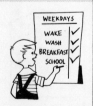

Needs the comfort of a regular but flexible routine.

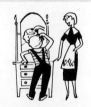

Start his training in habits of personal hygiene but . . .

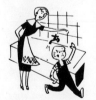

Try to be tolerant toward rowdiness and personal sloppiness characteristic of his age.

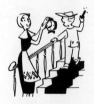

Needs about 11 hours of sleep every night.

377

meeting the needs of
the child
FROM 8 TO 10

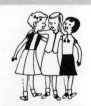

Needs to feel accepted and approved by his own age group—dislikes being alone.

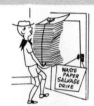

Enjoys feeling important and useful. Likes club activities, Scouting.

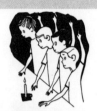

Relishes the tribal excitement of membership in a tight and secret group.

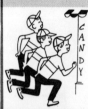

Conforms to his gang's standards of dress, speech, games and manners.

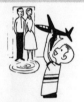

Looks for the reassurance of parents' understanding and support.

Allowance or earnings helps him learn value of money, independence.

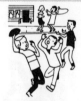

Running, jumping, other strenuous, hard-on-adults activities are necessary.

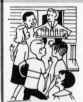

But adults must be watchful to forestall exhaustion or overstimulation.

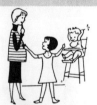

Parents who answer sex questions frankly are helpful.

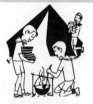

Activities away from home give scope to his yen for adventure.

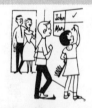

Helping with household tasks gets him used to shouldering obligations.

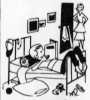

Needs realization by parents that he's not yet ready for adult conduct.

*Less home centered, more social minded,
your child meets new responsibilities
in these years. Here's a cross section
of research on his special needs*

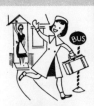

Wants freedom to visit alone and to play host to friends at home.

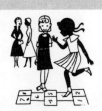

Needs adult example and guidance on tolerance, morals, life goals.

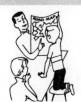

Likes to participate in family planning and activity.

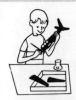

Needs satisfaction of starting projects, completing them.

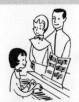

Must know that parents are sympathetic to his creative interests.

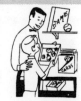

Needs patience with his rash of special and usually short-term interests.

Broadens mentally with practice in discussion, arguments, reasoning.

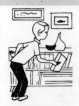

Has to develop his own taste in literature. Needs good books readily available.

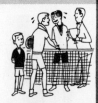

Unobtrusive aid helps him to develop his own standards of decency, fair play.

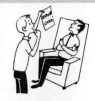

Needs tolerance of his nervous gestures —and a parental review as to their source.

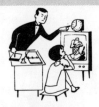

Should have an agreement with parents about time for homework, TV, movies.

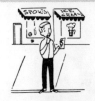

Matures when allowed to make decisions and face non-serious consequences of mistake.

prime needs of
11-13 YEAR OLDS

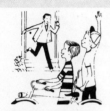

They need to feel accepted by their age group and to take an active role within it.

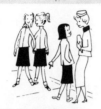

Want to conform to group's standards for dress, activities, possessions.

Begin to develop friendships with opposite sex and need to feel at ease with them.

An understanding of his own body, its changes and its capacities is important.

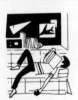

Appreciates moments of privacy and—if possible —a room of his own.

Generally needs eight to ten hours of sleep a night.

Wants enough money from odd jobs and his allowance to finance his personal projects.

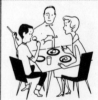

Looks to adults for guidance as to what is considered good manners and behavior.

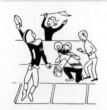

Thrive when they shine in some activity admired by their group.

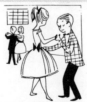

Welcome opportunity to learn social dancing —though boys may be reluctant to admit this.

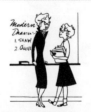

Should be spoken to and directed on the basis of mutual respect.

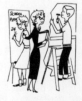

Chooses some admired adult for her model of dignity and good sense.

Conformity to the group, independence toward parents, mark this as an important self-testing period. But tactful guidance is welcome

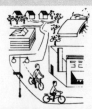

Should have chance to broaden their first-hand experience with the world around them.

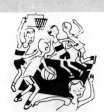

Like to play games which require high degree of teamwork and organization.

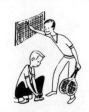

They should be encouraged to try their skill with new sports.

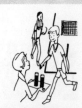

Require supervision to make sure they don't get too tired from strenuous play.

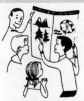

Wants to feel that his views play an important role in family discussions.

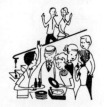

Must have the freedom to organize social activities on grown-up lines.

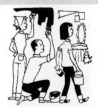

Gains family status by being given family responsibilities within her capabilities.

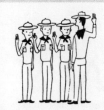

Need the goal of a high minded moral code such as religion, Boy Scouts.

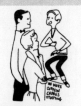

Needs tolerance toward his revolt against adult ways and standards.

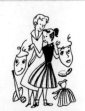

Assurance and guidance foster a positive attitude toward sex roles.

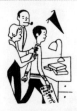

Parents' open recognition that he is a worthwhile individual is essential.

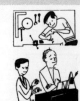

Careful attention must be paid to development of individual potentialities.

14 TO 16
are crucial years in growing up

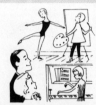

Needs active encouragement for steadily broadening intellectual and aesthetic interests.

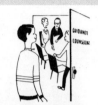

Should have expert counsel on his future course toward a vocation or higher education.

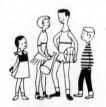

Wants a chance to excel in sports or some other activity.

Needs chances to earn money and decide how to use his own earnings.

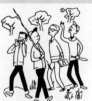

Requires freedom to choose leisure time activities and to enjoy them in his own way.

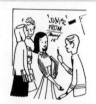

Needs confidence in his attractiveness for the opposite sex.

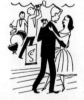

Appreciates instruction in and opportunity for social contacts with opposite sex.

Must have factual knowledge about sex and reassurance that feelings are not to be feared.

Must be made responsible for personal possessions and hobby equipment.

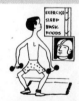

Should be encouraged to accept responsibility for his own health and general well being.

Looks for worthy projects on which to expend abundant physical and emotional energy.

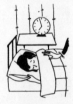

As a rule requires 8-10 hours sleep a night.

Mid-teens is a training ground for responsible adulthood. Understanding parents will alternate their helping hand with a hands-off policy

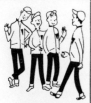

Acceptance and approval by his gang are very important to him.

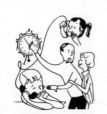

Needs the freedom to develop deep friendships.

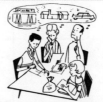

Appreciates opportunity to share in family planning and family responsibilities.

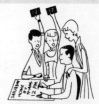

Wants a part in making decisions as to the degree of freedom which he may have.

Asks for tolerance through those long inactive periods of the "figuring things out process."

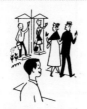

Wants his parents to be models of appropriate behavior.

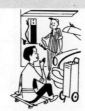

Must have friendships with adults other than his parents to gain insight into other points of view.

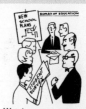

Wants encouragement and goals in his growing awareness of social and community problems.

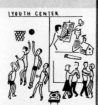

After-school and holiday youth center program foster interests, curb delinquency.

Tolerant attitude toward his need to be rough, tough and noisy is essential.

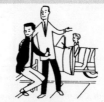

Especially needs parents' realization that his aggressiveness and rejection of them are only temporary.

Thrives on family relationship which balances understanding, affection, freedom.

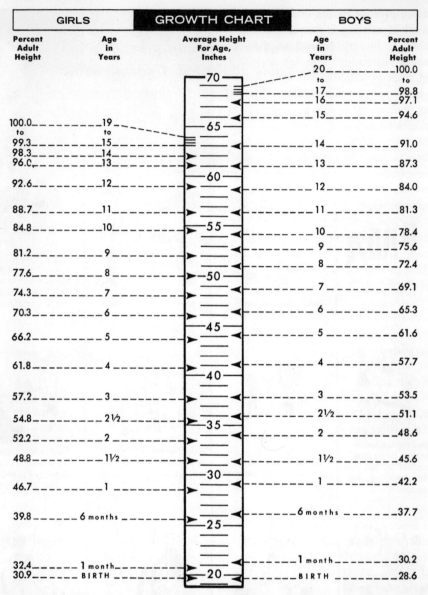

| GIRLS | GROWTH CHART | BOYS |

Growth—This Growth Chart shows (in the middle column) the average height, at different ages, of girls from birth to nineteen years as shown on the left, and of boys from birth to twenty years as shown on the right. This chart can be used for predicting probable adult stature by taking the height of a child at a given age and figuring from the percentage indicated. A seven-year-old girl, for example, has already attained about 74.3 per cent of her growth in height. If she is an inch taller than the average (49 instead of 48), she may grow to be almost 66 inches tall. An eight-year-old boy has attained about 72.4 per cent of his adult height. If he is an inch shorter than the average for his age (50 inches instead of 51), he may grow to be 68 inches tall. All such predictions are speculative.

more profuse by the end of the first week if nursing is frequent and the child is hungry enough so that he sucks vigorously. The first secretion of milk is actually not milk, but a cheesy protein-rich substance known as *colostrum* which appears about the third day and is nourishing for the baby. Later the true milk begins and is pale bluish white in color, resembling skim milk. This color is normal and does not mean that the milk is weak.

By the end of the first week, the average mother should have no difficulty secreting a pint of milk daily. This gradually increases and by the sixth month she is producing a quart of milk daily. The amount produced usually parallels the demands of the baby. Complete emptying of the breasts at nursing time is desirable to encourage good milk production. Nursing from both breasts at each feeding is recommended until maximum production is established. Then alternate the breasts to avoid over-production.

Mature milk which is secreted by the mother after the first month is about 87.5 per cent water, 1.25 per cent protein, 7.5 per cent sugar, and 3.5 per cent fat. Breast milk is considerably sweeter than cow's milk, though somewhat lower in protein. It is also much more digestible and breast-fed babies are less apt to regurgitate or have gastrointestinal upsets. Through the mother's milk they also receive protective antibodies against disease which are not found in cow's milk. If the mother's diet is insufficient, the milk will be poor in quality. Vitamins should be taken

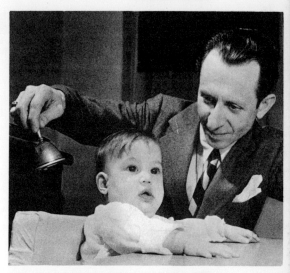

Responsiveness—Physician is testing the baby's response to a ringing sound. As unresponsive as they sometimes seem, babies are nevertheless capable of showing a great variety of responses indicative of their ability to comprehend simple situations.

by the nursing mother to enrich the milk.

Smoking does not affect the milk, and alcohol may be taken in moderation while the mother is nursing since it does not pass into the milk except in small amounts.

Hygiene during nursing. The nursing mother should keep in good physical condition and eat properly, and allow for a good night's sleep with a rest period in the midafternoon and, if possible, before nursing periods. Worry and overfatigue are to be avoided.

The size of the breasts does not seem to be linked to supply of milk and women with smaller breasts often produce the most milk. Determining in advance whether or not a mother will be able to nurse her baby is not possible. Certain women

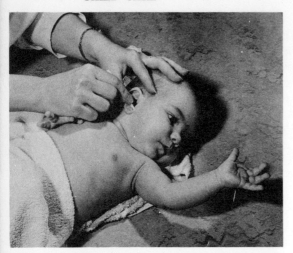

Ears—The baby's ears should be cleaned regularly. Photograph shows the correct technique for this operation. The movements should be gentle and the swab is never inserted deep into the canal. After the ear has been washed, the head may be turned on one side and any extra fluid allowed to run out. The ear is then wiped dry with cotton. Antiseptics may be applied if prescribed by a physician.

should not nurse, however. These include those women who are not in good health, those who have active tuberculosis or other infections, those who have had arduous labors, and those who have previously had tumors of the breast or breast infection. If the breasts become infected while nursing, it should be discontinued. Premature babies thrive on mother's milk, but often their sucking power does not permit nursing. In some hospitals the mother's milk is drawn off by a breast pump and then fed to the baby with an eye dropper or small tube until it is strong enough to nurse by itself.

If the baby begins vomiting or fails to gain weight, the mother probably should stop nursing. How-

ever, she should consult the doctor first. Failure to nurse one child need not signify that future attempts will be unsuccessful.

Frequency of feeding. Babies are usually given their first feeding about twelve to twenty-four hours after birth. The feeding is started at about four-hour intervals. If the mother does not have milk, sugar-and-water solutions may be fed to the baby.

Although opinion as to how often to feed the baby varies, most doctors seem to favor a three- or four-

Examination—Baby undergoes a thorough ear, nose and throat examination. Note that the doctor and nurse wear masks to prevent spreading germs. Young babies are very susceptible to infections.

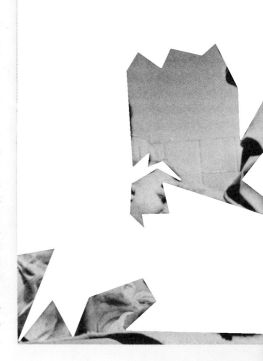

hour schedule. During the first few days it may be necessary to nurse the baby more often but the interval should not be less than two hours. In short time, most babies seem to wish to be fed every four hours and by the sixth week sleep through the night and do not wake up to be fed. Babies should never be awakened just to feed them unless their sleep pattern becomes set in such a way that the entire household is upset. One theory favors letting the baby get hungry before feeding him, since usually he will not only nurse more vigorously but also take more at each feeding. Generally, after being fed, the baby will sleep for several hours. When he awakens he may be wet or need to expel gas and cry, which does not necessarily mean that he has not received enough to eat.

Nursing should take place in a quiet surrounding. The mother should lie down on her bed or sit in another comfortable position during the feeding. Prolonged nursing is not desirable and may lead to irritation of the nipples and not more than ten or fifteen minutes should be allowed for nursing. Studies show that the food obtained after the first six to eight minutes is hardly sufficient to be significant. Breast-fed babies develop strong sucking powers and can empty the breast rapidly. Mothers should be sure to "burp" the baby about halfway through the feeding. Once the baby is on a regular feeding schedule, it is desirable to try to maintain it, except in unusual cases.

Overfeeding and underfeeding. If the baby seems fretful after nursing and does not rest or sleep, the mother's milk may be insufficient. In such cases, the doctor will prescribe a supplementary formula to be given after the regular nursing period.

Most babies stop nursing when they have had enough and seldom does a nursing baby overfeed. Occasionally, however, a baby getting too much milk too fast may vomit or regurgitate, or have an upset stomach afterward, but this is rare. If it does occur, the nursing time should be shortened.

It is not advisable to weigh the baby before and after the feeding to see how much milk he gets; this is not only bothersome but may also disturb the mother unnecessarily. The behavior of the baby after the feeding is the best indication of whether or not he has received the proper amount. After nursing, hold the baby for a few minutes until he is ready to sleep. If he sleeps satisfactorily for two or three hours, he has had enough to eat.

Cow's milk. Generally the formula for babies is based on cow's milk, which should be pasteurized to remove harmful bacteria and purchased from a reliable dairy or market. In country homes where milk is obtained directly from cows, the milk must be boiled immediately after being drawn, then strained through cheesecloth into thoroughly boiled and sterilized bottles, cooled promptly, and placed in the refrigerator. In cities, these precautions are not necessary since milk is produced and pasteurized under the supervision of a health department. Heat-

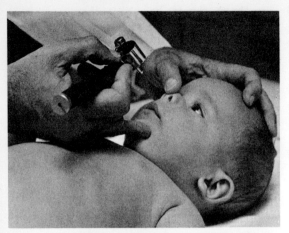

Examination—The physician examines the baby's nose and throat carefully on every office visit. Babies are especially susceptible to respiratory infections. Every precaution should be taken to keep the baby from catching cold.

ing milk does not remove any nutritional factors but does kill bacteria which may cause infections with streptococci or transmit tuberculosis, typhoid, diphtheria, or scarlet fever. Heating also helps to increase the digestibility of cow's milk. Because the vitamin C in the milk, essential to the child, may be destroyed by heating, it is customary to begin giving the child diluted orange juice or vitamin drops at two weeks of age.

Directions for feeding a baby with cow's milk should be obtained from the doctor. Cow's milk varies in composition from human milk, but in the formula must simulate breast milk. Ordinarily the baby cannot digest plain cow's milk until he is six months old and should receive it only upon suggestion and supervision of the doctor.

Preparing the baby's formula. When preparing the formula, all equipment needed should be washed thoroughly and boiled daily. The top of the bottle or can containing the milk must be washed with hot water and soap and rinsed thoroughly. Mix and measure the ingredients in sterilized containers, wash and boil the bottles to contain the formula, and close with sterilized rubber nipples. Individual bottles for each feeding are preferable to one large bottle from which the milk is measured. To provide for accidents, such as breakage or contamination, make one extra bottle. It is usually easier to make the whole day's supply in advance, preferably in the morning. After the feedings are prepared, the formula should be placed in the refrigerator. Nipples should be made of thin rubber, washed and boiled daily, and rinsed after use to extend their life.

Before feeding the baby, the mother should wash her hands well with soap and water. The bottle can be warmed by placing it in a pan of water on the stove. To test the temperature, shake a drop or two of the formula on the inside of the wrist. It is best to let a spray of milk run out until the drops fall one by one. In some cases, the holes in the nipple may need to be enlarged, which can be done by heating a pin over a flame and plunging it into the top of the nipple.

Cleanliness in the care of the baby's feedings is essential when he is young to protect him against serious infection. Sterilization is not essential after six to nine months, but the equipment should continue to be carefully cleaned before use.

Changes in the formula should be made only on the advice of the doctor because the baby's stomach and digestive system are extremely sensitive. If the baby seems healthy and continues to gain weight, there is ordinarily no need to change the formula. If he fails to gain weight, or if diarrhea or constipation occur, the doctor may prescribe a new formula with an increase or decrease or adding or elimination of some ingredient.

A baby's weight gain is not always continuous. If he drinks greedily and rapidly, cries for more, or gets fretful long before feeding time, he probably needs more food. But the baby may be crying for other reasons and the mother should be sure that underfeeding is the reason before increasing his food, or overweight may occur. At one time, fat babies were considered the healthiest babies but this idea has been disproved and in fact the opposite may be true. The baby should never be deliberately overfed. He can handle so much food a day and beyond his limit will become upset and nauseated.

Water requirements. In relation to his weight, an infant needs about three times more water than an adult. His output of heat is greater and his body metabolism requires more water. Therefore, he occasionally ought to receive a bottle of lukewarm water. In winter, especially in dry apartments, he may awake fretful, with a dry throat, and need a few swallows of water to quench his thirst. The total fluid intake, including milk, water, and juice, of a growing baby should be about three ounces per pound of his weight, and a little more in hot or dry climates.

Feeding with spoon and cup. Food or a few drops of juice or formula on a spoon may be given to the infant when he is just a few weeks old. This will prepare him to use a spoon for solids later. At first he may appear to spit out the food because he cannot control his tongue. To prepare the baby for drinking from a cup, let him sip his daily orange juice from a small glass. Some babies do this easily, others find it difficult. By the sixth to ninth month, many babies can drink successfully from a cup. If, during the first few attempts, the baby shows any reluctance to drink from a cup, further attempts should be discontinued for a few weeks. Even if he cannot drink from a cup by one year, the parents should not be alarmed. He will learn to do this by imitating those around him, and forcing will only disturb him.

Solid foods. At the end of the first month, most babies can begin to take solid foods mixed with formula or water. The baby may begin with bran, rice, or oat cereal; avoid cereals containing wheat until he is nine months old. The foods should be given in small amounts, thinned with formula or water so that the baby can swallow them more easily. After the cereals are well established in his diet, vegetables are tried one by one, carrots, peas and string beans first. It is usually cheaper and more convenient to purchase the vegetables already cooked and strained and ready to eat after

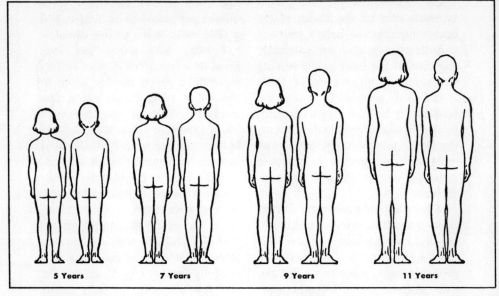

5 Years   7 Years   9 Years   11 Years

Growth—At five years, girls and boys are about the same height. The boy gains in height until about nine years. At eleven the girl has overtaken him.

a slight warming. At three months, the baby can begin to eat fruit; at four to five months, meat. When the baby is seven or eight months old, if he has teeth, he may begin on the junior foods, which are coarser and must be chewed slightly. They should not be given until the baby's teeth appear and he is able to eat the foods without fuss. A new food should be introduced in a small amount, only a teaspoonful, and then increased according to the baby's appetite. A boiled potato may be given when the child is seven months old; crackers, zwieback, dried bread or toast added when the teeth appear. Substances eaten by the baby may appear in the bowel movements, and this should not cause alarm. By ten or eleven months, the baby may eat many of the easily digested foods that the rest of the family are served, if they are cut up or chopped.

Schedule for the one-year-old child. When the child is a year old, he will be eating approximately as follows.

Upon rising, he should have from 7 to 8 ounces of milk. About 8:30 he receives breakfast of cereal, fruit and, if the doctor recommends it, egg yolk.

At noon, the baby should have 4 to 6 ounces of vegetable or meat broth, or one egg, or as a third possibility some scraped or chopped meat. To this may be added some white vegetables, such as 2 tablespoons of potato or rice, and from 2 to 4 tablespoons of a green vegetable, such as string beans, peas, or spinach. He may also drink more milk.

In the evening, around six, he

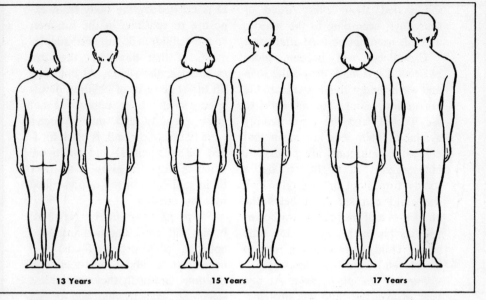

13 Years   15 Years   17 Years

Growth—At thirteen the boy is taller. After this age the girl tends to grow little, but the boy usually continues to grow until he is seventeen or older.

should have cereal and milk, and also a cracker or small piece of toast, and 1 or 2 tablespoons of cooked fruit, which has a slight laxative quality.

Babies thrive best on a strict daily schedule. Occasionally exceptions must and should be made in his daily routine, but they should be kept to a minimum.

Self-feeding. At the end of the first year, babies ordinarily show an interest in self-feeding and can pick up pieces of carrot, potato, or toast. Actual self-feeding should be accomplished by the end of the second year. Rarely is there need to feed a child after this time. The child should eat a variety of foods at mealtime, and the mother see to it that the diet is well-balanced and the food attractively prepared. The child should drink water several times be-

tween meals, but soft drinks and candies should be avoided.

Most pediatricians recommend that food be given at regular intervals, and removed if not eaten in a reasonable time, about twenty minutes, and the child not given more food until the next regular meal. Coaxing the child to eat does little good and should be avoided.

Cleanliness. The child should have a complete bath at least twice a week after the first year and preferably one every day, before bedtime. Washing the hands should be encouraged during the second year. The child, if he plays as he should, is likely to get dirty and disheveled. The mother should not badger the child to remain clean, although it is wise if the mother teaches the child to clean up following play and meals.

The young child's hair should be

shampooed about every three or four days, according to the season, and oils need not be used afterward.

Cleanliness will become more habitual if it is made easy—the soap and washstand within easy reach, the mirror low enough for the child to see himself, and the towel readily available. This does not mean that child-size bathrooms are necessary, but perhaps it might require a steady firm stool or box on which the child can stand. It helps the child if one of his parents washes or brushes his teeth at the same time as the child, since children love to imitate and learn best this way.

Feeding the older child. At one year of age, the child will probably be able to eat some of the foods that the family is eating, unless he has an allergy to one of them or does not have enough teeth to chew his food well. Eggs should be taken easily in all forms by one year. While egg yolk is started at six months, egg white should not be given until the end of the first year.

Cod liver oil. In the United States, cod liver oil or vitamin compounds in liquid form are practically universally given to children daily. Cod liver oil contains large amounts of vitamins A and D, which prevent or help cure rickets. In rickets, softening of the bones occurs due to failure of the body to use properly the mineral substances calcium and phosphorus. Vitamin D is the essential material involved in utilization of these minerals and so should be added to the diet in plain or mint-flavored cod liver oil, or through other vitamin preparations. Vitamin D is created by the body from exposure to sunshine in the summer, so most children do not need supplements at that time; but they are essential in the winter. At one time 50 to 80 per cent of children developed rickets; their bones did not grow properly and their muscles were flabby. Now milk is often fortified with vitamin D and additional vitamins are also given. Cod liver oil in straight form is also prescribed by some doctors.

Sleep for the baby. Newborn babies with good digestion and good appetite, plus proper foods, will usually sleep about nine-tenths of the time. Gradually they require less sleep, so that by the age of six months they sleep only about fifteen hours a day; from then until they are six, about twelve hours; from seven to ten years, ten hours a day; from eleven to fourteen years, nine hours a day. Seven hours of sleep are needed by older teen-agers. Up to six years, a child should also have a nap during the day, lasting from 45 minutes to an hour and a half.

A baby should sleep in a room that is darkened and away from routine household noises. Hunger, pain, sudden noises, flashes of light, and sudden changes in temperature will awaken a small baby. The child will sleep soundly if he is warm, but not overly warm, well fed, and in a quiet darkened room. A baby often tends to wake up at a slight sound, and so the mother should not rush into his room every time he whimpers, even at night.

A baby should be put to bed at a reasonably early hour, usually

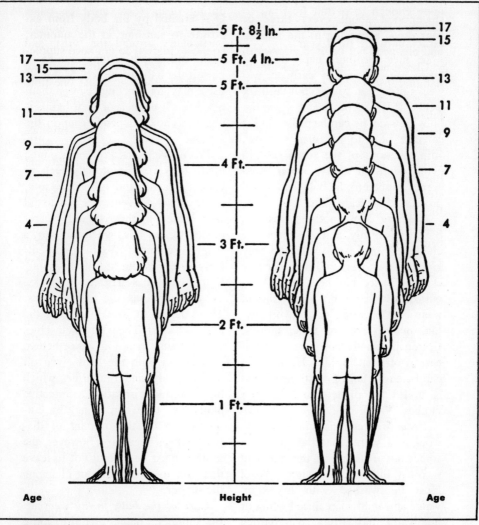

17
15
13

11

9

7

4

5 Ft. 8½ In.

5 Ft. 4 In.

5 Ft.

4 Ft.

3 Ft.

2 Ft.

1 Ft.

17
15

13

11

9

7

4

Age   Height   Age

Growth—Based on photographs taken over a period of years, this drawing of one girl's growth (*above left*) depicts the rate at which most girls grow and develop and shows how it slows as they approach maturity. Boys, as shown in this drawing of one boy's physical maturing (*above right*) usually grow steadily from the age of four to ten with a brief period of slowing down around ten to twelve years, followed by a two-year period of rapid growth, with a slower growth after fifteen or sixteen years.

around six o'clock, and not kept up late, unless for a good reason. Frequently an overtired child has difficulty going to sleep and will be cranky and irritable the following day.

The mattress on which a baby sleeps should be firm, but soft enough to be comfortable. The child should be lightly covered and his room comfortably warm, but not hot. In good weather, the window may be open enough to permit fresh air to circulate freely. Pillows are not necessary until the third year.

In nice weather, naps may be taken out-of-doors as early as two weeks of age; in winter, not until six weeks. If it is inconvenient to put the baby outside, he can be placed in his carriage next to an open window, with the door of the room shut to avoid draft. In cold weather, cold cream applied to the baby's face will protect its delicate skin.

Clothing. Most mothers dress the baby too warmly, and as a result the child perspires excessively and may kick off his covers and then become chilled. There has been much discussion whether or not a baby should wear cotton, wool, silk, rayon, nylon, or mixtures of these fabrics. Cotton is usually not warm, since it carries off heat rapidly. However, it can be easily boiled or sterilized and is useful for diapers and summer clothes.

Because it conducts heat poorly, wool is a warm material, but it is somewhat irritating to the skin and is often difficult to launder. Wool must be washed with lukewarm water and mild soap since boiling or hot water and strong soap harden and otherwise harm its fibers.

Silk is not a warm material and some babies are sensitive to it. Rayon, too, is not particularly warm and must be washed with some care.

Sleeping bags. The sleeping bag is very useful for the baby. Correctly sized and constructed, it is loose enough to permit plenty of motion and warm enough to prevent loss of heat. Also, it cannot be kicked off during sleep. Care must be taken that the sleeping bag fits loosely, particularly around the wrists and neck, and that it is long enough to permit the baby to stretch. Materials used may be sheeting, canton flannel, French flannel, or light blanketing, the choice depending upon the season.

Protective pants. Protective pants, made of various materials such as rubber, plastic, and rubberized silk, are a great convenience. To avoid skin irritation, they should be replaced by dry ones when the baby's diaper is changed. Washing immediately prolongs the life of the pants. If the child has irritated buttocks, avoid continuous use of the pants. They should fit loosely around the legs and waist. The pants themselves do not cause irritation; nevertheless, they retain both the heat given off by the body and the urine, which may produce irritation. Protective pants save time and money by cutting down on the amount of diaper changes necessary; however, the mother must be careful not to leave them on too long without changing the diaper.

Care of the baby in hot weather. In summer, babies require more fluids and should be offered plenty of water to drink. The need for solids diminishes and the baby may seem less hungry. Since fats produce heat, the baby's diet should contain less fat than during the winter.

In hot weather, if the baby vomits or has loose stools, all food must be stopped immediately and boiled skimmed milk substituted for the formula. If the symptoms cease, the formula may be given again in weakened amounts until full strength is attained. When older children have stomach upsets, fluids—juices, weak tea, skimmed milk, clear soup—only are to be given.

During the summer, a baby can be clothed in very thin cotton underclothes and diapers. He will need more clothing early in the morning and late in the afternoon. A cotton sunsuit is sufficient clothing for a hot day. The baby's clothing should be a little lighter in hot weather than an adult's.

If the baby's skin is moist in hot weather, he is probably wearing too many clothes; and if his lips, fingers, and toes are cold, he needs more clothing.

Frequent baths are comforting to the baby in hot weather. The bath water should be tepid, not cold. One teaspoonful of baking soda to a pint of water soothes and helps cool the skin. After the bath, the baby may be powdered lightly. Cornstarch is as good as any other powder.

Exposure to sun. Moderate exposure to the sun is not dangerous to the baby's eyes or skin. In summer, the baby may take a nap in the sunlight in the morning or late in the afternoon, avoiding the extreme of heat at midday. Exposure to sun should be gradual, beginning with just a few minutes and increasing to about half an hour in direct exposure. A child may become ill or sunburned if exposure to sun is excessive. Various lotions are available which help to prevent an excessive reaction to the sun.

Traveling with the baby. Travel is not recommended or desirable for a very young baby. But short trips are often possible when the baby is slightly older and, if adequately planned in advance, can be done with a minimum of difficulty.

Car beds are obtainable and can be placed in the back seat of an automobile or taken on a train, bus, plane, or ship. They provide a comfortable resting or sleeping place for the baby. Extra diapers, fresh water, and canned formula or evaporated milk should be taken along in case of emergency. Refrigeration for the baby's formula bottles is sometimes possible on trains and other public transportation. If refrigeration is not available, a thermos bottle is a handy container for juice, formula, and other drinks for the baby, or an ice container may be used to keep the drinks cold.

Travel will be less taxing for the mother and child if it is done at a time when the roads or the transportation system are least congested.

The child's teeth. Development of teeth differs among children, as do the time of eruption and the reaction to teething. Even very healthy children may become fretful, sleep poorly, and refuse meals during teething periods. Teething often causes drooling of saliva, and looseness of bowels and slight fever. The doctor should be consulted; he may prescribe some medication to ease the baby over the teething period. Eruption of the child's teeth usually proceeds as follows: the two central lower teeth during the sixth to ninth month; the four upper central teeth during the eighth to twelfth month;

the other two lower central teeth and the four front double teeth during the twelfth to eighteenth month. Altogether twenty teeth are in the first set. Most children have six by the end of the first year, although it is not unusual for a child not to have any teeth the first year. The rest of the teeth come between the eighteenth and twenty-fourth month, except the four back double teeth, which usually appear between the twenty-fourth and thirtieth month, but may come even later.

Because the teeth begin to form before the child is born, the pregnant woman's diet should be nutritionally adequate, including sufficient vitamins, minerals, especially calcium which is found in milk, and fresh vegetables, eggs, cooked fruits, cereals. Calcium supplements are often recommended.

To build healthy teeth, adequate food materials are essential in the child's diet, especially calcium and phosphorus, and the vitamins A, C, and D. The diet should include a sufficient quantity of milk each day, or its equivalent in butter or cheese, and eggs, leafy green vegetables, and fresh fruit. For growing babies, the diet is often supplemented by cod liver oil. Milk and cheese are the best source of calcium. Foods rich in vitamin A are eggs, butter, carrots, and other vegetables. Vitamin C is abundant in citrus fruits, and D is found in fortified milk, in cod liver oil, in beef liver, salmon, butter, and in most vitamin preparations.

Many physicians feel that coarse foods strengthen the jaws and help to harden the gums. When a new tooth is coming in, coarse foods serve as a resistance against which the gums may work to permit the teeth to cut their way through. Heredity is also significant in determining the type and quality of the child's teeth.

Special mouth care is not essential during the first two years. Some time in the beginning of the third year the child may be shown how to use a toothbrush by having him imitate the actions of the older person. During his third year the child should see a dentist, who will note any difficulties and plan for future care.

The sick child. Since children are not as articulate in drawing attention to their needs as adults, most mothers soon learn how to detect the first signs of illness. The child who is listless, drowsy for no apparent reason, flushed, and breathing with difficulty is obviously in need of medical attention. A child who looks and acts well and has plenty of energy probably is well. The child should get regular checkups at frequent intervals during the first two years, and after that twice a year. Most communities have public health services where a child may receive a checkup without charge if a private pediatrician cannot be consulted. Medicine should never be given to a child unless ordered by a physician. Unused portions of medicine should always be destroyed after the illness for which they were prescribed has been cured. If, months after an illness, the child develops what seems to be the "same" condition, under no circumstances should he be given the original prescription unless ordered by a doctor.

The child in the hospital. If a child must be hospitalized, for an operation or a protracted stay, there are a number of things to know and to be done which can help the child through the experience. The child should be intelligently prepared for his stay in the hospital. Confidence in the doctors and nurses should be established by suitable explanations; visits to the child planned as periods of happiness rather than of worry. The child will reflect his parents' attitudes so it is important that they appear hopeful, confident, and encouraging throughout the entire experience. The homecoming should also be carefully planned.

Prevention of infection. Some diseases can be prevented by inoculation or vaccination, including smallpox, diphtheria, whooping cough, scarlet fever, measles, typhoid fever, tetanus, and poliomyelitis.

Although smallpox is rare nowadays, every child should be vaccinated against it, and in most parts of the country this is mandatory before the child can be admitted to school. The child may be vaccinated when he is from three to six months of age. Ordinarily vaccination is not done during the summer months, and it should be postponed if the child is not well or if other children in the family have infectious diseases.

Vaccination is best performed on the outer side of the upper arm. Although many parents of baby girls demand vaccination on the thigh, this is not always a safe technique because of difficulty in keeping the area clean and free of infection.

Usually, after a week, a small pimple forms at the site of the vaccination and in a few days the area around the vaccination may swell and become black and blue. This is the normal process of a vaccination and should not cause alarm. The vaccination must be kept dry until the crust falls off. To prevent scratching the area, the child may wear a long-sleeved shirt day and night. Occasionally the vaccination will not "take," and must be repeated. Smallpox vaccination is usually repeated at age six, just before the child enters school, and again at the age of twelve.

For protection against diphtheria, toxoid is given in three doses, once a month, starting at the age of three months. Booster injections should be given at eighteen months and again at the age of three or four. Whooping cough vaccination is usually given at the same time.

Polio vaccination should be given when the child is six months old, repeated two weeks to a month later and again in about six months. Inoculations against other illnesses, such as measles, scarlet fever, and typhoid fever, can be given as the need arises according to the physician's judgment of the individual case.

Hygiene for the sick child. If the child has an infectious disease, all unnecessary draperies, carpets, pictures, and other articles such as books and toys should be removed from the sickroom before the child is put into it. Occasionally, in a

397

serious illness, objects with which the child has been in contact must be destroyed. Hardwood or metal pieces of furniture are preferable for the sickroom rather than stuffed furniture, because they are easier to clean. When possible, the child's room should be near the bathroom to lessen the amount of work.

The person who cares for a child with an infectious disease should wear a washable smock over her clothing. She should also wear a cloth mask and wash her hands thoroughly after leaving the child.

A large paper bag is useful at the side of the sick child's bed. In this can be placed soiled towels, used gauze, cotton, and other sickroom items. The entire bag and its contents can then be conveniently disposed of daily. If the infection is contagious, it is best to burn the waste.

The sick child should be dressed in a loose-fitting, easily washable garment and the room should be well ventilated, although free from unusually cold drafts. Bathing the sick child is preferably done by a careful sponge bath rather than immersion in a tub. After the sponge bath, the child may receive an alcohol rub, or, if he is too young for this, talcum or cornstarch may be patted over his body. If the child has much fever, cold cream or petroleum jelly applied to the lips helps to overcome dryness and crusting.

Fever. A fever usually indicates that the child is ill, although occasionally a slight variation in temperature is not a sign of illness.

Every parent should know how to read a thermometer and both rectal and oral thermometers should be on hand in the medicine chest. A small child's temperature is best taken with a rectal thermometer. The normal range is between 99°F and 100°F when taken rectally (one degree higher than an oral temperature). To be certain of a correct reading, the thermometer must be shaken down well and left in position for three to five minutes. After use, it should be washed in lukewarm, not hot, water, rinsed with alcohol if possible, dried, and put away in a safe place.

A variety of disorders may cause elevations of temperature in children. Simplest and most common is the ordinary cold, which may give a high temperature. A sore throat, stomach upset, or infection will cause fever, as will the onset of the common childhood diseases, scarlet fever, measles, whooping cough, or chickenpox. When the temperature is above normal, the doctor should be consulted and no home treatment, such as laxatives or enemas, should be given until they are prescribed.

Many feverish babies feel better after a sponge bath with lukewarm water. Ice-cold rub-downs or alcohol should not be given to babies under two years of age. Occasionally the doctor may order a cool-water enema for a high temperature, or prescribe a small dose of aspirin. These treatments are soothing, but usually do not cure the cause of the rise in temperature. The doctor should always be consulted about what to feed the sick child. In most instances a poor appetite follows a high temperature and parents should not force the child to eat. Fluids may be encouraged, but solids are to be avoided during the first few days of the illness.

The common cold. The most frequent illness in babies is the common cold. It is usually not serious, even when the temperature is elevated, but because of the danger of the cold's developing complications such as pneumonia, bronchitis, or ear infection, the doctor should be called promptly. The best way to avoid contracting colds is to avoid exposure to persons with colds. Other factors, such as chilling, poor nutrition, and fatigue are probably also significant in making the child more prone to the cold. The child with a cold is more comfortable in a moist environment. This does not mean a damp room, but rather a properly humidified room.

Enlarged tonsils and adenoids seem to make children more susceptible to sore throat. If the tonsils are found to be infected, the doctor should decide whether or not they should be removed.

Babies may have tub baths in winter, but the room in which it is given should be warm and free from drafts. A brisk, gentle rub-down afterward is also helpful. Preferably the bath is given at night, just before the baby goes to bed.

Use of vaccines to prevent colds is as yet not established as effective. Nose drops may be prescribed to clear the nasal passages and permit easier respiration. At the first sign of a cold with nasal drip, cough, or rise of temperature, the child should be put to bed, and his food intake lessened. If the child runs a fever, of more than 102°, the doctor should be called.

Hernia. Frequently a child is born with a weak spot in the muscles of the belly wall or groin. This condition is commonly known as a rupture or hernia. Swelling is caused when the intestines or other tissues are pushed through the weak spot in the wall. Often the spot appears around the navel in newborn babies. When the child coughs, cries, or strains, the rupture is seen more easily because of the increased pressure within the abdominal cavity. Usually the lump disappears on lying down. Operation is not immediately necessary in these instances and often the doctor may just tape the navel hernia for a few months in the hope that scar tissue will seal over the defect. Hernias in the groin are less likely to disappear without surgery.

Tonsils and adenoids. Apparently tonsils serve to take care of infectious germs. The tonsils frequently become inflamed, swollen, and infected in children, and may cause pain on swallowing, earache, difficulty in hearing, breathing, or talking, and high temperature. The organism which causes most tonsillitis, the *streptococcus,* is similar to the organisms that lead to rheumatic fever, erysipelas, scarlet fever, and other disorders. Penicillin is effective in curing tonsillitis in most cases and removal is not always necessary unless sore throats are

399

particularly recurrent or resistant to penicillin, or the tonsils are enlarged.

The child with tonsillitis should remain in bed. If he is able to gargle, salt water will help to shrink the throat tissues. An ice collar and aspirin may give relief of pain. The doctor may use injections of penicillin or pills to help cure the infection, or he may prescribe other medicines such as terramycin, achromycin, or one of the other antibiotics. These drugs must never be administered without doctor's orders. Because of the serious nature of complications from neglected tonsillitis, the doctor should be consulted if the parents suspect the child has a sore throat.

The adenoids lie in the cavity behind the nose. Like the tonsils, they are prone to infections. When they are enlarged or infected, breathing and talking is difficult and the child's voice has a nasal twang. Typically he keeps his mouth open at all times. Eventually this may even lead to a change in facial expression: the upper lip is shortened and turned out, the lips are thickened, and a line between the cheeks and lips is formed as a result of the narrowing of the dental arch of the upper jaw.

Infections of the ear may follow adenoid infection and, if neglected, can lead to permanent deafness. Enlarged adenoids should be removed; this may be done at any age. Usually further trouble will not be encountered after tonsils and adenoids are removed, but in 10 to 15 per cent of cases they grow back and a second operation may be required.

Care of the ears. The ears do not require special care. Syringes should not be used to wash out the ears, nor should cotton-tipped sticks be employed to remove wax or other objects. When a small child has a pain in his ear, he will usually indicate his discomfort by putting his hand to his ear or by crying when the ear is touched. Infections of the ear frequently follow infectious conditions in the nose or throat and acute infectious diseases.

When the doctor examines the child with a painful ear, he routinely takes the temperature, which is usually quite high, even in simple ear infections. Next he will look directly into the ear canal with a special instrument, the *otoscope.* If infection is present, and the condition warrants, the doctor may make a small opening in the eardrum to release accumulations of fluid or pus. Otherwise, simple antibiotic treatment may be all that is required. Relief of pain is usually prompt following drainage or other therapy. Sometimes the pain of earache may be relieved by ear drops prescribed by the physician. Such treatment should not be used unless a doctor has seen the child.

Before the introduction of penicillin, ear infections often caused more or less permanent deafness. Mastoid infection too was frequent. In mastoid infection, severe pain and tenderness are noted in the mastoid bone which is just behind the ear. Opening the mastoid bone to free it of accumulated pus, the so-called *mastoidectomy,* was a common operation twenty-five years ago, but is relatively rare today.

Puncture of the eardrum by the doctor to release pus is not a dangerous procedure. If it is done early, hearing will not be impaired because the eardrum will heal promptly and hearing be as good as before. Puncture of the eardrum is far less dangerous than postponing the operation too long.

Cuts and bruises. Little children frequently suffer cuts, bruises, burns, and similar injuries to the skin which can possibly become infected. In such instances, first aid given at home is of the greatest significance in preventing complications from simple injuries. Many different antiseptic substances are available to kill germs located on the skin around a skin injury. The area affected should be washed immediately with plenty of soap and water. A suitable antiseptic may then be applied, but a clean cut usually requires only a finger-bandage such as the Band-Aid®. Children often object to iodine solutions or alcohol because of the burning sensation, and other non-burning antiseptics may be used.

Occasionally a bruise to the fingertips may result in a painful swollen area of blood clot under the nail. The doctor should be called. Most likely he will make a small nick in the nail to permit free drainage and relief from pain. This should never be done by anyone but a physician. Bruises which are painful often can be relieved from pain by cold compresses.

Convulsions in babies. Babies have convulsions much more frequently than adults. The nervous system of a baby is so sensitive that frequently an infectious disease or high temperature will give rise to a convulsion or extensive shaking. In ordinary convulsions, the child loses consciousness and becomes rigid. Then there may be a spasmodic jerking of the face and of the arms and legs. It may be difficult for the parent to differentiate between a simple convulsion and one due to epilepsy. In only about one-fifth of convulsions in children is the cause epilepsy. Convulsions should be promptly reported to the doctor. During a convulsion, the child should be placed gently on his side. Usually the child will sleep following a convulsion. *See also* ADJUSTMENT PROBLEMS OF SCHOOL-AGE CHILD; ADOPTION; BED WETTING; COLIC; EYE; FEEDING, BREAST; HEAD BANGING; HEAD ROLLING; IMMUNIZATION; CHILDBIRTH AND PRENATAL CARE; PUBERTY; THUMB SUCKING.

CHILL, a sensation of cold, accompanied by shivering and usually with teeth chattering, throbbing, and trembling. It is frequently a prominent early symptom of acute infection. Any severe chill during a fever is a danger signal and a doctor should be called at once.

A chill results from an increase in the chemical activity going on in the body and therefore a rapid rise in the production of heat by the body. The ultimate result of a chill is increased body temperature. A person with a chill is usually quiet, lies doubled up, has a pale cool skin and sometimes "goose flesh," due to the constriction of the superficial blood vessels under the skin which is sometimes so great that the skin appears blue. A mild chill can usually be controlled to some degree by the person; however, a severe chill cannot. Warm blankets and clothing, hot drinks, hot-water bottles, and electric pads will help relieve the discomfort of the person with chills.

A chill can be induced in patients by injecting certain nonspecific protein substances. It can also be prevented by drugs which act as sedatives and as controls of body temperature. The action of these drugs, which are known as *antipyretic* and *antifever drugs,* is to depress the activity of the center in the brain which controls chills and shivering.

The chill is being studied to gain further knowledge as to its cause and significance. Many physicians feel that a chill is often of real importance in helping to overcome a disease since it raises the body temperature through muscular movement. *See also* FEVER.

CHIROPRACTIC, a therapeutic system based on the theory that the bones of the spinal column, by pressing on the spinal nerves, cause an interruption of the normal function of the nerves. The result of this pressure is said to be eventual damage to the tissues. Extensive medical investigation has failed to show any scientific foundation for this theory. Chiropractors are nevertheless licensed to practice in most states. Practically all chiropractors are in the United States.

CHLOASMA. *See* LIVER SPOTS.

CHLOROFORM, *trichloromethane,* a heavy colorless liquid with a typical ether smell. Chloroform is best known as an anesthetic, and has been used for that purpose since 1847 when Dr. James Simpson, an Edinburgh gynecologist, dissatisfied with ether, discovered the narcotic qualities of chloroform. It became fashionable as an anesthetic in childbirth when Queen Victoria permitted its administration during the delivery of her seventh child.

Too large quantities and habitual use of chloroform may result in poisoning, injuries to the liver and kidneys, a condition of transient *albuminuria* (albumin present in the urine) and other diseases. *See also* ANESTHESIA; POISONING.

CHLOROSIS, a form of anemia, characterized by a large reduction of hemoglobin in the blood, but with only a slight diminution in the number of red cells. Some decades ago, chlorosis, or "green sickness," was common among girls and young women, but today it has almost completely disappeared because of increased knowledge of the role of iron in the diet. The symptoms of this iron deficiency are a greenish color to the skin, and menstrual and gastric disturbances. *See also* IRON; HEMOGLOBIN; ANEMIA; RED BLOOD CELLS, DISEASES OF.

CHOLECYSTITIS, the scientific name for inflammation of the gallbladder. *See also* GALLBLADDER.

CHOLECYSTOGRAPHY, roentgenography, x-ray diagnosis, of the gallbladder after it has been made visual by substances not transparent to the x-ray.

Gallstone attacks have characteristic symptoms, yet differences in related symptoms and severity of pain often makes a definite distinction from other diseases difficult. The introduction of cholecystography has been a great advance in the diagnosis of gallstones. *See also* GALLBLADDER.

CHOLELITHIASIS, a condition associated with *calculi,* stones in the gallbladder or in a bile duct. *See also* GALLBLADDER.

CHOLERA, an acute infection which chiefly involves the small intestine. The main symptoms are severe, constantly flowing diarrhea, vomiting, collapse, cramps in the muscles, and suppression of the flow of urine from the kidneys.

Cholera spreads most rapidly in moist warm climates. From time immemorial it has existed in India, from where at one time it spread throughout the world, probably traveling along caravan routes into Europe and along water trade routes.

The cause of cholera was described some fifty years ago by the German researcher, Robert Koch. A germ, the *comma bacillus,* gains entrance into the body through polluted drinking water. The organism then gets into the bowel where it causes acute infection. Cholera spreads in much the same way as typhoid fever does, the germs escaping from the body with material that is vomited or defecated.

To prevent the spread of cholera, the cholera patient must be isolated. Material that is passed from the patient must be destroyed by fire. Only food that has been cooked, and boiled—or preferably chlorinated—water should be used by people in an area where cholera exists. The food and water should not be permitted to stand for any length of time since they may become recontaminated. Those who live or travel in cholera-ridden areas can be partially protected against this disease through vaccination with a serum made from the killed bodies of the specific cholera germs. The incidence of cholera among inoculated people has been low.

About five or six days after a person has been infected with cholera, a severe diarrhea begins, with violent purging, and eventually practically pure mucus and water are passed. Then vomiting begins, followed by collapse. The skin loses its elasticity, the muscles cramp, the eyes are sunken, and the voice is feeble. As more and more water is lost, the thirst becomes intense, the pulse becomes rapid and weak, and the blood pressure falls. The face becomes sunken and the skin develops a blue, cyanotic tinge, as the blood gradually loses its oxygen. As the patient's condition improves, the reverse of the process occurs.

Whenever large amounts of fluid are lost from the body, danger of death from *acid intoxication* ensues. Therefore, the chief step in the treatment is restoration of the fluid. Large quantities of normal or physiological salt solution are given to the patient by injection into the veins. Delay may be fatal, and frequently it is necessary to give one or two quarts of this solution, every six or eight hours, for two or three days. The acidosis may be overcome by giving large doses of *sodium bicarbonate*. Usually the person with cholera is content to remain in bed. Warmth is sustained by blankets, hot-water bottles, and electric pads. The physician can help to control the vomiting by prescription of proper remedies.

In the United States, cholera has ceased to be a serious problem, although it still occurs in many other parts of the world.

CHOLESTEROL, a fatty substance, a basis for hundreds of chemical processes in the body. Animal meat, cream, butter, and eggs contain large amounts of cholesterol and its presence in excess amounts in the blood stream is believed by some medical investigators to be responsible for *arteriosclerosis*. In this disease, cholesterol plaques in the inside wall of arteries cause the wall to thicken and roughen. Ultimately the flow of blood through that portion of the artery is restricted, or a piece of the roughened wall may tear away and block the flow of blood to those tissues served by the artery. When this occurs in the arteries that supply the heart muscle with blood, the condition is called *coronary thrombosis*.

It has been proposed that a definite correlation exists between severe coronary attacks and excess blood cholesterol. Other medical investigators have produced arteriosclerosis in animals by feeding them diets high in cholesterol. Certain heart specialists advocate a low-fat, low-cholesterol diet to prevent or control coronary heart disease, but others believe that since the body produces its own cholesterol, dietary restriction of it will not help appreciably. Sometimes high-protein, moderate fat and low carbohydrate diets have been employed with some success. Investigations indicate that factors other than the existence of excess cholesterol may be responsible for arterial hardening. These may involve the body's ability to metabolize the cholesterol, or its ratio to other substances, such as protein and phosphatides, in the blood stream, the size and number of the cholesterol molecules, and the effect of exercise on the amount of circulating cholesterol. In one experiment, it was reported that a definite correlation between exercise and a reduction in certain types of cholesterol molecules existed.

A potent anticoagulant, *Dipaxin* (*diaphenadione, Upjohn*), has been developed which will reduce cholesterol, triglyceride, and phospholid levels by from 25 to 38 per cent. This drug has been successful in reducing serum and aortic cholesterol levels.

CHONDROMA, a slowly developing tumor growing from tissues or cartilage. In the chest this tumor tends to spread toward important organs. Generally benign, chondroma may recur after removal by surgery.

CHORDEE, a painful hardening and deformity of the penis sometimes arising in neglected cases of acute gonorrhea.

CHOREA, more familiarly known as *St. Vitus' dance,* a disease of the nervous system which causes involuntary twitching of various parts of the body. Children prior to puberty are most often affected. Girls are affected more frequently than boys.

Unlike many diseases of the nervous system, St. Vitus' dance normally lasts a relatively short time, often no more than twelve weeks. Sometimes relapses occur, and in other instances the disease may endure for one or two years, although not usually.

Chorea is believed to be the result of a general streptococcus infection which in some apparently indirect way, perhaps through toxic substances developed by the germs of the infection, strikes at the brain and the nervous system. Children may develop a temporary, habitual twitch from imitating the movements of other people, but this is completely different in origin and in character from the involuntary twitching that is seen in St. Vitus' dance.

The onset of the disease, which often accompanies *rheumatic fever,* may appear as a generalized illness with fever, vomiting, and headache, along with dizziness and weakness. The first disturbances of bodily movement are often mistaken for clumsiness of the child. However, the true nature of the ailment soon becomes apparent.

When fully developed, the movements are rapid, of short duration, and distinctive; none exactly duplicates any that preceded. Muscular coordination becomes difficult and approximately 25 per cent of the cases are so severe as to disturb the speech function. The child becomes irritable and restless, and his memory, attention span, and emotions may be mildly disturbed.

The treatment of chorea, a disease implicating the whole system and not just isolated parts, begins with prolonged bed rest of three to six weeks at least. Because of the close relationship to streptococcus infection, the child should be kept under close observation. Any infection of the throat, in the tonsils or adenoids, in the teeth or elsewhere should be eliminated quickly and the child kept in bed. Both in streptococcus infections and in chorea, attention must be given the heart, which may be particularly affected. The use of penicillin or sulfa is recommended by the American Heart Association to prevent streptococcal infection and to protect against a recurrence of rheumatic fever.

Baths and sedative drugs directed at alleviating the symptoms of chorea are frequently quite helpful. Both heat and drugs striking at the infection itself are often beneficial, but neither are specifically effective.

Convalescence of the patient with chorea should be gradual, with a nutritional diet assuring plenty of vitamins and minerals. Exercise and play should be resumed in moderation, but the child must relax and not overdo. *See also* ATAXIA.

CHORION, the outermost of the fetal membranes which covers, nourishes, and protects the developing ovum. Later it becames the fetal part of the placenta.

CHROMOBLASTOMYCOSIS, a rare skin infection caused by a fungus which grows on plants and trees in warm humid areas. Only a few cases have been reported in the United States, but the disease occurs more frequently in South America.

The infection usually starts on the feet or legs. The skin turns purplish red and develops colored, warty, cauliflower-like growths. X-ray, used externally in combination with appropriate drugs, has successfully disposed of the fungus and the growths. A potential danger, however, in any such disorder is that the offending organism will reach the lung or some other vital part where it may cause death.

CHRONIC signifies long-continued or of long duration. A chronic disease is prolonged, often slowly progressing and never completely cured —as, for example, chronic bronchitis or chronic arthritis.

CHRYSAROBIN, an orange powder, derived from the bark of a Brazilian tree, which stains the skin a deep brown. It is used to treat *psoriasis,* and is also effective in fungus infections called *gym* or *jockey itch,* involving the skin of the groin, perineum, and perianal regions. *See also* RINGWORM.

CILIA, fine, hairlike appendages which cover the surface of mucous membranes and the sensitive lining of the respiratory tract. The cilia are also filtering organisms which keep harmful particles out of the lung. They move upward and downward, and through the more pronounced upward movement, mucus, dust, and other infectious particles are swept and propelled toward the mouth, so that they are not breathed into the lungs. Eyelashes are also cilia, and protect the eyes from foreign particles.

CIRCULATORY SYSTEM. The heart pumps the blood through a "pipeline" of closed tubes or vessels. This pipeline forms two major circular routes in the body, the *systemic circulation* and the *pulmonary circulation,* with the *heart* acting as a central pump. The circulatory system, with its major and minor routes, reaches every cell in the body, bringing the blood with its life-sustaining products from the organs where they are manufactured to the tissues where they are needed. It also carries away the waste products to other organs in the body, where they are broken down and either converted to be used again or excreted as waste. In addition, the circulatory system takes care of the more active organs by bringing them an increased flow of blood, whereas those organs which are less active, or temporarily at rest, receive less blood.

The heart is divided into a *right side* and a *left side.* Each side is further divided into two chambers: an *auricle* and a *ventricle.* The

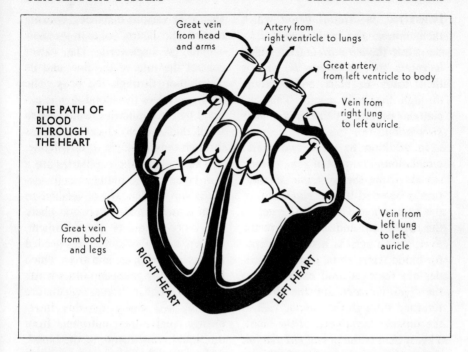

THE PATH OF
BLOOD
THROUGH
THE HEART

Great vein
from head
and arms

Artery from
right ventricle to lungs

Great artery
from left ventricle to body

Vein from
right lung
to left auricle

Great vein
from body
and legs

Vein from
left lung
to left
auricle

RIGHT HEART

LEFT HEART

Circulatory System—Chart shows the path of blood through the heart as it comes in by the veins and goes out through arteries. Large veins bring the blood into the right heart, then the pulmonary arteries conduct blood from the right heart to the lungs. Blood from the lungs goes to the left heart through the pulmonary veins and subsequently goes out of the left heart to the body through the great artery (aorta).

auricles are the collecting depots for the blood, while the ventricles pump the blood out of the heart into the blood vessels.

In the *systemic circulation,* the blood is pumped from the *left ventricle* into the *aorta,* or large *artery,* passing through a series of smaller arteries which branch from it, then continues through the *arterioles,* or smallest arteries, which end in a fine network of tiny vessels called the *capillaries.* The capillaries transfer the blood, with its oxygen and nutriment, to the various tissues of the body and then conduct it from the tissues into the *venules,* or tiny *veins,* on through larger veins until

it finally reaches the *inferior vena cava,* one of the two great veins on the right side of the heart. From here, it passes into the *right auricle,* and thus completes the systemic circle. The *venous blood,* dark in color, which enters the right auricle, has deposited most of its oxygen, and has picked up the carbon dioxide from the tissues.

Before the blood can resume its systemic flow, it must secure a fresh supply of oxygen. The *right ventricle* now pumps the blood through the *pulmonary artery* into the *capillaries* of the *lungs,* where it deposits its carbon dioxide and gathers up the new oxygen. This blood, now a

407

bright red, is *arterial blood* which then enters the *pulmonary vein,* flows into the *left auricle* from which it enters the *left ventricle,* and is then ready to start on its route through the body again. This circuitous routine is the *pulmonary circulation.*

In addition to these two major circulations, some of the blood stream from the systemic circulation is diverted by the *capillaries* of the *stomach* and *intestinal tract* to the *portal vein* and is carried to the *liver,* which acts as a storage depot for blood. Here some of the impurities are removed and excreted into the *digestive tract,* and the blood is returned through the *hepatic vein* to the *superior vena cava* of the heart. This system is the *portal circulation.* Another accessory circulation from the systemic feeds blood to the *kidneys* and is called *renal circulation.* The *coronary arteries, veins,* and their *capillaries* supply the heart itself with oxygen and nutriments and remove waste material, and constitute the *coronary circulation.* The *brain* and *head* are served by the two *carotid arteries* which bring the blood supply, and also by the *jugular veins* which carry away the blood and waste materials.

The circulatory pipeline consists of the three types of blood vessels described: the *arteries,* the *veins,* and the *capillaries.* The capillaries connect the ends of the smallest arteries to the beginnings of the smallest veins. Valves inside the heart and also in the veins keep the flow of blood continuous and in one direction. In the veins they are

spaced at various distances, opening toward the heart, so that the flow cannot go backward. The valves control the rate of the flow and its distribution through the body. The final control of the blood flow is exerted by the capillaries, which are so small that the blood cells can pass through only in single or double file.

The walls of the capillaries are a thin layer of fine platelike cells, *endothelium,* which are dovetailed to form a membranous network where the blood deposits its nutriment, oxygen, and other substances needed by the body tissues, and from which it picks up the gases and other waste products. Those tissues which are not reached easily by this interchange receive their nutriment from the liquid constituents of the blood, which also filter through the capillary network and carry food and oxygen to the tissues. The clear fluid filtering out of the capillaries is called the *tissue fluid.* The capillaries are found throughout all tissues and organs of the body, and are more numerous where the body organs are most active. Over a million capillaries may run through a square inch of muscle tissue, and if all the capillaries were joined in a single tube it would stretch for thousands of miles.

The walls of the arteries must be thick and strong to accommodate the stream of blood within them which is pumped by the heart under great pressure. They consist of three layers, the *endothelium,* or fine *inner layer*; the *middle layer,* on which the strength and caliber of the vessel depends, which is a thick coat of strong *muscle fibers* and heavy elastic tissue permitting expansion and contraction of the artery; and the *outside coat,* or *adventitia,* a thick layer of connective tissue which gives the vessel elasticity and enables it to act as a reservoir for the blood flow, and at the same time prevents the blood from oozing into the tissues.

The walls of the veins are structurally similar to the arteries, but they are thinner and their diameter is much larger since the flow of blood through the veins and into the heart is under less pressure.

In the course of normal routine, and more so in disease, much strain is placed upon the structures that constitute the circulatory system. As cells deteriorate, new cells replace them. Fortunately not all the cells wear out at the same time, and the process of replacement continues throughout life, so that a steady balance is maintained between the removal of wornout cells by the circulating blood and the regeneration of new cells. *See also* CORONARY THROMBOSIS; EMBOLISM; HEART; LYMPHATIC SYSTEM. *See* MEDIGRAPHS pages 93, 127, 129, 229, 231, 283, 449, 735, 1035, 1229.

CIRCUMCISION is the surgical removal of the loose fold of the skin, the *foreskin* (*prepuce*), which covers the head (glans) of the penis.

Circumcision originated as a religious rite in ancient Egypt and was also observed by the Hebrews, Moslems, South Sea Islanders, and American Indians. The Book of Genesis interprets circumcision as a blood covenant, and it is still practiced as such by Jews.

Today the operation is recommended by many doctors as a hygienic measure, or to diminish the possibility of contracting venereal diseases. It is performed routinely in many hospitals on infants.

The best time for the operation is before the infant is ten days old, when it represents a minor procedure. Circumcision should always be done under strictest surgical or aseptic conditions. Proper repair of the tissues after the extra skin has been removed is essential. If the doctor's instructions regarding protection and cleansing of the wound are carefully followed, complications are rare.

Circumcision is recommended when the foreskin is unusually long so that it retains urine which might cause infection. Inflammation and irritation under the foreskin are also associated with various nervous manifestations. *See also* PENIS.

CIRRHOSIS, a chronic progressive disease, essentially inflammatory, with a pathological hardening of tissue brought about by an increase of connective tissue elements. The lungs, ovaries, heart, or stomach may be affected with cirrhosis, but it occurs more often in the kidney and liver.

Cirrhosis of the kidney, *chronic interstitial nephritis,* is a chronic inflammation of the connective tissue elements of the kidney. *Cirrhosis of the liver,* the most frequent type, is usually a disease of adults but may occasionally occur in younger people, and is three times more common among men than women. It in-

the disease and its causes Cirrhosis of the liver is a chronic disease of the liver which results in its hardening because of scar formation. Its causes and the exact mechanism of its development are uncertain. The disease is believed to be the result of chronic alcoholism and poor diet. Occasionally it is a complication of other diseases where malnutrition is a factor, as for example, diabetes, chronic dysentery, and some thyroid disorders.

A form of cirrhosis is also caused by the hepatitis virus.

symptoms The disease usually develops very slowly and the initial complaints are generalized, as illustrated in the Medi-Graph. The specific symptoms of the advanced stage may not appear for months or even years. As the disease advances, signs of liver failure develop. Jaundice, swelling of the feet and abdomen, and bleeding tendencies are seen. The skin is sallow and the veins over the face are larger, presenting the typical "alcoholic" face. There is also loss of hair in the armpits and pubic areas. The breasts in the male may enlarge and impotence may develop. As the disease progresses further, the patient becomes more anemic, his abdomen swells further and, in the final stages, he is likely to fall into a coma. The liver, which is enlarged when the disease begins, shrinks as it progresses.

complications Varicose veins can develop in the esophagus (the passageway between the mouth and stomach). This can result in bleeding from the intestinal tract. There can be severe secondary infections. Cancer of the liver can develop. Other complications are pancreatitis and peptic ulcer, but these are more likely to be related to the alcoholism and poor diet than to the liver cirrhosis. Liver coma is the most serious complication. It occurs late and may end fatally.

prevention (or lessening of impact) As with so many other diseases, early recognition and vigorous treatment can give good results. The approach includes control of drinking, adequate diet, and vitamin therapy. Secondary infections which appear must be dealt with and eliminated. Where there is abdominal fluid to be drained or bleeding to be stopped or any other specific symptom to treat, the signs and symptoms will determine the kind of treatment to be given. If the patient is in a coma, the attending physician will issue specific instructions for his care.

Again it is important to emphasize the grave consequences of indifference and delay in treating this disease.

Cirrhosis of the Liver

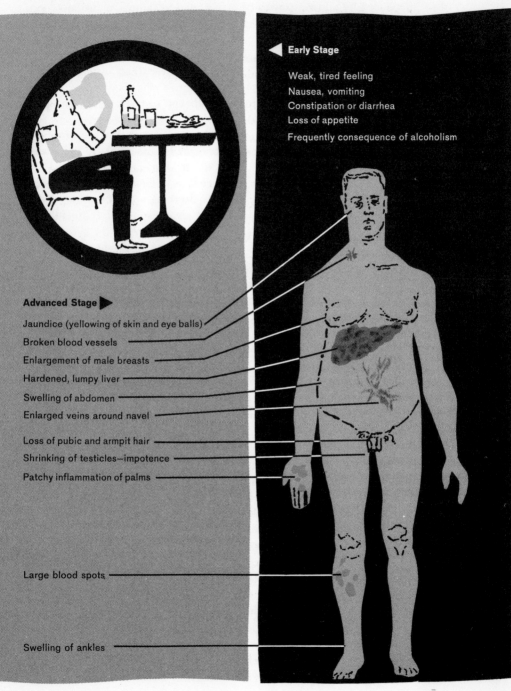

Weak, tired feeling
Nausea, vomiting
Constipation or diarrhea
Loss of appetite
Frequently consequence of alcoholism

Advanced Stage ▶

Jaundice (yellowing of skin and eye balls)
Broken blood vessels
Enlargement of male breasts
Hardened, lumpy liver
Swelling of abdomen
Enlarged veins around navel

Loss of pubic and armpit hair
Shrinking of testicles—impotence
Patchy inflammation of palms

Large blood spots

Swelling of ankles

411

volves a scarring or hardening of the liver, produced by an overgrowth of the connective tissue elements to the neglect of the true hepatic cells.

Heavy consumers of alcohol are often victims of cirrhosis, but moderate drinkers may become affected. The disease may also be caused by bacterial infection, particularly from bacteria of the colon, *infectious cirrhosis*. *See also* LIVER. *See* MEDIGRAPH page 411.

CITRIC ACID, a tribasic acid occurring in the juice of many fruits and in various animal tissues. It appears as translucent crystals or a white crystalline powder, soluble in water, and is employed as an acid flavoring and in effervescent drinks. Citric acid has an alkalizing effect, but is without vitamin value and is not an effective substitute for citrus fruits.

CLAUSTROPHOBIA, an intense fear of being in confined area. *See also* AGORAPHOBIA; ACROPHOBIA.

CLAVICLE, or *collarbone,* the curved bone which extends from the top of the breastbone out to each of the shoulders. Because the two clavicles are thin and small and support much weight they are frequently and easily broken. While mending, a small bony disfigurement is likely to occur, unless the person will lie motionless on his back, without a pillow, so that the two parts can remain in perfect adjustment to each other until they have completely grown together. *See also* FRACTURES.

CLEFT PALATE, a congenital defect, due to failure in fusion of embryonic facial processes, which results in a fissure through the palate. This cleavage, starting in the soft palate, may extend forward all the way across the bony roof of the mouth and even reach to the upper lip, resulting in *harelip*.

A person with this deformity is abnormally susceptible to inflammations in the area of the palate. Speech is difficult, as well as sucking, drinking, and chewing. Food being swallowed will frequently go through the roof of the mouth into the nostrils, and special feeding techniques become necessary.

A cleft palate can usually be corrected by an operation in which the tissues in the roof of the mouth are loosened and then fitted together. This operation is sometimes performed as early as the third month, or as late as the third year. If done before the child begins to talk, undesirable speech habits can be prevented. Even after a successful operation, however, some physical defect may remain. New techniques employing braces or plate or other prosthetic devices, along with intensive training, can significantly benefit persons with cleft palate. *See also* HARELIP; LIPS; PALATE.

CLIMATE, the average weather condition of an area over a period of years, as indicated by the temperature, rainfall, barometer, and other measurements. The connection between climate and health is a subject which has interested people for centuries. Greek and Roman physicians recognized that malaria affected persons living in low marshy areas, but they believed the cause of malaria was sleeping in night air. Hippocrates, the father of medicine who lived in the third century B.C., wrote, "If there be no rivers and the water that the people drank be

marshy and stagnant, the physique of the people must show protruding bellies and enlarged spleens." He did not know that the protruding belly and enlarged spleen are results of malaria, prevalent in marshy areas. In his book *Air, Water and Places,* he notes that "...

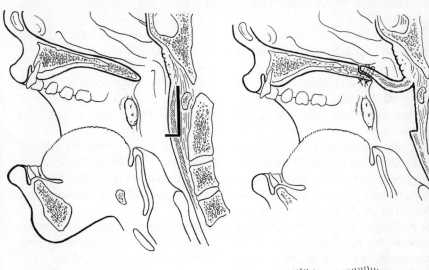

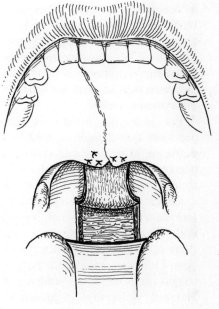

Cleft Palate—Cleft palate is the most frequent of congenital anomalies. The baby is born with a defect of the roof of the mouth. The opening in the roof of the mouth allows direct communication with the nose. Feeding is the major problem encountered with cleft palate. Sucking is difficult or impossible, and the milk tends to run out through the nose instead of being swallowed. Eventually, dentition and speech are affected. Drawing (A) shows the opening in the roof of the mouth. Part of the posterior pharyngeal flap will be brought forward and attached to the posterior end of the short soft palate. (B) shows the flap attached. (C) View of the roof of the mouth showing the repaired fissure.

the inhabitants of a region that is mountainous, rugged, high and watered, where the changes of the seasons exhibit strong contrasts, are likely to be of big physique, with a nature well adapted for endurance and courage." This is the first recorded recognition that the temperate zone is a region conducive to good health.

More recently, persons with "consumption" or tuberculosis went to dry, high-altitude areas in an attempt to cure their illness. However, today it is felt that climate is not important in treating tuberculosis, and emphasis is place on drugs, food, rest, and competent medical care.

Persons with rheumatic conditions frequently feel better when they are not exposed to cold and dampness. Research on rheumatism has shown that changes occur in the composition of the body tissues, including the blood, when there are changes in barometric pressure. Changes in blood supply to the joints are associated with sudden changes in temperature. While climate cannot cause rheumatic conditions, it may lower the resistance so that a rheumatic inflammation results.

For years the belief has been prevalent that dampness, cold, and drafts are associated with colds and pneumonia. However, statistics seem to indicate that, unless a person has a tendency to respiratory ailments, inclement weather does not provoke such illnesses. For example, students at Stanford University at Palo Alto, California, have about as many coughs and colds as students at Harvard University in Massachu-

setts, despite the fact that the California climate is mild and the Massachusetts climate rigorous. However, persons whose resistance is generally low will be more susceptible to inflammation of the nose, throat, and sinuses during cold weather, and will benefit by a change to a warm dry climate.

Persons with heart disease do not do well at high altitudes, because of increased difficulty in getting oxygen for circulation.

Generally a mild climate is most beneficial to those persons with chronic diseases, and a specialist may propose that a change of climate be made to relieve their symptoms. But it is wise to check with a physician before assuming that another climate will be more beneficial.

CLINITEST, a commercially available kit by means of which persons having or suspecting a diabetic tendency may check the extent of sugar in the urine. *See also* DIABETES.

CLITORIS, the organ in women which is homologous to the penis of the male. This small tubelike body is located in the angle at the top of the vulva, the external sex organ of women. Like the penis, the clitoris is composed of tissue which becomes engorged with blood, and hard and erect during sexual excitement. *See also* REPRODUCTION SYSTEM; VULVA.

CLOTHING. The fundamental needs of the human being include food, fuel, clothing, shelter, medical and dental care. Much is written about the hygiene of the body from the point of view of housing, nutrition, and warmth. Seldom is serious consideration given to the hygiene of our clothing.

Some scientists insist that human beings first adopted clothing for decorative purposes in order to call attention to themselves or to certain portions of their bodies. Others insist that clothing came because of the development of a sense of modesty. A final view says that we wear clothing to protect us against exposure to cold and the elements.

Probably clothing came first as a decoration; exactly as various animals have highly colored plumage to attract the opposite sex, primitive man probably began fastening things to his body as a means of attraction.

In earlier days most men lived in warm climates, so that clothing was not needed for protection against the elements. It is reasonable to believe that human beings could not have spread from these warm areas to the cold areas without the development of clothing. Man is a warm-blooded animal. He must sustain the warmth of his body if he is to live. Clothing is one means by which the warmth is held within his body. The coverings do not create heat; they do diminish the rate at which heat is lost from the body.

We lose water from the body through the skin. By the evaporation of this water we also lose heat. When there is too much heat lost from the surface of the body, chilling occurs; hence clothing must be changed from one season of the year to another to meet the conditions necessary for health and comfort.

Various fabrics vary in their ability to retain heat and moisture and to permit ventilation. Cotton and linen garments permit heat to pass off rapidly and thus help to keep the body cool. Silk and wool do not conduct heat rapidly and are, therefore, better suited to winter than summer wear.

Of special importance is the choice of underclothing. In summer all cotton or lightweight silk or mixed silk and cotton garments are more suitable than woolen garments. Some types of clothing permit ultraviolet rays to pass through them more easily than others. A fabric with open mesh not only permits the circulation of air and irradiation of heat but also permits more sunlight to pass through than a fabric with closed mesh.

From the health point of view garments should in general never be so tight as to constrict the tissues. Any garment that is so tight as to prevent circulation of the blood and a free expansion of the organs of the body is not a healthful garment. Garters, belts, and bands which are so tight that they leave red marks on the skin and dents in the flesh interfere with the circulation of the blood and should not be considered suitable.

One of the chief difficulties in modern clothing is the necessity of adapting its use to both indoor and outdoor conditions. In winter women wear fur coats for outdoor use but customarily wear thin clothing both summer and winter for indoor use. The average man wears heavy clothing both indoors and outdoors.

Most hygienists are inclined to recommend to both men and women that all clothing not necessary for warmth or modesty should be eliminated for indoor wear. Nevertheless fashions have much more to do with the choice of clothing by both men and women than hygienic considerations. When it is the custom for men to wear jackets indoors, they will do so; when it is the custom for women to do without protection to the feet, legs, and chest, they will go without the clothing necessary for warmth.

Change of clothing according to the season of the year is much less necessary in the modern city than was the case in a previous generation. The use of the automobile for transportation, the heated street-car and bus, the heated and air-conditioned schoolroom, assembly hall, and theater make it possible for most people to wear clothing that is reasonably light and to plan only for a single heavy garment for protection against the elements.

The growing boy and girl may well be cautioned against following every foolish fad in clothing that comes along. Students are often responsible for beginning unusual fads. The intelligent student will consider carefully whether or not the wearing of clothing of a conspicuous appearance for the attraction of momentary attention is worth while. Cleanliness, orderliness, neatness, and the most nearly perfect fitting that is possible are what is most important in producing attractiveness.

CLUBFOOT, a deformity of the foot, present at birth or caused subsequently by muscle paralysis or injury, in which the heel or the ball of the foot or one edge of it does not touch the ground.

In three-fourths of the cases noted at birth, the heel and inner edge of the foot are raised. This condition occurs once in every thousand births, and considerably more than half of those affected are male children. Also, in more than half the deformity occurs on only one side.

Treatment must be started at the earliest possible moment. The later therapy begins, the longer it will take to remedy the deformity. Children under a year can be treated in twenty-three weeks, whereas those of six years or more require almost forty-two weeks. One of the signal achievements of modern medical science has been the development of treatment for club foot.

The doctor, usually an orthopedist, will outline a routine of the manipulations of the parts involved to get them into the correct position and then make the position secure with one or more of the devices designed especially for the purpose, such as adhesive bindings, plaster casts, or braces and splints. After the proper position has been firmly established, special exercises, shoes, massage, and other measures which may be beneficial will be prescribed. Active treatment often continues for several months, and follow-up supervision is necessary for years.

Manipulation alone may not be satisfactory. Then surgical rearrangement of the affected tissues and parts becomes necessary.

The cause of clubfoot is un-

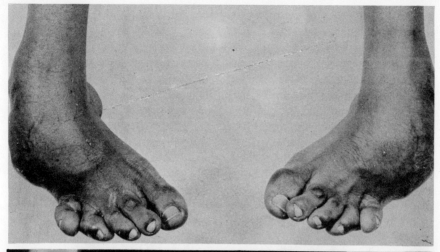

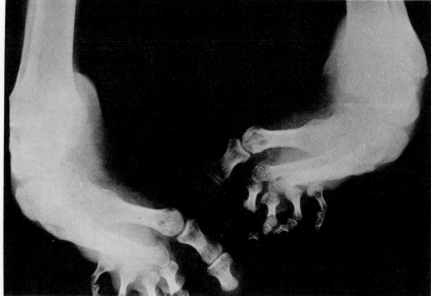

Clubfoot—Condition of clubfoot. X-ray shows the malformation of the bones in the foot.

Surgery, if done early, can often correct much of the deformity in infants born with clubfoot.

known. Heredity is suspected by some persons, because approximately 5 per cent of cases occur in families in which the deformity has appeared previously; others believe that an incorrect position of the child before birth is responsible.

COAGULATION, the formation of a *coagulum, clot,* or *curd* as in blood or milk. When bleeding is present, threadlike fibers called *fibrin* are produced by a substance in the blood, the *fibrinogen.* These fibers trap *white* and *red blood corpuscles* which form a clot. Contraction of the fibrin squeezes out the liquid portion of the blood, the *serum,* and a *crust* develops. The system of clotting is counteracted by agents, including *heparin* and other *anticoagulants,* which keep the blood fluid. The power of coagulation of the blood varies with different persons. In people with *hemophilia,* a hereditary disease, the clotting is so retarded that they bleed profusely from minor wounds and may even bleed to death.

Formation of a blood clot in a *coronary artery* may obstruct the flow of blood to the heart muscle and produce *coronary thrombosis.* The incidence of clotting may be increased when the person is under stress. A blood clot blocking an artery of the brain, usually where a weak spot has resulted through *arteriosclerosis,* may induce a *cerebral hemorrhage.* Coagulation of blood in the lower body regions can cause serious complications if particles of the blood clot reach the lungs and obstruct the major blood vessels.

Heparin, dicumarol, Tromexan, and other anticoagulants have been developed and the administration of anticoagulants has become a significant medication. *See also* BLOOD; CORONARY THROMBOSIS; EMBOLISM; HEMOPHILIA; MENORRHAGIA. *See* MEDIGRAPHS pages 127, 129, 1035.

COCAINE, an alkaloid derived from the coca bush, in use for centuries. Inca priests in Peru, for example, were aware of its anesthetic effect and chewed coca leaves in an attempt to improve their physical endurance.

Medically it was first used as an anesthetic in eye operations in Vienna in 1884. Cocaine is now employed as a local anesthetic. It produces temporary insensitivity to pain when applied to the surface of mucous membranes or injected by hypodermic needle.

Cocaine is habit-forming and poisonous, and should never be used in any way except when prescribed and administered by a physician. The amount of cocaine required to poison varies greatly; some people react unfavorably even to small doses. New synthetic compounds have been developed which are similar to cocaine but less toxic. *See also* DRUG ADDICTION.

COCCIDIOIDOMYCOSIS, also known as *desert fever, San Joaquin fever, valley fever,* or *the bumps,* a disease with pulmonary symptoms caused by one of the fungi, *Coccidioides immitis,* which thrives in the dry dusty areas of the San Joaquin Valley and in the southwestern states. During World War II, thousands of servicemen stationed in camps throughout this area became ill with coccidioidomycosis after inhaling the tiny invisible particles of spore-laden dust. Spores may also enter the skin through open wounds.

The first symptoms, which resemble the symptoms of tuberculosis, are generally chills, fever, headache, general malaise, night sweats, and coughing. These symptoms usually subside after a week or two and small bumps may then appear under the skin, which also disappear in time. In severe cases, x-rays show changes in the lungs and occasionally thin-walled cavities which may persist for years.

Recovery from a simple lung infection is usually rapid and complete even without treatment, but in cases where deep lung cavities have developed, surgery may be required.

The growing prevalence of coccidioidomycosis has made it a public health concern. About 90 per cent of the people living in these arid regions have had the infection within a ten-year period as a result of inhaling the spores of the fungus. Droughts in this area add to the disease hazards. Residents or visitors who show signs of a chronic infection resembling any of the serious respiratory diseases should have chest x-rays and skin and blood tests. *See also* HISTOPLASMOSIS.

COCCYX, from the Greek meaning "shaped like the bill of a cuckoo," the last bone at the lowermost end of the spine.

CODEINE, an alkaloid derived from opium and closely allied in chemical constitution to morphine. Though weaker, its action is similar to that of morphine, and it is used medically to diminish sensitivity to pain.

COD LIVER OIL, the partially destearinated fixed oil, obtained from the fresh livers of cod. The liver of the cod (and also of the halibut) is one of the richest sources of vitamin A and D, and cod liver oil has been

known for many years as an effective treatment for malnutrition. Mild cases of rickets improve quickly with cod liver oil. Diets which do not contain enough fat-soluble vitamins are a basic factor of sinusitis in children, and cod liver oil is recommended by many physicians as an effective preventive measure against this infection. Every growing baby and child should have cod liver oil or its equivalent in vitamins A and D, and nursing mothers are advised by physicians to take it regularly. The amount of cod liver oil usually recommended is a teaspoonful daily of the more concentrated preparations, or two teaspoonfuls of the less concentrated. *See also* CHILD CARE.

COFFEE, a beverage made by an infusion or decoction from the roasted and ground or pounded seeds of a shrub, small tree, or other species of the madder family. Although coffee has no nutritional value, taken in moderation it does have some pharmacological worth.

An average cup of coffee contains about one grain of *caffeine,* an alkaloid which stimulates the brain, kidney, and circulation. It increases the force and beat of the heart and the flow of urine and thus helps cleanse the body of metabolic end-products. This action has made coffee valuable in cases of edema or dropsy, conditions in which fluid accumulates excessively in the tissues. In these cases, it is vital to increase the heart rate so that more blood is pumped into the blood vessels, thus promoting greater flow through the kidneys with elimination of fluid.

Generally a cup of coffee after dinner may have a good effect on the digestion since it increases the gastric juice. However, an excess of coffee can easily have toxic effects, such as rapid pulse, nervousness, irritability, and insomnia. In some persons, too much coffee may even bring on attacks of dizziness and faintness, or palpitation from an overaccelerated heart rate and force. The amount of coffee that can safely be drunk varies among people. For some people a few cups a day may be excessive. People should discover what is the correct amount for them.

Tests made in 1955 by the American Medical Association established that a cup of regular ground coffee has almost twice as much caffeine as a cup of instant coffee, and a cup of regular decaffeinated coffee has about one-third the amount of caffeine as a cup of regular ground coffee.

COITUS, a technical term for sexual intercourse. *See also* REPRODUCTION SYSTEM.

COLCHICINE, a water-soluble, pale brownish alkaloid derived from the meadow saffron which has been used as an efficient pain reliever in gout for more than a hundred years. However, it has proved of little value in other types of arthritis and rheumatism. *See also* GOUT.

COLD. *See* COMMON COLD.

COLD CREAM, a mixture in an ointment of petrolatum, lanolin, and rosewater, which is useful for soothing dry, inflamed, or irritated skin, and also for removing cosmetics. *See also* COSMETICS.

COLD SORE. *See* HERPES SIMPLEX.

COLIC, the abnormal and violent contraction of certain internal muscular tissues. *Intestinal colic* is caused by a sudden contraction of the intestine. When the bile ducts contract abnormally, *biliary colic* results, and *renal colic* is caused by a tightening of the tube, the ureter, which passes between the kidney and bladder. Alternate contraction and relaxation is the normal behavior of these organs, and pain occurs only when this contraction becomes spasmodic.

Intestinal colic is the most common. The pain is noticed usually around the navel, and is often accompanied by a clogging or loosening of the bowels. If the cause of pain is doubtful, cathartics and laxatives should be avoided but an enema may be given if necessary. A simple chill, infected food, or a nervous condition are a few of the many possible causes of colic. Colic may be easily confused with a serious disorder, such as *appendicitis*. If the pain does not respond promptly to simple treatment, such as an electric pad or a hot-water bottle, or bicarbonate of soda, a physician should be called.

Intestinal colic, produced by gas, is commonly seen in infants. Often this condition results from the air taken in with the child's milk or food. Occasionally, however, it may

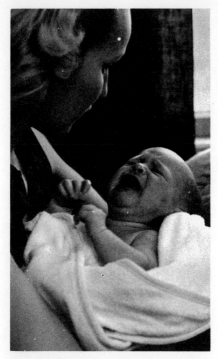

Colic—This intestinal cramp is common in babies of about two to four weeks and up to four months. The exact causes are unknown, but they probably include tension, under- or over-feeding and swallowing air. A doctor should be consulted if colic occurs frequently. Extra care in burping, and soothing the baby are recommended. Colic usually disappears after four months.

be generated by the fermentation of food in the bowels. Regardless of the source, this gas can often be relieved simply by placing the baby across one's shoulder after every feeding and tapping it lightly on the back until it "burps." If the pain persists or is severe, a doctor should be consulted.

A special type of *stomach colic,* afflicting adults, which involves spasmodic contractions of the large bowel, is known as *mucous colic.* The pain occurs characteristically

after meals, and is located chiefly in the right section of the lower abdomen. Such symptoms should be carefully investigated by a specialist who may take x-rays, inspect stools, and study the person's diet. Occasionally psychiatric observation may be necessary.

Renal colic, distress after meals and in the lower right abdomen, is usually caused by a stone in the kidney trying to descend to the bladder. The pain almost always starts in the kidney area and moves to the abdomen, leg, and genitals. Nausea and a frequent desire to urinate appear. In attempting to walk, the person will experience a pronounced tendency to tip his body to the side affected, depending on which of the kidney areas is affected. The pain may fluctuate and may even be severe enough to induce delirium.

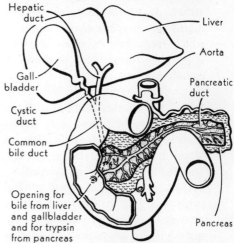

Colic—Here are shown the relationships between the liver and the gallbladder and the tubes known as the hepatic duct, the cystic duct, and the common bile duct, which carry the bile to the intestines. From the pancreas comes another duct which carries a digestive fluid called *trypsin* into the intestine.

421

Renal colic can be subdued by proper drugs. The pain will sometimes persist for days, but usually is limited to twelve hours or less. The stone is sometimes passed spontaneously in the urine, but frequently surgical treatment is required. *See also* CONSTIPATION; DIARRHEA; INDIGESTION.

COLITIS, inflammation of the *colon,* the part of the large intestine extending from the *cecum* to the *rectum.* Various forms of colitis can occur. Simple colitis is an acute irritation or infection of the colon, accompanied by diarrhea. Some types of colitis are caused by infection of the colon by specific organisms.

Mucous colitis is a condition in which the mucous membrane of the colon is inflamed, with symptoms of colicky pain, and constipation or diarrhea. It would seem to be primarily a psychosomatic ailment, which frequently becomes chronic.

Another form which is probably usually nervous in origin is *ulcerative colitis,* characterized by ulceration of the mucous membrane of the colon. The symptoms may range from only painless excretion of blood in stools to dysentery, fever, and death as a result of exhaustion, perforation of the colon and general peritonitis. Less critical cases usually recover completely, although frequently there are periods of relapse. Sometimes the disease becomes chronic, but without producing any severe disability. The entire length of the colon becomes scarred and thickened with ulcerations, and at this stage such complications as per-foration, malignant disease, nutritional deficiency, and intestinal obstruction frequently occur.

Treatment of ulcerative colitis requires patient medical care, including bed rest, proper diet, sedatives, control of infection, and, if necessary, blood transfusions. Cortisone and ACTH have been used in treatment, but it is too soon to determine their value. Occasionally surgical removal of the colon is advised; and when emotional factors are thought to be involved in any way, psychotherapy is recommended. *See also* INTESTINES; ILEITIS; PEPTIC ULCER. *See* MEDIGRAPHS pages 301, 1295, 1297.

COLLAGEN DISEASES, the name for certain diseases of the connective tissue. They are rather unusual and rare diseases and are often grouped together under the general term of collagen diseases. Their names are *polyarteritis nodosa, diffuse lupus erythematosus, scleroderma, and dermatomyositis.* They resemble each other in that all of them represent disturbances of connective tissue in the body in contrast to glandular tissue or surface secreting tissue. An important fact about the collagen diseases is the discovery, made in 1950, that all of them are benefited, at least temporarily, by ACTH or cortisone. Arthritis, which also responds to the drugs mentioned, occurs commonly in connection with each of these diseases.

Polyarteritis nodosa. Polyarteritis nodosa is a disease in which the blood vessels are chiefly affected. Because this disease is primarily associated with serious damage of blood vessels, it may occur in any part of the body. The condition affects men four times as often as women and mostly those between twenty and forty years old. Arthritis and many of the reactions associated with hypersensitivity are observed in this disease.

Lupus erythematosus. Disseminated lupus erythematosus is a chronic, usually severe, disorder occurring mostly in females fifteen to forty years old. A characteristic is a butterfly-shaped inflammation over the nose. Other symptoms involve the joints and the heart.

Scleroderma. Scleroderma is a disease that affects the connective tissue of the body and particularly that in the skin, where there is hardening. Chiefly women between thirty and fifty years old are affected. The swelling in the skin may be followed by calcification. This disease comes on slowly and insidiously, but as it progresses, changes occur in the skin of the face, neck and arms. The skin looks waxy and tight and loses its color and hair. When the face is involved there may be difficulty in moving the jaw. Fortunately this is not a common disease; certainly it is not as serious as *polyarteritis nodosa* or *diffuse lupus erythematosus,* which are similar. In the older forms of treatment emphasis was placed on the use of thyroid extract and vitamins. Great care was given to prevent secondary infections. More recently attention is being focused on the use of ACTH and cortisone.

Dermatomyositis. Fourth in this group of collagen disorders is one called dermatomyositis. This is a common and often fatal disorder involving the skin and the muscles. The exact cause is still unknown. It affects people of all races, both men and women, and in general those between the ages of ten and fifty years.

Characteristic of this condition is the involvement of the muscles. As they deteriorate, the organs concerned show effects, as in the eyes, throat, diaphragm, or muscles between the ribs. The symptoms then are difficulties of vision, swallowing, breathing, speech, etc. These symptoms are accompanied by weakness and loss of weight. *See* MEDIGRAPH page 869.

COLLARBONE, the common name for clavicle. *See also* CLAVICLE.

COLLODION, a coating or film used to protect and dress wounds. It is produced by dissolving gun cotton in ether and alcohol.

COLOR BLINDNESS. *See* EYE.

COLOSTOMY, a surgical operation, usually on the left side of the lower abdomen, creating a more or less permanent opening in the colon to permit evacuation after the normal rectal and anal opening is lost (usually because of operation to remove a tumor or cancer).

COMA, a state of complete loss of consciousness from which the person cannot be aroused even by the most powerful stimulation. The forms of coma most frequently seen

Causes of coma in a large city hospital

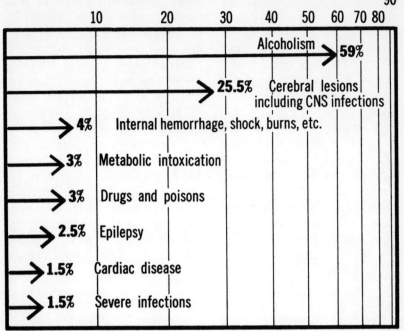

are those following gross alcoholic intoxication and in diabetes. The treatment of such forms of coma is so serious that it should never be undertaken except by a physician. *See also* DIABETES.

COMEDOS, the scientific term for blackheads. *See* ACNE.

COMMON COLD, an acute inflammation of the upper respiratory tract, involving the nose and throat. It is one of the most familiar ailments which afflicts mankind yet its specific cause is little understood. Susceptibility to colds is almost universal, particularly among children. The cold is highly contagious, especially indoors, and places where groups of people congregate are excellent transmission spots for the infection.

When one has scarlet fever or diphtheria or measles, a single attack seems to protect against a second attack, at least for many years. However, the immunity of resistance to another similar infection following a cold is short. Studies made on animals show that it lasts less than a month. An extensive investigation made in human beings indicated that it was probably between two and three weeks.

In large urban communities where the climate is temperate, the general population averages about three colds a year. This median is higher among susceptible adults and children. The incidence is lowest in the summer, rises in the autumn, reaching its peak in midwinter and declines in the spring.

Several peak periods occur in smaller urban communities. The first is in early autumn when schools re-open and children are brought into greater proximity indoors. In addition to the winter rise in incidence of colds, a smaller rise often appears in the spring.

Colds are definitely communicable and are transmitted either by direct contact or by spread of the infected droplets of discharge. A practical method to control the spread of colds has not yet been developed. The common cold is due to any of several viruses. Scientists believe that these viruses are generally present in the throat but become active only when the body resistance is lowered. When the activated cold virus attacks the mucous membranes of the nose and throat, these tissues are weakened and become susceptible to infection by bacteria which are also generally found in the body. It has been demonstrated that sudden changes in temperature and excessive chilling or wetting of the skin promote conditions of the mucous membranes in the nose and throat that permit the virus to invade some individuals and from them to spread throughout the community. Chilling alone will not produce a cold, since the organism necessary for the infection must also be present.

The bacteria are secondary invaders and the virus paves the way for their entry into the mucous membranes. Although they are not re-sponsible for the common cold, the bacteria may initiate a secondary infection which either intensifies the local inflammation present, prolonging the cold, or causes new complications such as *purulent sinusitis* or *otitis,* an inflammation of the ear. Infants and young children appear to be more susceptible to these secondary infections than adults.

A cold usually begins abruptly, with a sense of soreness and dryness in the nose or back of the throat. Within a few hours the nasal passages feel congested, sneezing develops and a colorless watery discharge comes from the nose. After forty-eight hours the cold is usually at its peak, and is accompanied by excessive watering of the eyes, huskiness of the voice, and difficulty in breathing as the congestion spreads. The nasal discharge becomes thick and sticky and some coughing may develop. The cough does not usually bring up much discharge unless the person has a tendency to *chronic bronchitis.* Frequently a headache, a sense of lethargy and malaise, and vague pains in the back and limbs accompany a cold. A fever is not always present, although in children a temperature of 102° F or even higher often develops.

The uncomplicated cold generally lasts from one to two weeks and terminates without special treatment. Colds which persist or recur repeatedly, or in which there is a steady prolonged fever or chills, particularly in children or susceptible adults, may indicate complications and a physician should be consulted.

As yet, a specific agent has not been developed to control the common cold and treatment is confined to relief of symptoms and control of complications. Treatment of the cold is not very different today from the treatment used by past generations. Bed rest should be enforced whenever possible and as much isolation as is practicable. Plenty of liquids, hot or cold, a light diet, and keeping warm promote greater comfort. Aspirin in small repeated doses generally gives relief as does gargling in cases of sore throat. An aspirin tablet or a teaspoon of salt dissolved in hot water is beneficial. In the latter stages of a cold, when the discharge has thickened, an atomizer or nose drops or inhaler helps clear the nasal passages. They should not be used more than once in four hours and if the person has a tendency to nasal inflammation should be employed sparingly.

Cold vaccines, which are suspensions of dead bacteria collected from the discharge of a cold, have not been found to be significantly effective either when taken by mouth or when given as an injection or nasal spray. However, continued research is being done. The routine use of *sulfonamides* or *antibiotics* for colds is definitely discouraged. These drugs should be given only in cases with a definite bacterial secondary infection—for example, in *bronchopneumonia, sinusitis,* or *otitis media.* Persons who have a consistent history of recurrent colds with accompanying complications may use antibiotics or sulfonamides, but only on the advice of a physician.

Although little is known about curing a cold, measures can be taken to ward off the infection and decrease its incidence. A well-balanced diet, sufficient rest, proper dress both indoors and out, all help to keep the body resistance high. Undue exposure to sharp changes in temperature should be avoided. Proper ventilation of rooms, with sufficient humidity in the air, helps to keep the mucous membranes in healthy condition. If humidifiers are not used, adequate moisture can be maintained by keeping a pan of water on a radiator or stove. Particular care should be taken to avoid contact with persons who have colds. Simple hygienic measures like washing the hands before eating or covering a sneeze all help to decrease the occurrence of colds.

In summary the common cold is an infectious disease caused by any of several viruses. Other incitants such as allergic or traumatic factors may produce conditions indistinguishable from the common cold. The viruses are about the size of the encephalitic viruses and measure about half the diameter of the influenza virus. They are infective only in human beings and chimpanzees. These viruses induce a poor immune response and apparently do not produce demonstrable antibody response. The occurrence of a cold increases resistance to reinfection with the same material for two weeks but not for three weeks. The incubation period in volunteers inoculated intranasally with bacteriologically sterile filtrates of nasal secretions from patients with typical colds is from one to six days with an average of two to three days.

Attempts to demonstrate contact transmission, even by the most intimate contact, have failed. This does not necessarily mean that the common cold is not contagious, but suggests that artificially induced colds may differ from colds occurring naturally.

Complications of the common cold occur because of the loss of the normal protective mechanisms in the mucous membranes, especially of the ciliary mechanism. The pain associated with sinusitis arises from changes in the turbinates and other structures in the nasal chamber rather than from the sinuses themselves.

Antihistaminic drugs such as Coriciden, Anahist, Pyrabenzamine, Benadryl and a host of others do not affect the common cold. Excessive use of antihistaminics may actually prolong and intensify a common cold. *Tonsillectomy* and *adenoidectomy* as such will not lessen the incidence of viral infections. If the tonsils or adenoids are manifestly infected their excision will remove a reservoir of secondary infection and thereby lessen the incidence and possibly the severity of secondary bacterial complications. *Antimicrobial therapy* (antibiotics or sulfa drugs) as a preventive measure to be given by any route to patients with the common cold in order to lessen the incidence or severity of complications is frequently inadvisable since such complications are few and since sensitivity to the drug or development of resistance by the bacteria

may thereby be produced. Exceptions to the general rule are those patients in whom by past history one can anticipate serious bacterial complications if antibacterial agents are not given.

Vasoconstrictors applied to the mucous membranes must be used cautiously. Many such agents available produce more harm than good since they cause vasodilatation and irritation following their initial constrictor action. Two per cent *ephedrine* in normal saline is relatively free from untoward effects and is more useful than proprietary agents widely advertised. It is well established that diet, fruit juices, ascorbic acid, and other vitamins do not significantly influence the incidence or course of the common cold. Oily sprays or drops are not recommended for use because of the hazard of *lipoid pneumonia,* particularly in youngsters. Otolaryngologists object to jellies of any sort, such as neosynephrin jelly. The jelly acts as a mechanical blocking agent obstructing nasal drainage. There is no evidence to suggest that vitamins of any sort are of value in preventing or treating any infectious disease unless there is coincident obvious undernutrition. *See also* BRONCHOPNEUMONIA; CHILD CARE; OTITIS; SINUSES. *See* MEDIGRAPH page 1183.

COMMUNICABLE DISEASES, those which are transmissible from one person to another. The distinction, often disregarded, between *infectious* and *contagious* diseases consists of the fact that while infectious diseases are caused by the invasion of an infective agent such as a fungus, bacillus or virus, the agents are not necessarily transmitted by another person as is the case with contagious diseases.

COMPOUND FRACTURE. The breaking of a bone is a fracture. In a compound fracture, the point of the fracture is in contact with the outer surface of the body—for example, through a wound. If the break is covered by the skin, it is a simple fracture. *See also* BONES; FIRST AID; FRACTURES.

COMPRESS, a piece of folded gauze cloth, or a soft pad which is applied firmly to a part of the body to relieve inflammations, produce pressure, or prevent hemorrhage. It may be wet or dry, hot or cold, and is sometimes perforated for drainage or observation of the underlying skin.

COMPRESSION. The chief effects of high altitude and changes in barometric pressure are dependent on the way in which this affects the use of oxygen by the body. The most common symptoms associated with compression, as in diving or descending suddenly from high altitudes, is pain in one or both ears, particularly when the tubes are obstructed. To this the name of *aero-otitis media* has been given. After or during the breathing of oxygen this condition may develop during sleep because the Eustachian tubes, which go from the back of the throat to the middle ear, rarely open during sleep. The

rate of compression is important in governing the degree to which an individual suffers from high altitude. If descent is made reasonably slowly, the difficulties do not arise. In commercial passenger aircraft the rate of descent from high altitude is limited to 300 feet per minute. Under these circumstances pain in the ears seldom occurs. Sometimes people who have been exposed to compression develop pains in the frontal sinuses because of blocking. The pain is due to the same conditions that result in pain in the ears.

A remarkable condition is the expansion of abdominal gas that occurs under some circumstances. When helium was used in diving, the mouthpiece produced flow of saliva and considerable amounts of gas were swallowed. When the men came to the surface rapidly, the gas in the stomach expanded and the pressure brought about so much pain as to induce collapse. Now it is generally known that swallowed air or gas rather than food is the source of most abdominal gas. Certain foods, however, tend to produce abdominal gas, including melons, beans, and carbonated beverages.

The big problem of high altitudes is little oxygen and this, of course, is being governed in aircraft by the use of oxygen chambers so that oxygen is then released into the cabins and the pressure is kept at a proper level. Nowadays provision is made for a supply of oxygen on all flights above 10,000 feet and on all flights of more than four hours' duration between 8,000 and 10,000 feet.

When divers and compressed-air

workers are subjected to rapid decompression, air bubbles form in the blood and they may produce such symptoms as pain, which are called "the bends," asphyxiation which is called "the chokes," and paralysis. The most common manifestation is the dull throbbing type of pain in the joints and in the muscles and bones which is known as "the bends." Normal breathing becomes shallow, rapid and then the worker seems short of breath. This condition is called "the chokes." If this is not relieved the skin becomes cold and moist, the circulation impaired and the person may actually have symptoms like those of shock. The treatment includes prolonged recompression and the use of oxygen and fluids and then slowly decompression so that the worker does not suffer from these difficult symptoms. The condition is a serious one and should always be recognized and treated promptly. *See also* CAISSON DISEASE.

COMPULSION, defined in psychology as an irresistible, irrational desire to repeat certain acts. For example, a person may have the compulsion to wash his hands every few minutes, or to avoid stepping on the cracks in the sidewalks.

COMPUTERS. Computers are being used increasingly in the diagnosis, evaluation, and care of heart disease. They are used to measure various body functions and to detect abnormal electrocardiographic, electroencephalographic, and radiologic signals and indications. One computer system reads Papanicolaou smears used in the detection of cervical cancer, screening out the suspicious smears which can then be examined by the pathologist. Similar computer techniques are used to examine cells from the lungs, stomach, and other organs. Computer departments have been established at many of the leading medical centers.

CONCEPTION, the union of sperm and ovum, the male and female sex cells, resulting in the development of a new life. Conception is sometimes called *fertilization, impregnation,* or *fecundation,* and should be distinguished from *copulation,* which refers to the act of sexual intercourse between the male and female.

Since the egg cell of the female lives for only about twelve hours out of every month, the male seed must be deposited within the female genital tract during these few hours, or within two or three days of release of an egg. The sperm cells live about three days after ejaculation.

Conception usually takes place within the Fallopian tubes adjacent to the uterus and ovaries, and may occur within an hour of intercourse. Following union of the male and female sex cells, development is rapid, and eight to fourteen days later the embryo imbeds itself in the lining of the uterus where it remains until birth. *See also* REPRODUCTION SYSTEM; PREGNANCY, SIGNS OF.

CONCUSSION, a shock, severe shaking or jarring of a part of the body, usually resulting from a fall or blow. It also refers to the morbid state resulting from such a jarring. A concussion of the brain is actually a paralysis of its function, and symptoms are not due to any fracture or laceration. Signs of hemorrhage or loss of blood from the coverings around the brain may be present. Sometimes disturbances occur in the circulation of spinal fluid through the brain, and occasionally part of the soft white material of the brain is crushed or the connection cords between different portions of the brain are damaged or destroyed.

Brain concussion itself is seldom fatal. Necropsies (post-mortems) have shown that some apparent serious lesion of brain substance or vessels has occurred in fatal cases which had the characteristics of concussion but actually were contusions or lacerations. Whenever a concussion is suspected, a physician should be consulted. An x-ray examination should be made to determine whether or not fracture of the skull or other complications have occurred. While a slight crack of the skull is not critical, the pressure that may result from the bleeding inside the skull may be so.

Symptoms of concussion appear immediately after the injury and vary depending on the degree of injury. Probably there will be a severe aching of the head, a weak dizzy "stunned" feeling. Disturbances in vision, cold perspiration, and shallow respiration may appear. If the jarring has been severe, more extreme symptoms may develop at once. The victim may be in partial coma or unconscious. The body will be cold and respiration exceedingly weak. Often vomiting accompanies these symptoms.

The consequences of a concussion may be of short duration or last for days or weeks or longer. Often, after regaining his senses, the person is unable to remember anything that happened during the time when consciousness was lost. Frequently symptoms of contusion and hemorrhage may develop and with them serious brain injuries. When the symptoms are protracted, a more serious affliction is always suggested.

During emergency treatment, the person should lie flat and be kept warm and quiet. Attempts at stimulation should not be made. No pressure should be applied or strong antiseptics given. *See also* HEAD INJURIES; SHOCK.

CONDITIONING, the development of a better physiological condition through physical exercise and training.

A great football coach once said that "a true athlete developed from the inside out, from healthy blood circulation and healthy cells to healthy muscles and nerves." Athletes are thus in "good condition," if their whole body functions as well as it can. To reach this goal, good nutrition, exercise, fresh air, rest and sleep as well as other healthful habits must prevail. Athletic coaches check carefully on the weight of their charges and keep accurate records of their physical well-being. Thus they can establish whether or not an athlete works out too much or needs additional assistance to get into top form. Psychologically, conditioning is the process of attaching a new stimulus to an old response, or a new response to an old stimulus. For example, in conditioning a dog to salivate at the sound of a bell, the salivation is an old response and the bell is the new stimulus which provokes the response.

CONDOM, a rubber or plastic sheath used to cover the penis during sexual intercourse to prevent the male sperm from reaching and fertilizing the female egg cell. It is a device for the prevention of infection as well as conception. *See also* CONTRACEPTION.

CONJUNCTIVITIS, inflammation of the *conjunctiva,* the mucous membrane covering the globe and lids of the eyes. Many types of conjunctivitis exist, including *allergic conjunctiva, catarrhal conjunctivitis,* the most common form which usually results from irritation or a cold, and *acute contagious conjunctivitis* or *pinkeye. See also* PINKEYE; EYE. *See* MEDIGRAPHS pages 433, 1331.

CONSTIPATION, the retention of feces within the bowel for an unusually long time, or undue difficulty in its evacuation.

The excretion of feces is the final step in the process of digestion. The waste material enters the colon as a loose moist mass, and there the excess water is absorbed by the body. The relatively solid mass of waste material then moves on into the rec-

tum, where it normally prompts the desire for a movement of the bowels by pressure on the muscles.

Evacuation ordinarily occurs once or twice every twenty-four hours, with a wide range of variation among individuals. With some persons greater frequency is common, while with others an interval of several days may often pass without ill effect. A fixed schedule for this function for all persons is unknown. Most doctors believe that the nature of the action, which should occur with some regularity and should produce well-formed stools, neither too moist and loose nor too dry and hard, is more desirable than the frequency.

Babies normally have three or four bowel movements a day, but the child who has less than three is not necessarily constipated. If the infant remains well and continues to gain weight, his digestion and elimination are probably normal for him. When constipation does occur, insufficient water, underfeeding, or an excessive amount of fat in the diet may be causative. Children who are weak or who have rickets may have difficulty in performing the necessary muscular actions associated with elimination.

Constipation is often the result of faulty habits and improper training. The habitual failure to respond promptly to the body's signal is often a basic cause. A lazy attitude, poorly developed habits, false modesty, or other extraneous factors often create a situation in which the signal is at first ignored and later not even felt. When such a pat-

the disease and its causes   This is an acute infection of the conjunctiva, which is the delicate lining of the eyeball and eyelids. A wide variety of bacteria and viruses cause this highly infectious and contagious disease. It is readily spread in families and schoolrooms by contact with towels, handkerchiefs, or fingers of patients who have it. Other forms of conjunctivitis are caused by foreign bodies in the eye, allergy, exposure to smoke or intense light, and certain contagious diseases.

symptoms   The eyes produce a secretion which is watery at first but soon becomes a thick, yellowish pus. Overnight this secretion dries and the patient's lids are pasted together when he wakes in the morning.
The eyelids usually itch and burn as if there were something in the eye. Sometimes there is sensitivity to light and blurred vision, depending upon how much infectious secretion is present. These symptoms tend to worsen toward evening. Usually one eye is involved at first, but conjunctivitis can and does spread to the other. The eyes get red and the lids swell.

complications   Conjunctivitis is usually a mild illness unless the cornea is attacked. In this event, there is corneal ulceration which can be serious and have a permanent effect on vision.
Treatment is important if the disease is not to become chronic and resistant to therapy. When it is caused by certain bacteria, as for example, bacteria responsible for gonorrhea, it can be quite serious and may even end in blindness.

prevention (or lessening of impact)   Since conjunctivitis is so very contagious, personal hygiene must be stressed. Every member of the family should use a separate towel. Hands should be washed frequently and thoroughly. It is well to avoid contact with the infectious eye discharge. Fortunately, this disease responds quickly to a simple routine of specific ointments and eye drops.

Conjunctivitis (Including Pink Eye)

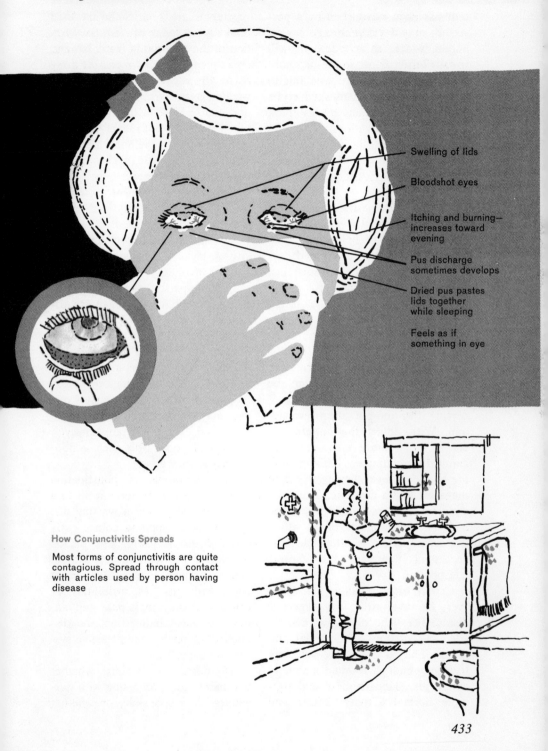

- Swelling of lids
- Bloodshot eyes
- Itching and burning—increases toward evening
- Pus discharge sometimes develops
- Dried pus pastes lids together while sleeping
- Feels as if something in eye

How Conjunctivitis Spreads

Most forms of conjunctivitis are quite contagious. Spread through contact with articles used by person having disease tern has been established by a person, he may develop chronic constipation, which, as an adult, he will usually attribute not to the bad habits which are actually basic but to nonexistent organic causes, which he will attempt to remedy by laxatives, enemas, and irrigations. These in turn may disrupt and interfere with the normal process of elimination and thus intensify his problem still further.

This type of constipation is commonly complicated even more by intricate chains of habits and misconceptions. Some constipated persons develop elaborate and mistaken notions about the shape, color, frequency, time, and consistency of the evacuation. A first step in overcoming constipation of this sort is to correct these mistaken beliefs. Thereafter new habit patterns can be encouraged. A baby can be trained so that the simple act of placing it on the pot causes evacuation. With adults the pattern becomes much more elaborate, and can include getting up, bathing, having breakfast, even having the right magazine and a cigarette. The principle nevertheless remains the same and the development of an effective habit pattern is often the most successful treatment for chronic constipation.

Certain organic factors can, however, be involved in this digestive disturbance. The diet must contain adequate amounts of essential materials. The bulk must be sufficient to supply enough residual matter to assure an adequate mass and promote normal activity. Fruits and vegetables are best. Sufficient fluid intake is needed to prevent dehydration of the material in the colon and consequent difficulty in passing a dry mass. Profuse sweating during hot weather or as part of an acute infection can so deplete the body's supply of moisture as to react adversely on the bowel. Without adequate residue and moisture, the bowel does not function properly.

Sometimes a defect of motor activity exists. Particularly in the aged and the undernourished, the intestinal wall may lose its tone and capacity. A lack of B-complex vitamins may be involved.

In some persons the nerves regulating the digestive processes are disturbed, so that the left half of the colon, its expelling section, does not function properly. Drugs are now available which overcome this condition. Other drugs which are given to combat certain conditions of disease may interfere with the action of the bowel. The physician, however, can usually deal with such contingencies as they arise.

The symptoms of constipation vary from a few or none at all to a condition resembling a wasting disease. Loss of appetite comes early and *halitosis* is likely. The person becomes depressed and dull without apparent cause, tires easily, cannot cope with his responsibilities as usual, and may look pale and unwell. Frequent indigestion and discomfort or pain in the digestive system are common.

The doctor can establish whether bad habits and overdosing with purgatives are responsible, or whether deep-seated organic disorders may be present. In any event, only the doctor can safely outline the measures to be followed.

In most cases of *dyschesia,* or constipation involving largely the lower end of the digestive tract, actual re-education is necessary to start regularity and reliance on natural processes. Often, however, enemas, suppositories, or mild laxatives may be used to get new habits under way. Regular exercise is frequently advisable, especially for a sedentary person. A walk before breakfast or daily exercise of the abdominal muscles may be desirable.

Along with re-education, an adequately varied diet is probably more significant than any other factor. The major constituents of a normal diet, proteins, carbohydrates, fats, mineral salts, vitamins, and sufficient indigestible bulk, should all be assured. Fruit, especially stewed prunes and apples, are recommended for breakfast, and green vegetables and salad at both luncheon and the evening meal. Bran should be considered as a medicinal food, to be used only on the physician's advice, because it seems to accomplish little more than other bulk foods and may be irritating to the bowel.

Many drugs are available for treating various kinds of constipation. Vegetable and salt cathartics, organic and mineral medicines, substances which act mechanically, and water in various forms are among the most common. Cathartics of both the mineral and vegetable types irritate the bowel and are not ad-vised for long use. They include the strong salts, cascara, jalap, senna, rhubarb, and aloes. Among the substances that act mechanically are mineral oil, bran, agar-agar, flax seeds, and psyllium seeds which lubricate the digestive tract or work by pushing its contents before them. Mixtures of mineral oil and such materials as agar-agar or flax seeds form a mucilaginous mass. Caution is necessary in using mineral oil because it absorbs vitamin A and may lead to a deficiency of that vitamin, and also because of a tendency of mineral oil to leak out of the bowel. Phenolphthalein is the chief ingredient of many widely used laxative combinations.

Recently attention has been given to methods of assisting the body itself to prevent overdryness of the bowel. If the amount of *bile* discharged by the liver is increased, making it thinner and greater in volume, the contents of the bowel remain softer and evacuation is easier and more normal when there has previously been a difficulty with overdry elimination. *Bile acids* have been found to accomplish this better than bile salts, which doctors formerly gave, because they thin the bile in the liver and enable it to be secreted more profusely. This is a normal body process and advantageous when constipation must be treated. CARTER'S PILLS® is one widely used remedy which is often effective.

More than $50,000,000 a year is spent in the United States on constipation remedies. Cathartics, when taken habitually, end by defeating

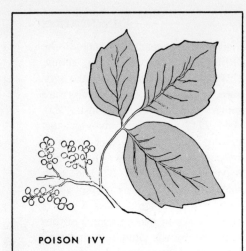

POISON IVY

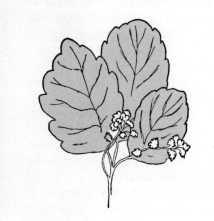

POISON OAK

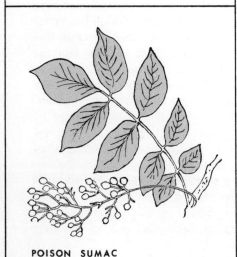

POISON SUMAC

their purpose and may make elimination more difficult rather than less difficult. Some have a useful function, but they are best prescribed by a doctor. *See also* CATHARTICS; INTESTINES; DIARRHEA.

CONTACT DERMATITIS, an inflammation of the skin due to a sensitization to a substance with which it comes into contact. As a permanent injury to health, contact dermatitis is not a serious disturbance, but this minor allergy is persistent and often exceedingly annoying. It affects all age groups from infants to old people.

Whenever the skin is exposed to *allergens,* substances to which a person is sensitive, rashes, hives, cracks, burning sores, and other irritations may develop. A good example is *poison ivy* in which an itchy rash is produced on the skin through contact with an oil in the poison ivy plant.

The substances to which a sensitive person may react on touch are numerous and include plants, wood, fur, silk, wool, dye, resin, plastic, rubber, metal, and many more. Some women have cosmetic contact dermatitis and cannot use ordinary beauty products such as soap, bleaches, deodorants, or powder. The active reaction of the skin to an allergenic substance makes contact dermatitis an occupational disorder too, and it frequently affects industrial workers who are exposed to certain chemicals, wood, metal, glue, or lacquer. In some instances, skin disorders spread to the nail bed and produce a condition called *onycholy-*

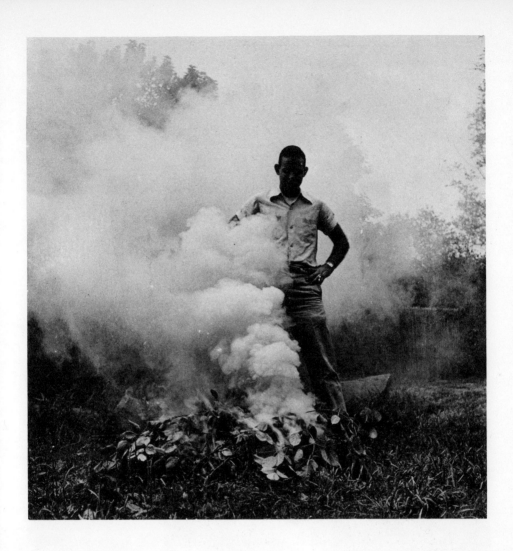

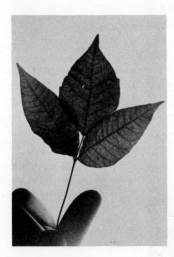

Everyone should learn to recognize the wild three-leaf poison ivy plant that causes an itchy skin rash at the slightest touch. The best protection against this plant pest is simply to avoid contact with it. If the skin should come in contact with the poison ivy plant, it should be washed immediately with cold water and soap—preferably a yellow laundry soap. This will remove the poisonous oil which is the cause of the dermatitis. The poison ivy plants can be eradicated from infested areas with various chemical preparations, or by burning. Above, a patch is being burned. Because the smoke from such a fire may contain the poisonous oils of the plant, the overseer should never stand in its path.

437

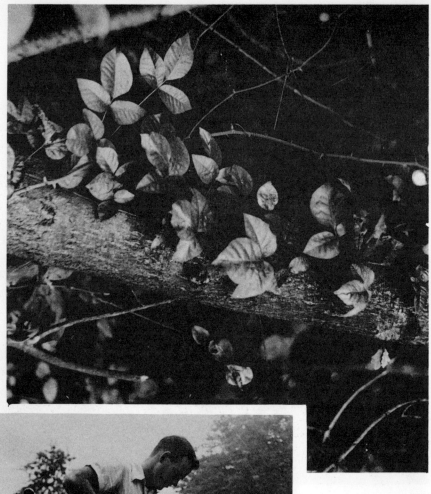

While poison ivy usually grows close to the ground, it sometimes assumes the form of a clinging vine, as shown above. A mixture of hormone-type weed killers —2, 4, 5-T, 2, 4-D—is effective in the eradication of poison ivy covering large areas. Mixtures can be purchased in concentrated solution under various trade names. They are sprayed on the foliage as a fine mist, as at left.

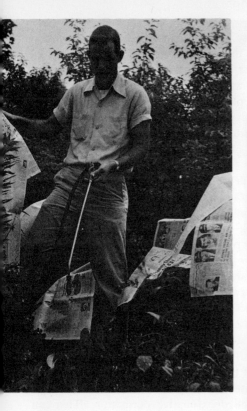

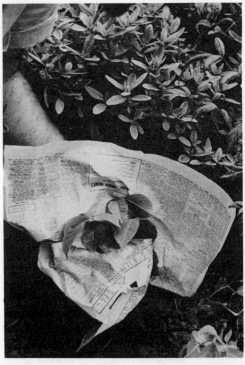

When spraying with weed killers, it is advisable to cover valuable plants in the vicinity with newspaper to avoid damage to them. Hand removal of poison ivy is sometimes advisable when it has infiltrated thick stands of valuable plants and weed killers might inflict indiscriminate damage. Newspaper or rubber gloves should be worn to protect the skin with contact with the poison ivy. Sometimes, weed killers in a solution of water are applied by means of an ordinary watering can.

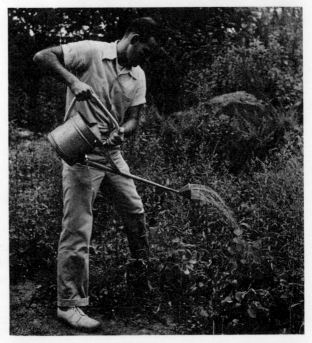

the disease and its causes   There are many possible causes of contact dermatitis and drug reactions—two allergic diseases of the skin. These causes include many chemicals used industrially, such as certain dyes, formalin, etc.; cosmetic preparations, such as lipstick, nail polish, and hair dyes; household items, such as paints, plastics, nickel, and even wood; many common plants, including poison ivy, oak, and sumac; externally applied medications, such as the penicillin and sulfa groups; certain drugs taken by mouth; soaps and detergents; clothing; starches and cleaning fluids.

symptoms   The severity of the symptoms depends upon each individual's sensitivity to the offending material. Generally, the reactions are of two types: *contact* reactions occur at the points at which the individual comes into contact with the material causing the reaction. The rash that results can, however, be spread to other parts of the body by the patient himself. *Drug* reactions tend to appear all over the body.

In contact reactions, a rash appears, accompanied by redness, swelling, blistering, and crusting of the skin areas involved. There is usually itching and burning. Secondary infections can be caused by scratching or rubbing. When this happens, the rash becomes pussy.

While drug eruptions may simulate any skin disorder, in general they are characterized by the even distribution of the rash on both sides of the trunk. Frequently, the skin of the hands and feet is involved.

Drugs taken by mouth can cause not only the dermatitis described above, but also a severe type called exfoliative dermatitis. This can begin suddenly, with or without fever, starting off with a slightly raised rash and followed by peeling. Loss of nails and hair is not unusual. The disease varies in severity depending on sensitivity. It can follow other skin disorders or be related to a generalized illness.

complications   There are usually no serious complications to contact dermatitis. Secondary infections are not unusual, but fortunately respond to treatment. Where large parts of the body are involved, there can be such symptoms of generalized illness as fever, weakness, and perhaps prolonged disability. Exfoliative dermatitis, when severe, can cause death.

prevention (or lessening of impact)   The offending agent must be found—a task that can be difficult in light of the many causes. Patch tests of skin reactions may be attempted by the doctor. The materials handled by the patient should be itemized and considered. The only form of desensitization that is at all satisfactory is for the plant contact group, including poison ivy, oak, and sumac. Both a vaccine and an oral preparation are available which tend to lessen the severity of the illness or prevent it entirely.

Once the cause of the reaction is found there are many forms of treatment available to lessen the serious effects. These include the use of anti-histamine drugs which, in many cases, give good results. Protective gloves and other clothing can prevent contact with allergy-causing industrial and household materials.

Contact Dermatitis and Drug Reactions

(Allergic Diseases of the Skin)

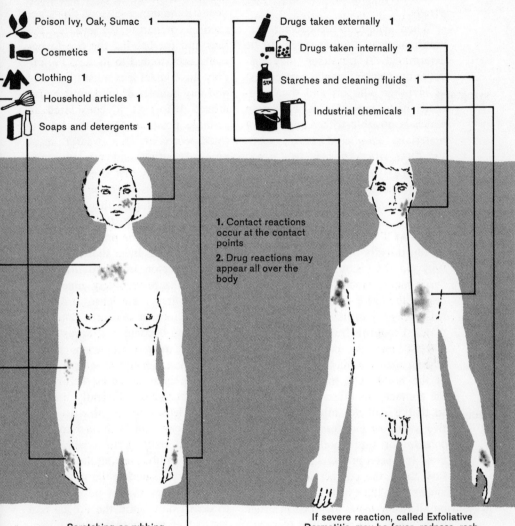

Poison Ivy, Oak, Sumac **1**

Cosmetics **1**

Clothing **1**

Household articles **1**

Soaps and detergents **1**

Drugs taken externally **1**

Drugs taken internally **2**

Starches and cleaning fluids **1**

Industrial chemicals **1**

1. Contact reactions occur at the contact points

2. Drug reactions may appear all over the body

Scratching or rubbing causes secondary infection

If severe reaction, called Exfoliative Dermatitis, may be fever, redness, rash, peeling, loss of nails and hair

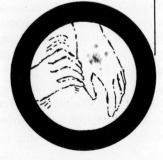

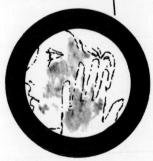

sis. Nails may become brittle, separate into layers, or fall out completely.

When symptoms of contact dermatitis appear, the cause should be determined. A physician may discover the source through a patch test as in other allergies and then proceed with special desensitization which is possible with a number of materials. *See also* ALLERGY; OCCUPATIONAL HAZARDS IN INDUSTRY; COSTUME JEWELRY SENSITIVITY; COSMETICS. *See* MEDIGRAPH page 441.

CONTACT LENSES, eyeglasses that fit directly over the eyeball and fully aid the vision. A mold of the eye is made, exactly as one makes a cast of the inside of the mouth when it is necessary to have false teeth on plates. From this fragile mold a permanent one is made with thin plastic; then the glass is modeled to fit the mold. The inner surface of the contact lens must fit the eyeball so that it will not injure the sensitive tissues or interfere with the circulation of the blood. Before the mold has been prepared, it is necessary to fit the contact lenses. This means that the eye must be studied by all of the usual methods in order to determine the difficulties of vision so that the lens will meet its needs.

The fitting of contact lenses is a procedure performed by experts in ophthalmology or optometry with the aid of the optician. In fitting the lens, the lids of the eye are separated by the thumb and forefinger of the left hand and the contact lens is then inserted between the eyelids and the eyeball, usually first beneath the lower eyelid and then beneath the upper. Special fluids are used in preparing the eye for the lens and for helping the eye to become accustomed to its use. Preferably the contact lens must fit closely and any bubbles of fluid must be removed before it is considered in suitable position. Once the lens is fitted correctly, the wearer must practice setting and removing the contact lens so that the placing of the lens and its retention become a habit. In developing this procedure, the optician who fits the lens is helpful in observing the practice.

Experiments have shown that the average person learns to insert the lenses in approximately nine minutes. At first, these lenses are worn only an hour or two at a time, but many who become well accustomed to them wear their lenses six to eight hours. Several months may be required, in some cases, before the person becomes sufficiently used to contact lenses to be able to wear them a long time without removing them and refilling them with fluid, and also without resting the eyes.

Those considering the wearing of contact lenses should be cautioned to do so only upon the advice and consent of an ophthalmologist. Not all persons are physiologically adaptable to such lenses. Several cases of serious eye disease and even blindness have been attributed to the improper wearing of contact lenses. *See also* EYE; EYE GLASSES.

CONTRACEPTION, the use of a device, substance, or method to prevent conception during sexual intercourse.

Perhaps the commonest of the various methods of contraception are the use of the *sheath* or *condom* of rubber worn by the man and, alternatively, the *pessary* or *diaphragm* worn by the woman. Chemicals, especially fixed in thick *creams,* which destroy or immobilize the sperm cell are also used. The American Medical Association has listed a number of such creams by name, as acceptable when prescribed by the doctor.

The physician's advice as to the proper use of such devices, materials, and methods is desirable, since not all are of equal effectiveness. The combination of pessary and cream, for instance, is probably 90 per cent or more effective; none is 100 per cent reliable. The pessary must be prescribed and fitted for the woman by the physician; otherwise, at best, its used will be haphazard protection. Creams and other chemicals are safe only on the advice of a physician. The use of *douches* is also common, but if they are to be effective and safe, should be employed only with medical advice. Many cleansing or sterilizing agents are dangerous to the body, or may alter normal bacterial growth undesirably in the parts where they are used.

Another method of avoiding conception is the so-called *rhythm technique.* The basis of this theory is the regular monthly cycle of ovulation. An egg cell or ovum passes from the ovary once every month, and consequently during the month the woman is more likely to conceive at one time than another. These intervals are commonly referred to respectively as the fertile and the safe periods. For the woman who menstruates regularly every twenty-eight days, the safe period is calculated as approximately a week before and a week after menstruation. More exactly, it lasts nine days, beginning the first day of menstruation. The fertile period, which normally is a maximum of eight days, follows, and then the next eleven days are again "safe." When the menstrual interval is shorter or longer than this, or is irregular, the physician's advice is desirable.

Another way of identifying the fertile period is to record the morning temperature, before any food is eaten or water or other fluids are drunk. Ovulation brings with it a fall in temperature, then a rise. Abstinence is practiced during the period of ovulation, and for three days before and three days after.

The latest development is a *steroid* called ENOVID® which prevents ovulation. Five days after the cessation of menstruation a pill is taken each day for twenty days. See a fuller discussion under BIRTH CONTROL. *See also* CONCEPTION; OVULATION; MENSTRUATION; RHYTHM METHOD; PREGNANCY, SIGNS OF; REPRODUCTION SYSTEM.

CONTUSION, a superficial injury or bruise, produced by impact, in which breaking of the skin does not occur. If the skin is punctured also, the term *contused wound* is used. *See also* BRUISES.

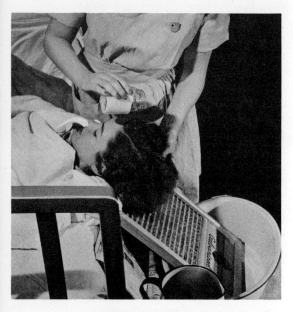

Convalescence—Patients confined to bed for long periods require shampoos. A washboard and metal tub make a satisfactory arrangement. This method allows the patient to rest comfortably while the home nurse washes her hair.

CONVALESCENCE, the period of gradual restoration to health following disease, injury, or operation.

During convalescence, it is particularly important that the patient receive a well-balanced diet. To encourage strong scar tissue to form and seal over a surgical incision, a high vitamin C level is required. Often after illness or surgery, the person may be anemic. To counteract anemia, which reduces the healing power, the diet should be rich in iron. Also important is protein, the building material of the body. The digestive tract may be sluggish at first, so food should be bland and low in residue to avoid overtaxing the digestive tract.

After diarrhea or infections of the intestines, clear fluids, such as soup, tea, juice, and plenty of water, should make up the bulk of the diet. Gradually the patient may take soft solids, such as eggs, toast, and custards.

Formerly a recuperating person was kept in bed for a long period of time. Physicians now tend to feel that fairly early ambulation is beneficial in speeding convalescence. Getting out of bed as soon as possible prevents dangerous blood clots in the legs and also boosts the spirits. However, just that a patient feels better does not mean the body is fully healed, and the physician should be consulted before increased activity is permitted. Damage to heart, kidneys, and other vital organs can result from overactivity following infectious diseases. As soon as possible, the patient should be permitted to sit in the sun and have fresh air. Visitors, provided they are not too frequent or the visits too long, are good for the patient's

Convalescence—A paperboard carton covered with muslin makes a convenient support for the patient's feet.

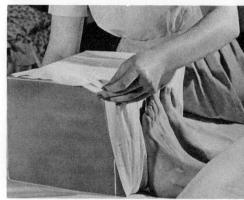

morale. Of course, persons with colds or other illnesses should never be permitted to see the patient.

Some persons appear to enjoy being invalids, an attitude which is enhanced by oversolicitous and oversympathetic friends and family. The convalescent person should begin to do things for himself, to engage in intellectually stimulating activities, and to plan for return to his regular life as soon as possible.

During convalescence, the temperature is taken daily, preferably in the morning. Until the person is able to take a shower or bath, he receives a daily sponge bath in bed by a qualified person. The room should be warm during the time of the bath and only a small part of the body exposed at a time. After the bath, the bed linen should be changed, making sure that the linen fits snugly on the bed without wrinkles which can irritate the skin of the bedridden patient. Although shampooing the hair is generally permissible in most illnesses, it is best to check first with the doctor.

A person who has been in bed for a long period of time will be weak when he first gets up, so before getting out of bed for the first time it is best for him to spend a few minutes each day sitting on the edge of his bed. Next he can be assisted to a chair placed next to the bed where he may remain for a short time. Someone should always help him the first few times he attempts to walk. If dizziness occurs, he should return to bed at once and try again later.

Constipation often occurs in bed-

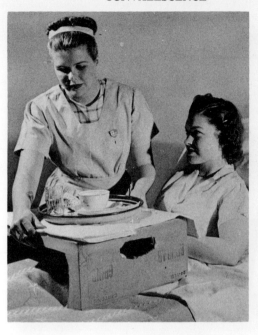

Convalescence—When a bed tray is not available, a fiberboard carton makes a good substitute. Handholds cut in each end permit easier handling. A smaller box can be cut in similar fashion for placing over leg to keep weight of covers off an injury, or to keep covers clear off a wet pack.

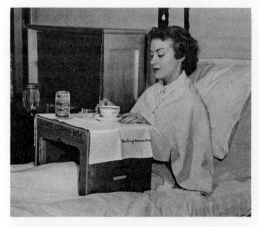

Convalescence—The back rest has been wrapped with a piece of old sheet, held with safety pins and padded with a pillow. The tray table also was made from a carton with sides cut out. Towel doubles as a bed jacket.

445

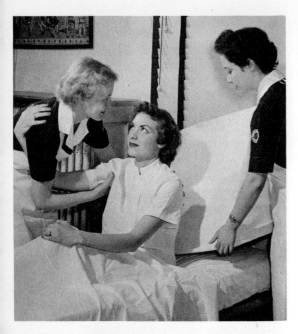

Convalescence—To give support, a back rest is put in place, the nurse places one hand behind patient's shoulders, grasps upper arm firmly. The patient braces herself by holding on to the nurse's shoulder. This method of support may be used to assist the patient in changing positions.

ridden persons. Generally the physician will prescribe a mild cathartic. Enemas should not be given without consulting the doctor. *See also* BED SORES.

CONVULSION, an involuntary general attack of muscle contraction. In a *tonic* convulsion, the contractions occur without relaxation; and in a *clonic* convulsion, alternate contractions of opposing groups of muscles take place. The convulsion may or may not be accompanied by unconsciousness. The word *fit* commonly denotes an attack of convulsions.

Convulsions occur in epilepsy, asphyxia, poisoning, lockjaw, rabies, apoplexy, meningitis, head injuries, nutritional deficiency, inherited tendency, and in slow-pulse diseases such as anemia of the brain. They may also appear, together with subsequent coma, as a disturbance of late pregnancy. Convulsion in infants is sometimes a reflex action connected with teething, indigestion, rickets, worms, diarrhea, breath holding (an emotional habit which some children develop) and, in particular, high fever, as in tonsillitis. When the convulsion is not brought on by high fever, it may be longer and more serious. Infant mortality rate from convulsions has dropped sharply; in 1900, 1 out of 1,000 births resulted in death from convulsions; in 1948, the figure had been reduced to 1 in 10,000, due mainly to advances in the care of infants.

Although convulsions are often frightening, especially in children, it should be remembered that a convulsion itself is not fatal. The patient should be prevented from injuring himself, but any use of force kept to an absolute minimum. A piece of wood placed between the teeth will keep the patient from biting himself. His clothes should be loosened, especially around the neck and across the chest, and he should be placed on his back, unless he vomits, in which case he is placed on his side. As the patient recovers, an effort should be made to communicate with him and to reassure him. *See also* CHILD CARE; ECLAMPSIA; EPILEPSY.

COPPER SULPHATE, bluish crystals or powder soluble in water, used in swimming pools to destroy fungi or bacteria. In medicine it is beneficial as an astringent and as an agent to induce vomiting.

CORNEA, the tough transparent membrane in front of the eyeball. It occupies about one-sixth of the circumference of the globe of the eye and acts as a kind of magnifying and protective lens for the eye. Various disorders of the cornea result in serious visual defects.

Astigmatism, or blurred vision, may occur when the central part of the cornea is more curved in one spot than in another. Light rays are thus not equally refracted and bent and some of them are focused on the retina and others in front or behind it.

If the cornea is too thin or exceedingly weak, a protrusion or bulge may develop and produce a condition called *keratoconus.* Vision will become increasingly dim as the cornea changes, and corneal transplantation may be necessary to restore sight.

Interstitial keratitis is an inflammation in which the entire cornea becomes hazy and almost completely covers the *iris.* Persons with *congenital syphilis* are often affected.

Traumatic keratitis is a consequence of wounds or injuries of the cornea. Even slight injuries may result in an inflammation which impairs vision. During the healing process of more severe injuries, opaque scar tissue may develop instead of clear corneal tissue and a curtain is drawn over the pupil of the eye, resulting in partial or total blindness. *See also* EYE; CORNEAL TRANSPLANTATION. *See* MEDIGRAPH page 1331.

CORNEAL TRANSPLANTA-TION, an operation in which a section of clear transparent cornea is substituted in places where opaque cornea has been removed. Corneal tissue is removed from the healthy eyes of persons immediately after death and shipped by air to "eye banks," where doctors can use the tissue as needed. The tissue must be used within thirty-six hours after its removal.

Corneal transplantation has been perfected and now brings great hope of restored vision to those blinded by corneal disorders. However, the success of corneal transplantations presupposes certain conditions. For example, the operation is rarely successful when the whole expanse of the cornea has been affected, and it is not attempted in cases of opaque corneas at birth. Other components of the eye must be in good condition; certain diseases of the eye, such as *glaucoma*, must first be eliminated before the operation. *See also* CORNEA; EYE.

CORNS. *See* FEET.

CORONARY THROMBOSIS, a rather loose term for a condition more accurately described as *acute coronary occlusion* or blocking of a coronary (heart) artery. This means that a clot of blood has formed within the heart or blood vessels, usually

the disease and its causes In coronary artery disease, there is narrowing or clogging of the coronary arteries which bring blood to the heart. As a result, the heart area supplied by the coronary artery is cut off both from its blood supply and from the oxygen and nourishment carried by the blood. The deprived area becomes severely damaged or destroyed (infarcted).

The narrowing or clogging of an artery is usually due to arteriosclerosis (hardening of the arteries): the inner walls of the artery are roughened or thickened, and fat deposits accumulate. Only a little, inadequate supply of blood can trickle through this hardened and roughened area— or the blood supply may be stopped completely. This is called coronary thrombosis.

The arteriosclerosis bringing on coronary artery disease may, in turn, have been brought about by a number of long-term factors, either singly or in combination: inheritance of a tendency toward hardening of the arteries and heart trouble; use of tobacco and other stimulants; inability to relax from the tension and stress of modern life; obesity, diabetes, high blood pressure. But a specific coronary artery attack may be precipitated by overeating, emotional upset, or unusual physical effort.

Coronary artery disease is a very common problem and occurs most often in the over-40 age group.

symptoms The symptoms—and severity—of coronary artery disease depend upon the size of the artery cut off . . . how big an area of the heart is injured or destroyed . . . the vigor and reserve power of the undamaged areas of the heart . . . the demands made upon the heart at the time, and many other factors. In 10% of the cases, there may be no pain.

As a result, the symptoms may vary. Some patients may have only a mild type of discomfort in the middle of the chest, similar to mild indigestion. In others, the pain may be very severe, starting from the chest area and radiating up into the neck and face, to the back, and down into the left arm. In the more severe forms, the patient may also develop shortness of breath, blue lips, and even enter a state of shock.

complications If the attack is severe or the patient not treated promptly, the complications are heart failure, change in rhythm and rate of the heart beat, shock, or death.

prevention (or lessening of impact) A life of moderation is the best way to prevent the occurrence of coronary artery disease. This means keeping one's weight down; avoiding overeating; taking regular exercise—but not to the point where one becomes overtired; avoiding tobacco and other stimulants; and making a conscious attempt to relax from the daily demands of work and the pressures of modern life. A patient who is already suffering from coronary artery disease will probably find his doctor prescribing an approach like this as he recovers from the illness.

Coronary Artery Disease (Myocardial Infarction)

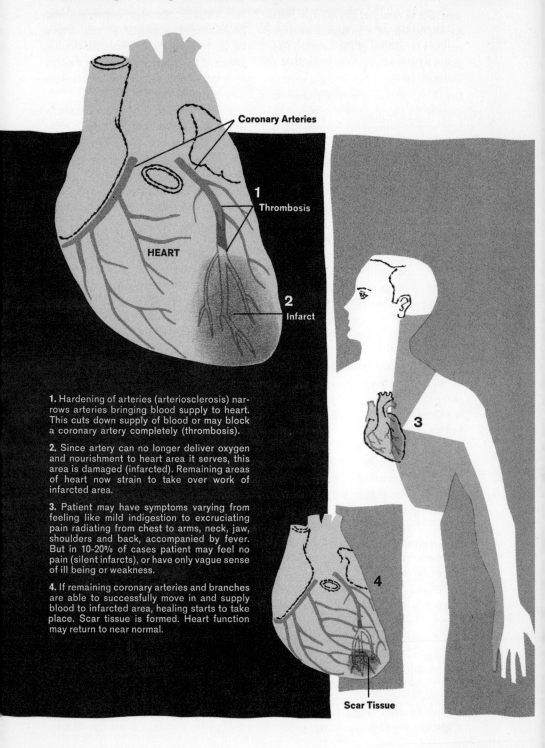

Coronary Arteries

1 Thrombosis

HEART

2 Infarct

1. Hardening of arteries (arteriosclerosis) narrows arteries bringing blood supply to heart. This cuts down supply of blood or may block a coronary artery completely (thrombosis).

2. Since artery can no longer deliver oxygen and nourishment to heart area it serves, this area is damaged (infarcted). Remaining areas of heart now strain to take over work of infarcted area.

3. Patient may have symptoms varying from feeling like mild indigestion to excruciating pain radiating from chest to arms, neck, jaw, shoulders and back, accompanied by fever. But in 10-20% of cases patient may feel no pain (silent infarcts), or have only vague sense of ill being or weakness.

4. If remaining coronary arteries and branches are able to successfully move in and supply blood to infarcted area, healing starts to take place. Scar tissue is formed. Heart function may return to near normal.

3

4

Scar Tissue

due to a slowing of the circulation or to alteration of the blood or vessel walls. The ability of the heart to function efficiently depends primarily on the state of the heart muscle or *myocardium*; thus, life itself depends largely on the state of the blood vessels which bring nourishment to the myocardium. These blood vessels are known as the coronary arteries.

Blocking or occlusion of a coronary artery may develop rapidly or slowly, and coronary disease may be mild or severe, sudden and fatal. If it develops slowly, the myocardium is gradually deprived of its blood supply and cannot function efficiently. The condition manifests itself as *angina pectoris* which is characterized by pain under the breastbone, produced by exertion and relieved by rest.

If the occlusion occurs rapidly as in acute coronary occlusion, one of two things may happen. Sudden death may result if the blocking involves a large artery or occurs in an already damaged myocardium. If a smaller branch of the coronary arteries is obstructed, the chances are good that the person will recover.

The primary cause of coronary artery disease, and therefore coronary thrombosis, is unknown, but is probably the same as that of *arteriosclerosis,* which is also not known. In a majority of cases, coronary thrombosis occurs in a coronary artery that has become thickened and hardened, or *sclerosed*, so that its channel is gradually narrowed. When this narrowing reaches a certain stage, the blood in that channel is liable to clot and completely block

the artery, thereby depriving the heart muscle supplied by this artery of its blood supply. This hardening process, or arteriosclerosis, is similar to that which occurs in arteries in any part of the body.

Coronary thrombosis is chiefly a disease of middle life, being relatively rare under the age of forty, and is more common in men than in women. It is found more frequently among professional workers than manual workers. In many instances, the victims are active high-strung people. Mental and emotional stress may precede attacks and persons with angina pectoris, high blood pressure, arteriosclerosis, nephritis, or syphilis are particularly disposed to coronary thrombosis.

Research or prevention of coronary thrombosis has established a link between the disease and a high level of cholesterol, a fatty substance in the blood that tends to clog the arteries. Some nutrition authorities and heart specialists urge that every adult male, particularly if he is obese and has a family history of heart disease, have a periodic cholesterol test. When the cholesterol level goes above the safety point, coronary thrombosis is more likely to occur. In the usual course of coronary thrombosis, the person, even at rest, is suddenly seized with excruciating pain over the heart, which rapidly spreads all over the front of the chest and sometimes down over the abdomen. Often the person will collapse. If efficient treatment is available, this alarming condition gradually improves, but even in the mildest cases a period

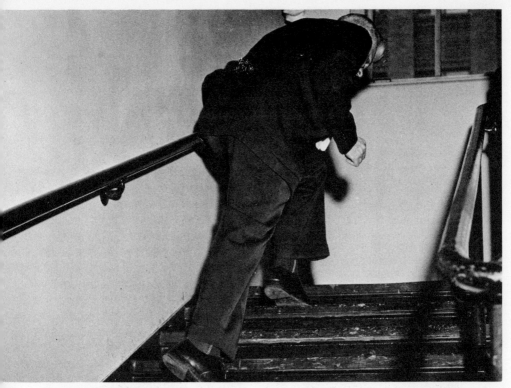

The heart may be likened to an automobile engine which puffs after climbing a steep hill. The heart likewise undergoes strain when subjected to extraordinary exertion, such as a run up a flight of stairs. If the heart is diseased, it may fail altogether under such stress. A periodic complete physical examination is essential in all persons over 40 to forestall or detect possible cardiac disease.

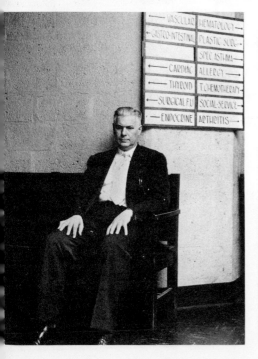

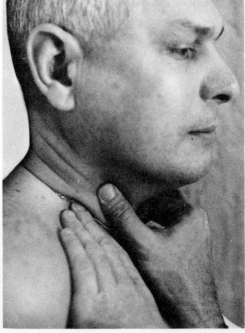

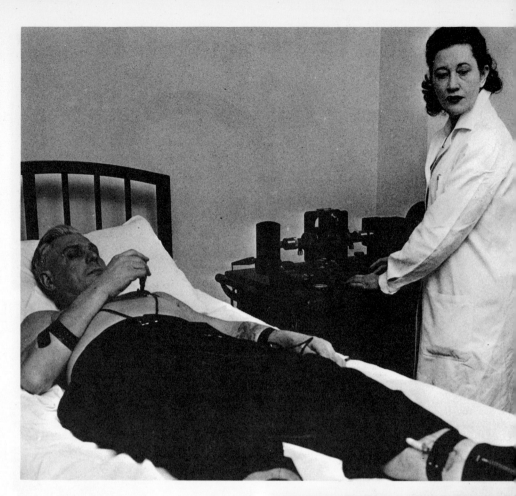

Electrocardiography and fluoroscopy are two methods used to diagnose heart disease. Electrocardiogram is graphic tracing of electrical currents produced by contraction of heart. Above electrocardiogram is taken; right a fluoroscope taken.

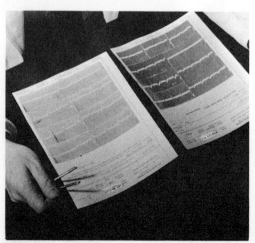

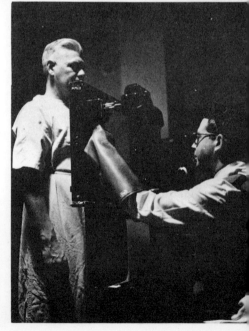

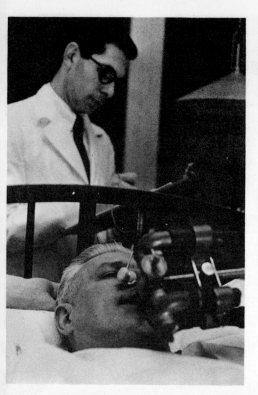

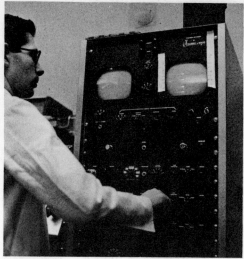

Other tests for diagnosis of heart disturbances include the lung function test, shown above left, used to study the interrelationships between heart and lung disorders, and the electronic recording of intra-cardiac pressures relayed by cathode ray tube to screen, shown above right.

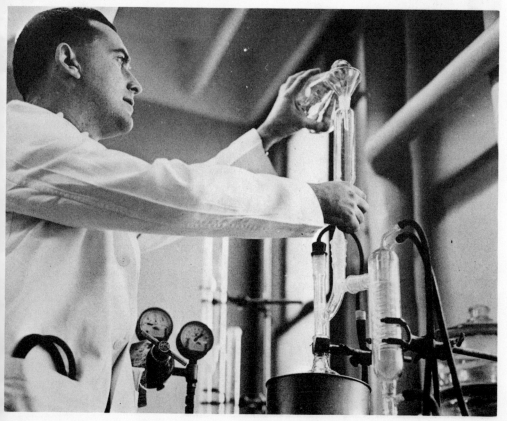

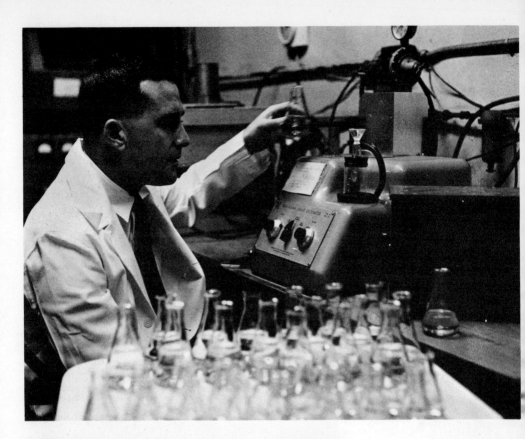

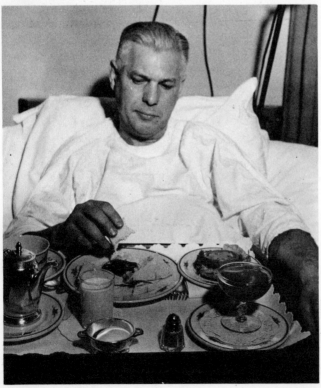

Chemical tests are conducted to determine the possible role of such glands as the thyroid, adrenals, and pituitary in heart disease, as in the lower photograph, preceding page. Salt holds water in the body and may contribute to heart failure. Above, the blood is tested for its sodium content. Since overweight is often a factor in heart disease, patients are put on a low-calorie diet. Special foods and fluids have been developed with a low sodium content for heart patients.

Rest is advised for the convalescing coronary patient. This does not mean an invalid's regimen for the rest of life, but rather an initial period of rest and limited activity. In time, the coronary patient is back at work and normal routine. He will know enough to avoid unusual physical or emotional strains as a safeguard against future attacks.

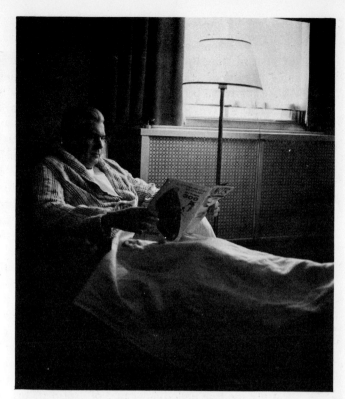

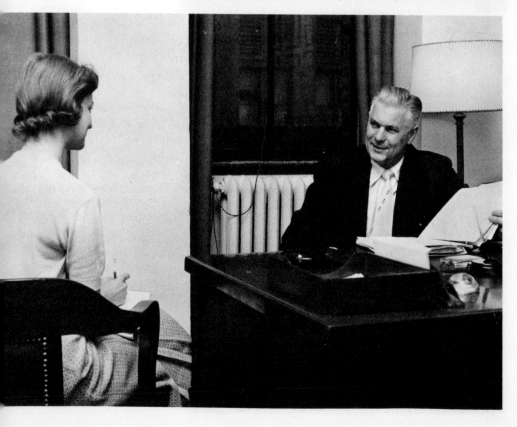

of at least three weeks' but preferably six weeks' rest in bed is considered essential before activities are resumed.

In the diagnosis of coronary thrombosis, electrocardiography is significant. The electrocardiograph is an instrument which records the electrical activity of the heart by attaching electric wires to the limbs and chest wall of the patient and then recording the heart impulse on photographic paper. When a coronary artery is occluded, the part of the heart muscle supplied by the obstructed artery is no longer able to transmit the impulse, and therefore an abnormal record is obtained. Occlusion of either of the two main coronary arteries produces a characteristic record.

Until the true underlying cause of coronary thrombosis is known, treatment consists in resting the heart as much as possible. The area of the heart muscle, deprived of its vital blood supply by the obstruction of the coronary artery, degenerates. If this degenerative process proceeds too far, the weakened area may rupture, which means death, or the process of healing may be so unsatisfactory that the normal muscle is replaced by fibrous tissues, a poor substitute for active muscle tissue. Therefore the heart is permanently crippled.

One of the most interesting reparative processes in the human body occurs when an artery is blocked. Junctions (*anastomoses*) develop between the occluded artery above the site of obstruction and neighboring arteries, so that in time the area, originally supplied solely by the occluded artery, is ultimately supplied by neighboring arteries. In some cases this brings the blood supply of the affected area back to normal, while in others an adequate supply is maintained even though it is less than it was originally. This explains why rest is so essential in coronary thrombosis.

Fluid is usually restricted, and a diet of not more than 800 to 900 calories per day is prescribed. Exceedingly difficult breathing may be relieved by oxygen. Formation of blood clots may be decreased by the drug *dicumarol,* or with other anticoagulants. (Vitamin K is given subsequently to stop the anticoagulant action.) Some surgical procedures are being tried experimentally. *See also* HEART; ARTERIOSCLEROSIS. *See* MEDIGRAPHS pages 231, 449, 713, 731.

CORTISONE, a highly complex chemical which is a constituent of *adrenal cortical extract.* Its formula is known, but the chief available basic source is the gallbladder juice of cattle. ACTH, not a synthetic like cortisone, is secreted by the pituitary glands of hogs.

Hydrocortisone, a derivative, has been found more effective than cortisone for local applications, such as to the skin, or for direct injection into joint cavities. These drugs are not a cure for disease; they only relieve and suppress its manifestations.

New preparations have been developed more effective than cortisone without such side effects as disturbance of the water-salt balance. Among them are *predniso-lone, Metacorten, Kenacort, Aristocort, Decadron,* and others.

Cortisone, quickly absorbed in the alimentary canal, is converted into hydrocortisone in the body and is thus a substitute for the natural hormone. It is used in certain acute conditions, such as the *collagen diseases* including rheumatic fever, rheumatoid arthritis, and polyarteritis. *Corticotropin* or *ACTH* stimulates the adrenal cortex to increase hydrocortisone production. An intact adrenal cortex must be present for ACTH to take effect. *See also* ACTH.

CORYZA, an inflammation of the mucous membranes of the nose, characterized by sneezing, discharge of watery mucus, and watering of the eyes. Translated from its original Greek, coryza means a "running at the nose." The term is used as a synonym for head cold, and hay fever is also called *allergic coryza. See also* HAY FEVER.

COSMETICS, preparations intended to beautify the skin, hair, and face. The American public spends almost a billion dollars on cosmetics each year and cosmetic manufacture is among the top twenty industries. The use of cosmetics has a long history. Four thousand years ago Egyptian women sought to beautify themselves in ways that would be familiar to the woman of today—with creams, oils, eye makeup. An Egyptian manuscript of 1200 B.C. gives treatments for gray hair, baldness, and moles. In ancient Rome, dyeing

and bleaching hair was common. Honey and barley were reputed to be good skin softeners, and preparations purporting to tighten skin and remove wrinkles were available. Breasts were padded, superfluous hair removed, and skin powdered.

Women of today employ a wide range of cosmetic products and treatments. Face powder is used by most American women and some men. Its practical purpose is to protect the skin against the weather, absorb moisture, cool, relieve irritation, and provide a faint pleasant odor. Esthetically it eliminates the shiny appearance of the skin.

In the past face powder has been composed of various ingredients: vegetable powders of rice, wheat, and corn flour, acadia and tragacanth; mineral powders of chalk, talc, kaolin, magnesium carbonate, bismuth nitrate, or carbonate and zinc oxide, with orris root frequently used to fix them. Today most face powder on the market is a combination of finely pulverized chalky minerals, fatty acids, and soaps blended with perfume and coloring matter. Face powder is more absorbent and adheres more evenly to the skin's surface than toilet powders which contain a large proportion of inert substances such as talc, boric acid, zinc stearate, and perfume and are designed primarily to absorb moisture and perfume the body. For example, talcum powder, developed in the United States in the 1890's as a protection against the weather, is magnesium silicate, slightly perfumed. Rouge is merely powder to which coloring matter and binders have been added. In the cream rouges, the coloring is in the waxes and oils.

Powder and rouge do coat the pores, but if used reasonably should not cause any particular enlargement. Pores are openings which are normally almost closed and occasionally open. With the passage of years, some elasticity is lost in these structures and they fail to close as completely as they once did, so that some enlargement of the pores is noted. The danger, although slight, in the use of face powder may be an allergic reaction to some substance in the powder. Some people are especially sensitive to orris root, now rarely used, and the use of face powders with this ingredient may cause sneezing, eruptions, eye inflammations, asthma, or hay fever.

Creams and lotions are another part of the modern toilette. Galen, one of the fathers of modern medicine who lived about 1800 years ago, developed the first formula for cold cream. It consisted of four ounces of white wax and a pound of oil of roses mixed with some water and perfumed. Today the creams do not differ radically from Galen's cream. They usually consist of mineral or vegetable oil, water in an emulsion brought about by the action of beeswax and borax, triethylamine, alkali stearates or a lanolin alcohol such as cholesterol. At one time some creams contained dangerous salts of lead or mercury.

Most dermatologists, or skin specialists, feel that creams are beneficial *in cases of exceedingly dry skin* and may help protect against chapping, cracking, and roughness, or soften lines and wrinkles, but not, however, prevent or eliminate them. In the application of cream, the face is usually massaged and, especially if heat is applied, a temporary swelling of the skin surface may occur with an ostensible closure of the pores; as a result, the skin may feel temporarily smoother and softer. Since the skin is a living tissue with certain automatic powers of regeneration, any improvement in its circulation will improve its condition. Proper diet and hygiene is the best way to encourage circulation and a good skin condition. Wrinkling is essentially due to a gradual loss of the elasticity of the connective tissues underlying the skin, which creams and lotions cannot correct. No method has been found for restoring elasticity to connective tissue. Face lifting does not do this; all that it accomplishes is a temporary smoothing by removal of a portion of the sagging skin, a process similar to taking a tuck in a loose dress.

Face creams can be useful as cleansing agents, but creams advertised as "skin foods" and "tissue builders" have no proven value. There is no evidence that vitamins can be absorbed into the skin to nourish it. The skin, like all other tissue in the body, must be nourished by food eaten, digested, and absorbed into the circulation.

Weight-reducing creams are also worthless for the purpose claimed, and creams promising to "rejuvenate" the skin are no better than any other cream. Hormone face creams, which contain estrogen, the female sex hormone, have been the subject of much discussion. Actually, if there is enough estrogen in the cream to restore elasticity to the skin, its use may be dangerous; if there is not enough to produce such an effect the preparation is misleading. So far it would appear that the creams available supply insignificant quantities of the hormone in comparison with medically recognized therapeutic doses. As yet there is no conclusive evidence that harm has resulted from their use although large doses of estrogen may disturb the menstrual cycle.

Vanishing creams are not entirely greaseless and usually contain potassium or sodium stearate and a little glycerin, plus some lanolin and mineral oil. The value of these creams is that in being rubbed in they serve as a slight massage which increases the blood supply to the face and produces a temporary filling-out effect.

Particularly dangerous are removers for wrinkles, freckles, moles, and warts, and bleaches and skin peels. Astringent substances produce a slight and temporary contraction of the cells around the pores but cannot remove wrinkles. Moreover, strong astringents should not be applied to the face. Egg white preparations have been made which stiffen the skin and give the impression that the skin is being straightened although actually it isn't.

Bleach creams have contained ammoniated mercury which acts as an irritant and speeds the peeling of the outer layer of the skin. They may have some bleaching effect, but cannot affect skin blemishes of internal origin. Furthermore, such bleaches can be injurious if applied excessively, too often, or to broken skin surfaces. Liver spots cannot be removed by bleach creams.

Freckles are pigmented areas of skin and freckle removers are designed to peel the skin slowly. The danger is that any preparation strong enough to remove this pigmentation may be strong enough to affect underlying tissues. Skin peels cannot remove skin blemishes of internal origin, and in addition often contain salicylic acid, resorcin, arsenic, and carbolic acid, any one of which may be dangerous to tender skin. Mole removers also generally contain a caustic which, again, if strong enough to destroy a mole can also damage surrounding tissue. The primary danger here is that every mole is a potential site of skin cancer which an irritant, such as a mole-remover preparation, can excite to malignancy. The only wise course in treating skin blemishes of any kind is to consult a physician, preferably a skin specialist or dermatologist. In the interim, harmless preparations are available which can be applied as a cover or a base for powder to diminish or conceal the defect.

Although occasionally women may be sensitive to dyes in rouges, lipsticks, or creams, more commonly a sensitivity exists to dyes for hair, eyelashes, and eyebrows. Practically all effective dyes contain ingredients that may be poisonous to some people, and may have effects ranging from serious eye injuries, skin inflammation, infection, chronic poisoning, and ulceration to baldness, fragility of hair, and loss of hair luster. Dyes which are completely harmless, the vegetable dyes such as henna or indigo, are also relatively ineffective. The metallic salts used in metallic dyes vary greatly in harmfulness. Bismuth and mercury are highly toxic. Dyes of the lead sulphur type may be poisonous and should not be used if there is a break in the scalp. Caution should also be taken against oral contact. Dyes containing a large proportion of copper salts can be poisonous, although dyes in current use contain only a minute amount of copper salts. Silver nitrate is less dangerous, but dyes containing it can produce skin irritations or blackened skin patches. Dyes containing pyrogallol, with metallic salts such as the sulphates of copper or iron, can irritate or poison. Metallic dyes act slowly, and do not penetrate the hair shaft but deposit a coating on the outside of the hair. For this reason, such preparations have sometimes been advertised as "hair-color restorers," but in general they reduce the tensile strength of the hair and tend to rub off, sometimes staining the scalp.

Aniline-derivative dyes, organic chemicals made from coal tar, act quickly and penetrate within the hair, and do not rub off or stain the scalp. Their danger is a tendency to produce dermatitis in some sensitive people and pave the way for serious infection. Some aniline-derivative dyes are safe as they are essentially nontoxic and nonsensitizing, but as a precaution a preliminary patch test is advisable before using them. This test should be repeated before each application since a person can be insensitive at one time and sensitive at another.

Dye should never be used for eyelashes and eyebrows. Mascaras or colorings with a carbon black base are harmless but preparations of aniline origin or metallic salt, particularly the former, can cause serious injury to the eyes if carelessly applied.

Chemical depilatories should be used with great caution since any substance capable of dissolving hair can also injure or irritate the skin. Even though a substance is safe for most people, there may be a few who are sensitive to it.

If reactions to cosmetics are apparent, a physician may diagnose the condition as allergic and try to discover the causative agent. Often this involves a patch test, the application of preparations to a sensitive part of the skin which is then covered with gauze. At the end of twenty-four hours, if no irritation or eruption is evident, the cosmetic can probably be used safely. Cosmetic manufacturers now produce a complete line of preparations designed for sensitive and allergic people. *See also* DEPILATORY. *See* MEDIGRAPH page 441.

COSTUME JEWELRY SENSITIVITY. Some women get red inflammatory reactions and even blisters on the skin when they wear costume jewelry. In some instances spots appear on the skin in spots touched by safety pins and the buckles of under-clothing. Dermatologists have found that these people are sensitive to the metal, nickel and chrome which can produce inflammations of the skin by uniting with proteins in the cells. They recommend avoiding the wearing of anything containing nickel or chrome; protective oint-ments may be put on the skin in the area where the jewelry touches. These protective ointments will unite with the metal and prevent the re-action to the proteins. Women have this type of sensitivity much more often than do men. *See also* ALLERGY. *See* MEDIGRAPH page 441.

COUGH, a sudden violent expulsion of air after deep inspiration and clo-sure of the *glottis,* the free margins of the vocal chords. It is a symptom rather than a disease itself. The most common cause of cough is irrtation or inflammation of the delicate lin-ing of the bronchial tubes or other parts of the respiratory apparatus. A foreign substance, allergy from inhaled substances, tumors of the lungs, or nervous disease may all cause a cough. The purpose of the cough is protective. The body tries by coughing to remove the irritation or obstruction from the breathing passages. Since coughing may spread germs it is advisable to cover the mouth and nose with a tissue or handkerchief when coughing. Cough-ing may occur in an asthmatic at-tack when the passageways of the lungs are constricted or narrowed.

By listening to the chest with a stethoscope, a physician may detect signs of mucus within the chest or abnormalities of breathing which point to localization of an obstruc-tion or infection in the chest. X-rays also detect obstructions or inflamma-tions of the chest which produce coughing. *Tuberculosis* or *silicosis* and other diseases which cause scar-ring in the lungs may aggravate coughing, and a cough is especially apt to occur in certain diseases such as *whooping cough.* A cough may persist as a habit after the infection has been eradicated.

Any cough should be taken seri-ously, especially one which con-tinues longer than two or three weeks or outlives the cold it origin-ally accompanied. In such cases, the doctor usually examines the sputum to determine the nature of the infec-tion causing the cough, or takes x-rays for signs of tumors. If simple infection is causing the cough, it should be thoroughly treated; an in-fection incompletely treated can lead to permanent lung damage. Surgery may be indicated when there is evi-dence of tumor growth, or special care in the case of tuberculosis.

Simple coughs are often relieved by medications designed to lessen phlegm within the bronchial pass-ageways and to relieve muscle ten-sion there. Inhalation of steam also loosens phlegm which can then be expelled by coughing. Hot drinks will relax lung tissues. Smoking and dusty atmospheres are irritating to these sensitive tissues and should be avoided. Allergic coughs can be re-lieved by antihistamines, but detec-tion and treatment of the source of the cough is necessary for long-range benefit. *See also* COMMON COLD.

COWPER'S GLANDS, two small glands attached to the male urethra which secrete substances serving to lubricate the urethra during sexual activity and to neutralize any remaining vestiges of urine in the urethral passage. They are also called the *bulbo-urethral glands. See also* REPRODUCTION SYSTEM.

CRAB LICE, the body lice which attach themselves to the hair of the groin and also to underarm hair, eyelashes, and eyebrows. They are square in shape with legs well developed and adapted to clinging. This parasite feeds from the skin near the hair to which it clings, leaving pin-point marks on the skin and causing severe itching. *Phthirius pubis,* the species which infests man, is ordinarily limited to the pubic region, though it may spread over the legs and around the anus, and is usually spread by direct personal contact. The female of the species, considerably larger than the male, lays eggs, ten to fifteen at a time, attaching them to hair at the site of contagion, and continues to lay eggs for fourteen days or until her death. The eggs hatch in about a week and there are three moultings in a period of about two weeks. Formerly difficult to eradicate, crab lice now succumb quickly to applications of DDT and other chemicals and ointments in a form suitable for application to the pubic area. These are obtainable by prescription. The venerable standard blue ointment is also satisfactory. Several effective preparations are now available without a prescription. These include A-200 PYRINATE LIQUID® and CUPREX®. *See also* LICE. *See* MEDIGRAPH page 851.

Cramps—Indigestion from unwise eating or contaminated food is a common cause of abdominal pain. Fear, unhappiness or tenseness can also produce stomachache. For repeated aches or pain persisting for more than an hour, a doctor should be consulted.

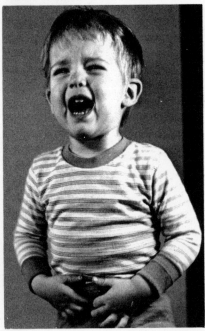

CRAMPS, sudden involuntary contraction of a muscle, or of a group of muscles.

Cramps in the calf of the leg, occurring especially during sleep, are frequent. They may be relieved by forcibly bending the knee as far as it will go, so that the muscular contraction can be released. The muscle should then be vigorously rubbed.

Nocturnal leg cramps in anemic girls sometimes occur because the leg is not receiving sufficient blood. However, the flow of blood to the legs will be increased if the person affected will get out of bed and stand up briefly until the pain departs.

Cramps of the stomach are much more painful and common than leg cramps. Application of heat is often beneficial and sometimes a drug to expel the gas from the stomach may be helpful. One teaspoon of bicarbonate of soda mixed with soda water, peppermint water, or plain water may be used for this purpose. The possibility of *appendicitis* should always be considered with abdominal cramps. If the cramps are not relieved within a reasonable time, a physician should be called.

When stomach cramps occur during the first day of a woman's menstrual period, the application of heat will often afford relief. Various drugs beneficial in relieving these cramps are now available. A woman who suffers persistently and severely from this type of cramp, however, should consult her doctor. *See also* ABDOMINAL PAIN; APPENDICITIS; COLIC; DYSMENORRHEA. *See* MEDIGRAPHS pages 119, 301, 779.

CRESOL, a poisonous substance that has antiseptic qualities. Its chief use in medicine is as a disinfectant.

CRETINISM, a condition originating during fetal life or early infancy in which mental and physical development are stunted due to a severe thyroid deficiency.

No one sign is typical of cretinism or insufficient thyroid but the combination is well nigh unmistakable. The child has physical and mental torpor. The circulation of the blood is poor. In fact, all the activities of the body are under par including the muscle tone, sweating, and the activity of the bowel. The growth, including bones and teeth, hair and brain, is stunted. The skin is thickened and coarse and fluid accumulates under the skin. The cretin is sluggish and shows little interest in what goes on around him.

The child with deficient action of the thyroid responds rapidly to treatment with thyroid extract. Almost immediately there is improvement in color and warmth of the skin. Within a few weeks there is loss of weight as the body gets rid of the extra fluid. Almost immediately growth begins again. Because of this prompt benefit there may be a tendency to give more and more thyroid and this will have bad results as shown in heightened excitability, nervousness and a rise in the blood pressure.

The earlier a diagnosis can be made and the sooner treatment can be begun the better. Sometimes the damage to the brain by just a few months deficiency may be so severe that it is difficult if not impossible to overcome. Such children may become irritable and unmanageable after treatment and the doctor must determine the amount of thyroid necessary to keep the child under control.

Cretinism is more common in regions where endemic goiter is severe; otherwise it occurs sporadically. *See also* FEEBLE-MINDEDNESS. *See* MEDIGRAPH page 465.

CROHN'S DISEASE. *See* ILEITIS.

the disease and its causes These diseases arise because not enough thyroid hormone is made available to the tissues of the body. The prime reasons for this are stated in the accompanying Medi-Graph. Other possible causes are glandular defects, particularly those of the pituitary, the use of radioactive drugs, and exposure to X ray.

The age groups involved are usually between 30 and 60, and the diseases occur more frequently in females than in males. When symptoms appear shortly after birth, the disease is called cretinism. In children and adults this disease is known as myxedema. The course of the illness differs, depending upon the age at which it starts.

symptoms The symptoms of cretinism and juvenile myxedema are quite similar. The effects of the disease on mentality and bone growth are determined by the age at which a child becomes involved. The effects of the hormone deficiency are more apparent in the cretin because it begins so much earlier. These patients are usually short and fat, as shown in the Medi-Graph.

Characteristic symptoms of the adult patient with myxedema are shown in the accompanying Medi-Graph. Some additional symptoms are anemia and premature graying. The outer third of the eyebrow may be missing. There are often vague muscle pains and weakness, and persistent upper respiratory infection.

complications In the untreated adult hypothyroid patient, heart disease may develop. There are occupational and emotional problems for the patient and family. Without adequate and early therapy, the loss of mental ability and bone growth in the infant and child may go beyond reversal.

prevention (or lessening of impact) Early diagnosis of this particular disorder is of extreme importance because bone growth and mental development can be stimulated by the proper use of thyroid hormone. Although the patient may be on medication all his life, the treatment is most effective, and he can at least be a functioning human being.

464

Cretinism and Myxedema

(Hypothyroid—Underactive Thyroid Gland—Diseases)

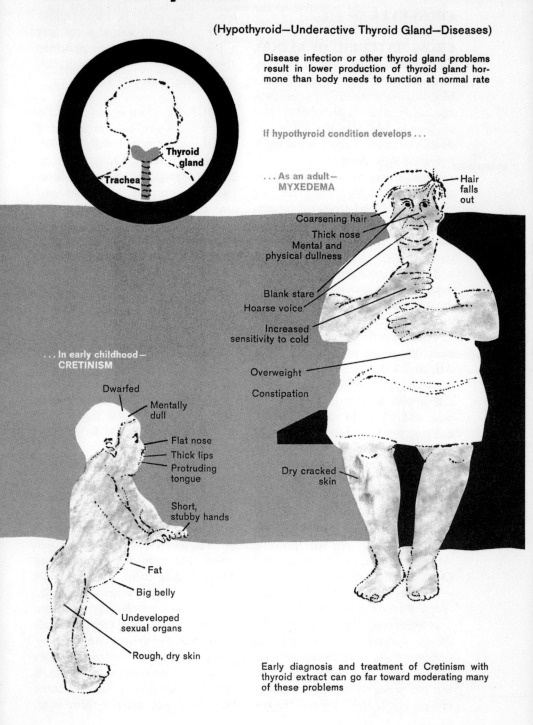

Disease infection or other thyroid gland problems result in lower production of thyroid gland hormone than body needs to function at normal rate

If hypothyroid condition develops . . .

. . . As an adult—
MYXEDEMA

Thyroid gland

Trachea

Hair falls out

Coarsening hair

Thick nose
Mental and physical dullness

Blank stare
Hoarse voice

Increased sensitivity to cold

Overweight

Constipation

Dry cracked skin

. . . In early childhood—
CRETINISM

Dwarfed

Mentally dull

Flat nose
Thick lips
Protruding tongue

Short, stubby hands

Fat

Big belly

Undeveloped sexual organs

Rough, dry skin

Early diagnosis and treatment of Cretinism with thyroid extract can go far toward moderating many of these problems

CROSS-EYES. *See* EYE.

CROSS MATCHING OF BLOOD, the technique used to determine before a transfusion whether or not the blood to be given to a patient will mix safely with his own blood. Not all human blood is the same and death can occur if cross matching is not accurately done.

Cross matching of blood deals specifically with the oxygen-carrying cells in the blood stream—the *erythrocytes* or red blood cells. A deficiency of red blood cells causes anemia when hemorrhage occurs and is dangerous because the body does not have enough cells to carry oxygen to primary structures such as the brain and kidneys.

The four main groups of red blood cells, discovered in 1900, are A, B, AB, and O. A person develops a certain type of cells through heredity just as he inherits the color of skin and eyes. In addition, each cell may carry a second factor called the Rh factor, present in 85 per cent of the population. In the absence of the Rh factor, the blood is typed as Rh negative. Therefore, blood may be grouped as A-Rh positive, A-Rh negative, B-Rh positive, B-Rh negative, AB-Rh positive, AB-Rh negative, O-Rh positive, and O-Rh negative.

During cross matching, several drops of blood containing the blood cells are mixed with blood from the donor, warmed in an incubator to simulate body conditions, and examined under the microscope to detect any tendency to form a clot or mix poorly. If this happens, the two bloods are said to be incompatible. Typing of blood cells requires only a few minutes and cross matching about an hour. *See also* BLOOD TRANSFUSION; BLOOD TYPES.

CROUP, a disease scientifically known as *acute obstructive laryngitis, diphtheria,* or occasionally *streptococcus sore throat.* Croup really refers to a single symptom of throat infection since it is used to describe any condition characterized by a harsh brassy cough and difficult respiration with a spasm of the larynx and a wheezing sound. Often caused by viruses, croup may be a secondary infection in cases of lowered resistance or other bacterial infections. Although it can affect adults, croup usually occurs in small children between one and six years of age. This age group is probably affected because it cannot easily cough up the bacteria-laden mucus which drips down the throat. The shorter channel to the larynx also permits easier infection.

In croup, the laryngeal cords or the vocal cords are inflamed and swollen so that breathing has a wheezy sound. The child coughs constantly, endeavoring to get rid of the obstruction. In *spasmodic croup,* spasm of the cords occurs which makes them red and pulls them toward each other without the presence of any obvious infection. A form of spasmodic croup in small children is *laryngismus stridulus* or "false croup." The infant breathes laboriously and respiration may even stop; the face flushes and then turns blue. However, after a short time, relaxation of the spasm sets in. During a crying spell, breathing will become normal again.

The most significant step in croup is to determine exactly what is wrong. The most serious form of the throat infection is that due to the *diphtheria* germ. In diphtheria, a thick adherent membrane forms in the throat. In severe forms of streptococcus of the throat, a membrane also forms, but usually is less thick and white. In the worst forms of croup, the fever is high, breathing excessively labored, and the child is exceedingly ill. In simpler cases of croup, the doctor usually advises that the child be put to bed promptly and given plenty of fluids. Steam inhalations, which may or may not be medicated with benzoin or other soothing oils, according to the doctor, usually provide noticeable relief. In cases of high fever, cool moist air may be preferred to hot steam. If coughing is severe, the doctor may prescribe sedatives which will relieve the spasms. An ice bag is sometimes used to relieve a sore throat.

The seriously dangerous cases of croup are those in which there is complete obstruction to breathing, and immediate medical attention is urgent. In these cases, the doctor may have oxygen supplied to the child through a small tube inserted into the opening remaining in the throat. A tube, known as an *intubation tube*, may be put into the throat which assures the passage of air through the larynx. In the most severe cases, a *tracheotomy* is performed; an opening is made directly into the windpipe from the outside which permits the patient to continue breathing while the inflammation is healing. Any case with severe swelling in the throat and difficulty in breathing should be regarded as serious, since stoppage of breathing for even a few minutes may be fatal. *See also* DIPHTHERIA; THROAT; SEPTIC SORE THROAT; TONSILS; QUINSY; LARYNGITIS. *See* MEDIGRAPH page 515.

CRYING. *See* CHILD CARE.

CUNNILINCTION, oral stimulation of the vulva. *See* HOMOSEXUALITY.

CURETTAGE, the scraping of a body cavity with an instrument, such as a *curette.*

CUSHING'S SYNDROME, a group of symptoms associated with *Cushing's disease,* which was first described in 1932 by Dr. Harvey Williams Cushing, famous American brain surgeon.

The disease, which seems to affect women primarily, is due to a tumor in the pituitary gland. Among its symptoms are excessive obesity of the abdomen and buttocks, color changes of face and hands which make the skin look bruised and stretched, brittleness of bones, and suppression or lowering of sexual functions. Diabetes often is a complication. Women with Cushing's disease develop excessive hair growth, such as mustaches and beards. *See* MEDIGRAPH page 469.

the disease and its causes   Cushing's syndrome is caused by the overproduction of the hormones of the adrenal cortex. The adrenal cortex, which is the outer sheath of a gland at the upper end of the kidney, is responsible for the formation and secretion of more than 30 steroid hormones, among which cortisone is the best known.

Cushing's syndrome is relatively rare, and is seen more often in females than in males. While it occurs most often in the third and fourth decades of life, it can occur at any age. In 60% of the cases noted, the disease is caused by an excessive growth of the adrenal cortex. A third of the cases of this disease result from benign or malignant tumors of the cortex. In 10% of all cases, there is no demonstrable cause.

This illness may be related to a tumor within the pituitary gland itself which, in turn, affects the secretions of the adrenal gland.

When, on occasion, the adrenal cortex is found to be the source of a cancer associated with Cushing's disease, it usually proves to be highly malignant and spreads quickly to adjacent structures as well as the liver and lungs.

symptoms   The earliest symptom is usually an increase in the weight of the patient, followed by the growth of hair over the face and other parts of the body. A high percentage of women patients stop menstruating. Some develop markedly masculine characteristics, as shown in the Medi-Graph (lower left).

The weight increase is marked by a complete redistribution of body fat, as shown in the Medi-Graph. The patient's face and neck redden. The skin becomes thin and fragile, and bruises easily. Red or purplish streaks may appear over the abdomen, breasts, and buttocks.

Other common complaints include backache and recurrent, severe headaches. There can be such mental disturbances as depression, confusion, and extreme irritability.

The diagnosis of this disease is established by means of examination, laboratory studies of 24 hour urine specimens, and blood chemistries and specific blood counts.

About a third of Cushing's syndrome patients develop diabetes and calcium deficiency in their bones. Fractures occur easily and frequently. Tumor in the adrenal gland is sometimes revealed by X ray studies.

complications   Patients with Cushing's syndrome do not always die, but the mortality is high. Causes of death include secondary infections, strokes, heart failure, and kidney failure. When there is a cancer present, death results from the spread of that cancer. Patients with this disease require care by a very competent surgical-medical team.

prevention (or lessening of impact)   If a diagnosis is made relatively early, before the onset of heart and kidney involvement, a patient can be helped. When the adrenal gland becomes enlarged, a cure may be effected with surgery. In a third or half of the cases where the pituitary gland is involved, X ray therapy can halt or slow the progress of the disease.

Cushing's Syndrome (Overactivity of the Adrenal Glands)

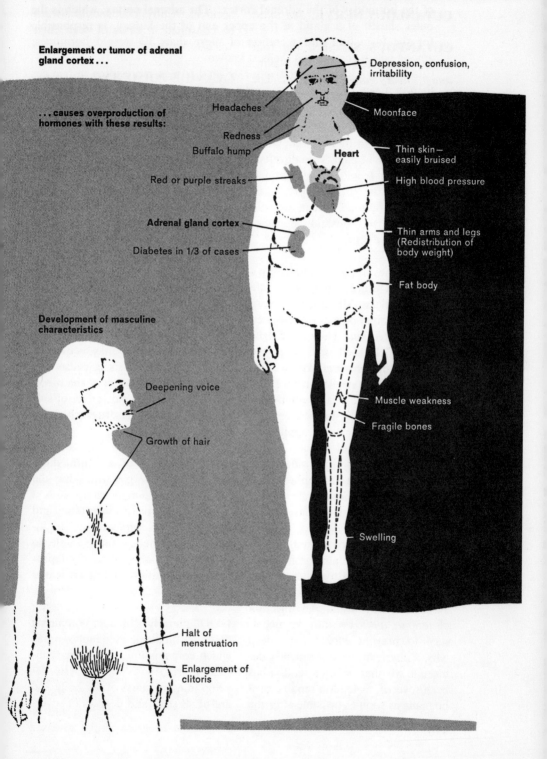

Enlargement or tumor of adrenal gland cortex...

...causes overproduction of hormones with these results:

Headaches

Redness

Buffalo hump

Red or purple streaks

Adrenal gland cortex

Diabetes in 1/3 of cases

Depression, confusion, irritability

Moonface

Heart

Thin skin — easily bruised

High blood pressure

Thin arms and legs (Redistribution of body weight)

Fat body

Muscle weakness

Fragile bones

Swelling

Development of masculine characteristics

Deepening voice

Growth of hair

Halt of menstruation

Enlargement of clitoris

CUTANEOUS NERVE. *See* SKIN.

CUTANEOUS SENSES, the four senses associated with the skin: *touch, heat, cold,* and *pain.* The sense of pain is especially well distributed over the surface of the body. The senses of heat, cold, and touch are responsive to lighter stimulation than the sense of pain. Pain develops as a sensation from stronger stimulation, and if the stimulus producing a sensation of touch, heat, or cold is increased, the sensation becomes pain. *See also* SKIN.

CUTS, gashes in the skin made by a sharp-edged object such as a knife or broken glass. All cuts, even very small ones, must be carefully treated to avoid infection. They should be thoroughly cleansed with soap and water, and then covered with a clean piece of linen or sterile gauze. If the cut bleeds profusely, as it often does when blood vessels have been severed, pressure must be applied to control the flow of blood. Strong antiseptics should be avoided, but tincture of iodine, metaphen, and other mild antiseptics can be applied to destroy surface bacteria.

If the wound is deep or dirty, a doctor should be consulted, or the person taken to the nearest hospital. Suturing or sewing together a deep cut will help the healing process and avoid unsightly scars. An injection of *tetanus antitoxin* may be necessary to prevent *lockjaw.* In deep cuts, a physician must frequently determine whether or not a tendon has been severed, as tendon repairs must be made as soon as possible after the accident. A physician should always be consulted in cases of deep cuts. *See also* WOUNDS.

CYANIDE POISONING. Cyanides are the most rapid poisons known. They produce death by asphyxia because of their interference with the carrying of oxygen by the iron in the blood. Cyanides are used as a gas to kill insects and rodents, and a few states use cyanide to execute condemned criminals. A variety of treatments are used designed to restore to the blood its ability to carry oxygen. *See* POISONING.

CYANOSIS, a condition which may occur during the course of certain disorders of the respiratory, nervous, brain, and circulatory systems. The face, lips, and skin may acquire a bluish tinge. Cyanosis is caused by defects in the oxidation of the blood and may also be a side effect of sulfonamides and other drugs which influence oxidation.

CYCLOPROPANE, a saturated cyclic hydrocarbon gas which has the odor of petroleum benzene. It is a potent but relatively nonirritating and nontoxic drug employed as an inhalation anesthetic—for example, to lessen intense labor pains. Cyclopropane works rapidly and rarely leaves after-effects.

CYST, literally a bladder containing fluid. In medicine it denotes a sac which contains fluids or other semisolid morbid substances. Cysts develop in many parts of the body and are of all sizes and degrees of severity. While their cause cannot always be determined, cysts are apt to form lumpy swellings beneath the mucous membranes or beneath the skin. A cyst is ordinarily movable, while a tumor, a new growth of cells and tissues, is firmly rooted in the tissues.

Some harmless or benign forms of cysts do not require medical attention; others do. The most frequent location of cysts which demand surgery are in the skin and glands. Whenever the opening of the glandular cell or organ is blocked, the accumulation of fluid produces a cyst. Cysts are also quite frequent in various parts of the female reproductive organs and in breasts with cracked nipples, which develop during nursing.

Among other substances, cysts may enclose foreign bodies (adventitious cysts), gas (air cysts), jelly-like substances (colloid cysts), and others. *See* MEDIGRAPHS pages 995, 1007, 1349.

CYSTIC FIBROSIS, a chronic disease of the glands of external secretion. It may seriously affect respiratory passages, pancreas and liver, and sweat glands. The disease, believed to have hereditary origins, is often fatal unless diagnosed early. Continuous medical supervision is required to prevent respiratory infections.

A study conducted in 1968 at the Harvard Medical School indicates that male victims of cystic fibrosis are sterile. This is because they lack the *vasa deferentia,* the excretory ducts of the testicles. Evidently, this congenital deformity was not previ-

ously noticed simply because medical treatment has only recently improved sufficiently to permit any sizable number of cystic fibrosis victims to live to adulthood.

Female victims of cystic fibrosis may be able to bear children, and their offspring do not necessarily inherit the disease, though they may carry a recessive gene which could transmit the disease to future generations.

Cystic fibrosis usually kills by chronic lung infections of ever increasing severity. It has been estimated that between one and ten in every 10,000 children born in the United States are afflicted with the disease.

CYSTITIS, inflammation of the bladder, acute or chronic, caused by bacilli. Women, especially during pregnancy, are more subject to cystitis than men.

One of the common symptoms of cystitis is a frequent urge to urinate. In many cases pus is found in the urine, and painful spasms during urination radiate into the upper parts of the body. A low fever may also be present, and in more severe cases a rapid pulse, chills, and urinary retention.

Bed rest, hot sitz baths, consumption of large quantities of fluid, evacuation of bowels, and a soft diet without spices, condiments, alcohol, and other stimulants are the first steps in treatment. Under professional supervision, cystitis responds well to antibiotics and sulfa drugs. Among the new preparations used are *furadantin* and *mandelamine.* Irrigation of the bladder and elimination of acid in the urine are helpful, and severe pain has been relieved by prescribed suppositories. Should the symptoms of acute cystitis persist, the condition may become chronic. As the kidneys may be damaged, it is advisable to have an x-ray examination to determine the extent of the infection. *See also* BLADDER DISEASES. *See* MEDIGRAPH page 1311.

CYSTOSCOPE, an instrument used in diagnosis and treatment of lesions of the urinary bladder, ureter, and kidney. It is inserted into the meatus of the male penis or the female urethra and permits the physician to look directly into the bladder. The outer sheath of a cystoscope incorporates a lighting system and room for the passage of operative devices.

D

DANDRUFF. *See* SEBORRHEA.

DDT, an acronym for *dichloro-diphenyl-trichloro-ethane,* a potent insecticide developed during World War II to combat malaria, yellow fever, and typhus among Allied troops. The use of DDT helped bring these diseases under control during the war, and the chemical was widely used in the United States and elsewhere as a pesticide during the succeeding 25 years. Because it could be manufactured cheaply, it became the most widely used of all insecticides.

However, DDT has extremely serious disadvantages. The chemical is very stable and does not decompose in the soil or in organic tissue until many years have elapsed. This can —and has—led to DDT poisoning in wildlife and DDT contamination of milk and various argricultural products.

DEADLY NIGHTSHADE POISONING. Deadly nightshade or *belladonna* is a plant whose roots and leaves are used medically in various forms. *Atropine* is a white crystalline alkaloid obtained from belladonna.

Symptoms of deadly nightshade poisoning are dryness in the throat and mouth with difficulty in swallowing, dryness of the skin, dilation of the pupils of the eyes, and blurred vision. The skin may develop a red rash, resembling scarlet fever rash. The pulse is more rapid and the person may suffer from delirium and hallucinations.

A doctor should be called immediately, and the victim induced to vomit. Afterward he should be given strong tea (the tannic acid acts as an antidote) or hot coffee as a stimulant.

DEAF MUTISM. A person who can neither hear nor speak suffers from

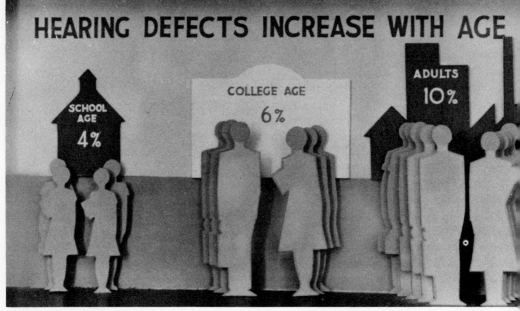

Deafness—Impaired hearing may result from severe emotional stress, damage to the hearing system by accidents, ear infections, and such diseases as mumps, scarlet fever, measles, and meningitis. Hearing defects increase as the person advances in age.

deaf mutism, or is "deaf and dumb." The term applies particularly if the inability to speak is due to congenital or early deafness. In other words, although he may have normal speech organs, the victim cannot form sounds because he has never heard.

Little can be done to cure such conditions. Surgical treatment of the ear and throat is of little value. However, the victim can be taught to understand a spoken language. Ordinarily the deaf mute can learn this skill by observing and imitating the lips of others. If the mastery of this technique (lip reading) should be too difficult, the manual alphabet can be learned with relative ease by any deaf mute of normal intelligence. The education of deaf mutes must begin in the home, with the help of the family. Schools and institutions are available which specialize in the training of the deaf mute, and a child may be sent to one nearest his home. Schools for deaf mutes admit all age groups, some beginning the training of children as early as two to three years of age. In recent years, new techniques of teaching have been progressing with exceptionally fine results.

DEAFNESS, the complete or nearly complete loss of hearing due to a variety of conditions which may affect the functions of the ear. Deafness is congenital or acquired. It may be caused by an infection in one or both ears; result from another infection in the body such as *meningitis, scarlet fever, measles, whoop-*

ing cough, or *pneumonia;* or be due to damage to the eardrum from a blow or accident. It is sometimes caused by *hysteria.* If the ear is subjected to incessant loud noise over a long period of time, hearing may be impaired, and a sudden violent explosion can cause instantaneous deafness.

Otosclerosis, one of the most serious forms of deafness, is caused by bony growths in the inner ear which hinder the conduction of sound and thus impair the hearing. As the person grows older, these growths become increasingly worse. An ear operation called *fenestration* has been successfully performed by ear surgeons in cases of otosclerosis. In this operation a window is drilled into the labyrinth of the inner ear, thus per-

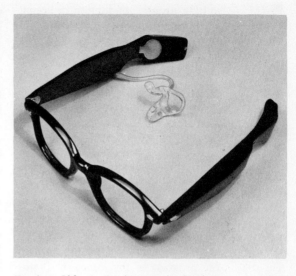

Hearing Aids—A development in hearing aids which minimizes their conspicuousness. This hearing air is concealed in the frame of glasses.

Hearing Aids—This hearing aid is worn entirely at the ear—no cord down the neck, nothing on the body. The transmitter, shaped to fit snugly behind the ear it assists, weighs only three-quarters of an ounce and takes up a cubic inch of space. A curved bridge connects the transmitter with the midget receiver nestled in the ear. The enclosed battery is smaller than a dime. Four transistors make possible this advance in electronic design.

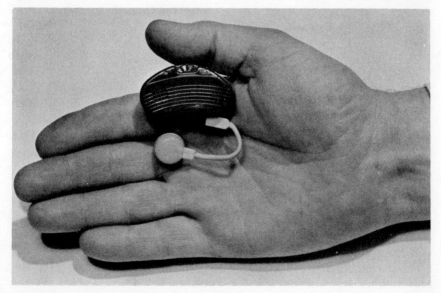

mitting proper conduction of sound waves and compensating for the loss of function of the small bones of the inner ear due to the growths. Another operation mobilizes the small bones of the ear.

One of the greatest problems in medical diagnosis is to determine the exact degree of deafness. Ear specialists give the deaf person a number of highly technical scientific tests. The audiometer is one of the devices used in testing defective hearing. When loss of hearing is due to infection, steps must be taken immediately by the doctor to stop the progress of the infection. If pus or infectious material forms in the external ear, the pressure should be released promptly. The eardrum may have to be punctured before permanent damage occurs. Infections in the throat or back of the nasal passages which connect with the internal auditory system should be given attention to prevent them from spreading. Any loss of hearing, however slight and regardless of cause, should be promptly attended to by an ear specialist.

A certain percentage of deafness is apparently due to inheritance of structure. The available evidence indicates that some deaf-mutism and the tendency to otosclerosis are inherited. Such inheritance is, however, recessive and tends to be bred out rather than in. If deaf persons are able to marry those who hear well, the tendency toward hardness of hearing will gradually disappear in successive generations. When people who are hereditarily deaf marry people who are also hereditarily deaf, many of the children are also likely to be deaf.

The development of the *hearing aid* has been a boon to the deaf and hard of hearing. Effective hearing aids at reasonable cost to fit various types of deafness have been developed. Generally the two types of hearing aids are (1) those which act by *air conduction* and (2) those which act by *bone conductions*. Tests must be made by specialists to determine the type of hearing aid best suited to the individual. In the case of children, the hearing aid should be fitted as soon as possible and the child taught to use it correctly so that he can adjust to his condition early in life.

Lip reading may also assist the deaf or partially deaf person to lead a normal active life, and schools are available where persons of all ages can learn to lip read. The person, whose hearing is defective should not retreat within himself and retire from the life about him. With the help of ear specialists, hearing aids, and lip reading, plus patience and courage, he can overcome his condition and live a full life. *See also* OTOSCLEROSIS.

DEATH RATES, FALL IN. The introduction of the sulfonamide drugs in 1935 followed by that of the antibiotics around 1940 has resulted in the great reduction of death rates from infectious diseases. Scarlet fever used to have a death rate in the United States of about two for each 100,000 living persons. Today the death rate for scarlet fever approximates zero. Erysipelas has become rare, streptococcal meningitis has practically disappeared, streptococcal sore throat is easily treated with low mortality and rheumatic fever is steadily declining. Once hospitals used to have 25 beds at all times occupied by little children who had had mastoid operations because of infection. Now a mastoid operation for secondary infection is actually rare. Pneumonia used to be one of the leading causes of death. Today the death rate from pneumonia is about one-fifth of what it was. Deaths from pneumonia at all ages throughout the nation vary between 5 and 7 per 100 cases of pneumonia.

Most amazing has been the effects of antibiotics on the two great venereal diseases, gonorrhea and syphilis, the latter of which was formerly a major killer. These conditions can now be controlled in most cases. Gonorrhea, which used to be a most difficult situation with many complications, can now be cured in a few days, and syphilis can be brought under control within a few weeks. Tuberculosis is another example which demonstrates the effectiveness of antibiotic drugs. There have been many new steps in the control of tuberculosis, notably the mass x-ray study which finds more minimal cases of tuberculosis subject to treatment, the use of the *tuberculin test* for identifying cases of tuberculosis, the *BCG vaccination* which has now been given around the world to more than 40 million children and the use of antibiotic drugs like *streptomycin, para-aminosalicylic acid, isoniazid* and *cycloserine* which are used to treat patients with tuberculosis while

they are ambulatory. The great public health movement which has developed for the control of tuberculosis involving isolation of open cases and the application of the new methods has brought about much greater confidence concerning the treatment of this disease. Even the more serious cases are now controlled by *artificial pneumothorax* which is the injection of air into the lung cavity in order to produce rest of the lung and surgical operations involving removal of portions of the lung.

Because of the much greater effectiveness in combatting infectious diseases, people are living to a longer average lifespan. As a consequence, the diseases associated with advanced age, notably heart disease and cancer, have become the principal causes of death in the latter twentieth century.

DECAY, DENTAL. *See* DENTAL CARIES.

DEFECATION, the act of elimination from the bowel. *See also* CONSTIPATION; DIARRHEA; URINATION.

DEFICIENCY DISEASES, abnormal conditions or diseases caused by the absence in the diet of certain essential substances, such as vitamins, proteins, amino acids, or minerals. The deficiency diseases include *rickets,* due to a lack of vitamin D; *scurvy,* due to a lack of vitamin C; *pellagra,* associated for the most part with a lack of niacin, one of the B-complex vitamins; *xerophthalmia* and *night blindness,* coming from a

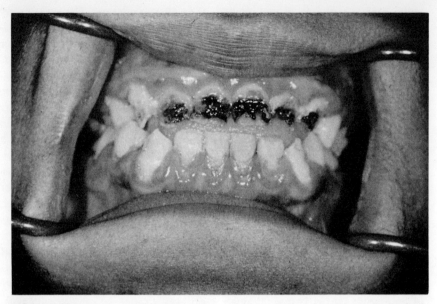

Deficiency Diseases—Severe defective formation of the teeth associated with *rickets*. In the child with a mild case of vitamin D deficiency, only the enamel of the teeth may be involved, but if the deficiency is of long duration there also may be imperfect formation of the dentin.

deficiency of vitamin A; *beriberi,* caused by thiamine deficiency; and *goiter,* related to a lack of iodine.

In order to produce a deficiency disease recognizable by its symptoms, the deficiency of a vitamin must be considerable. It is probable that deficiency states exist in which the food is not devoid of sufficient vitamin to produce a recognizable deficiency disease and yet is insufficient for normal nutritional needs. Perhaps such a state might more properly be called not a deficient state but one of failure of enrichment of diet by the vitamin. It seems to be true of vitamin B, as also of vitamins A and C, that the *optimal* amount is much higher than the *minimal* (actual) requirement: in other words, that the body is able to make good use of a much more liberal intake than can be proved to be absolutely necessary.

That is, there is a zone between the merely adequate and the optimal in nutrition. This is a relatively new and exceedingly important concept. Although we may be getting enough vitamins to give us "passable" health, we may not be getting enough for "buoyant" health. It seems reasonable that in the future we shall be concerned more with this idea than with the occurrence of advanced deficiency diseases.

Although diseases produced by deficiency of vitamins are distinct among themselves when clear-cut, in the earlier stages and in those states between passable and buoyant health it may be impossible to determine clearly which vitamin is deficient. As a rule, all deficiency states at first

478

lead to failure to gain weight, or loss of weight, exhaustion, lassitude, and weakness.

The knowledge of deficiency diseases gained through animal experiments has been indispensable in our understanding of their nature, prevention, and treatment. The dependability with which such disorders develop among certain animals on suitable diets, and the relative ease with which these experiments allow study of the various dietary-deficiency conditions, has advanced our knowledge further in proportion than in the case of many other diseases. If we were able to produce other diseases experimentally as readily as we do dietary deficiencies, the knowledge gained and the suffering saved would be immeasurable.

The average American dietary is adequate to prevent the development of dietary-deficiency diseases. It may not be adequate in all cases to maintain buoyant health. It is only under unusual circumstances, such as war, famine, floods, and other deprivations, that actual deficiencies are likely to develop. There are other factors which must be thought of in a consideration of the elements which enter into the development of deficiency diseases, such as differences or disturbances in the assimilation of vitamins from the digestive tract, due to disease, or variability in storage of a vitamin in the body.

The most gratifying feature about deficiency diseases, both to the physician and to the patient, is that they are not only curable but preventable. From the individual standpoint, therefore, their control is easy. From the standpoint of the community, the state, and the nation, the problem

Deficiency Diseases—*Angular cheilosis* associated with riboflavin deficiency. The lips appear dry and cracked. Oral tissues are frequently affected by vitamin deficiencies.

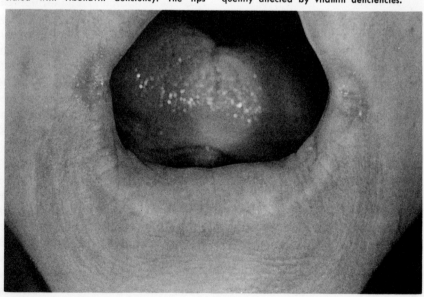

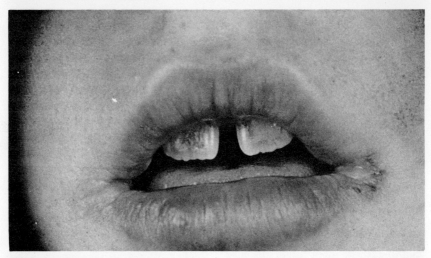

Deficiency Diseases—*Cheilosis* and *angular stomatitis* due to a diet deficient in riboflavin. The corners of the mouth are fissured and the lips are dry and cracked.

is one of public health and economics. *See* XEROPHTHALMIA; BERIBERI; SCURVY; RICKETS; PELLAGRA; ANEMIA; NUTRITION; VITAMINS; KWASHIORKOR; SPRUE; CHEILOSIS. *See* MEDIGRAPHS pages 195, 1019, 1149, 1167, 1331.

DEGENERATIVE DISEASES. The deterioration or breakdown of important organs of the body, such as the heart, liver, and kidneys, leads to disorders called degenerative diseases. A group of such diseases affecting the nervous system, such as various forms of *sclerosis,* both hereditary and nonhereditary, produces serious paralysis in various parts of the body.

DEHYDRATION refers to the loss of water from the body. Sometimes it occurs from perspiration due to overheating in warm weather or over-exertion. The remedy is an increase in the intake of fluids such as water, fruit juices, or milk. Abnormal dehydration may result from fever, diarrhea, vomiting, or other disorders. Such conditions may be serious and the intake of fluids should be supervised by a physician or nurse. Salt deficiency may accompany both normal and abnormal dehydration. This may be remedied by adding salt tablets to the diet or by the injection of saline solution in the case of severe illness.

The dangers of dehydration lie in the development of *acidosis* and the accumulation of waste products in the body. If the acidosis is severe as in *diabetes,* injections of an alkalizing solution are often given.

Much progress has been made recently in the development of techniques for correcting dehydration, and countless lives are saved by the prompt application of such measures.

DELIRIUM, a severe mental disturbance in which the sufferer is confused and disturbed by delusions and hallucinations. Extreme restlessness and excitement generally accompany delirium. The chief cause of a delirious state may be high fever, but it may result from mental disease or disorder as well as a variety of conditions stemming from structural damage of the brain.

When delirium is produced by high fever, the application of ice packs and cold compresses and other measures to lower the temperature and calm the patient are helpful. Low, muttering delirium may occur toward the end of a fever. *See also* FEVER; MENTAL DISORDERS.

DELIRIUM TREMENS, an acute disorder of the mind and body which results from *alcoholism*. Visual and auditory hallucinations as well as the physical symptoms of delirium tremens may follow abstinence after prolonged addiction, or may occur at any point in a long debauch.

Ordinarily an attack of delirium tremens lasts from two to ten days. The mind wanders and sensations of pain, itching, burning, and prickling of the skin torment the victim. His hearing and vision are disturbed and he may imagine he sees animals and loathsome insects of magnified size. In short, he has "the horrors." Muttering and muscular tremors are also characteristic of this state.

The control of delirium tremens is difficult. The mental aspects are important. The lack of food during a long drinking bout brings on deficiencies of such vital elements in the diet as thiamine and niacin which are important to replace in order to eliminate some of the nervous and muscular manifestations. Therefore, concentrated feeding of vitamins is essential in the treatment. Rest, too, is essential and if drugs and sleep producers are used these should be administered under most careful medical supervision.

Proper circulation of the blood must be maintained. Until recently the victims were often placed in straitjackets or otherwise forcibly restrained and the resulting blocking of proper circulation by tight straps frequently brought on collapse of the heart and even death. In present-day treatment, rest, nourishment, and a more positive approach to the total problem of the alcoholic yield improved results. *See also* ALCOHOLISM.

DELIVERY. *See* CHILDBIRTH AND PRENATAL CARE.

DELOUSING AGENTS. *See* DDT; LICE; CRAB LICE.

DELUSIONS, false beliefs manifested by victims of mental disturbances. A common type of delusion, occurring in melancholia, is one in which the person thinks that certain organs are missing. Frequently a delusion is the first sign of mental disorder, and calls for prompt professional attention rather than futile attempts at reasoning with the victim.

DEMENTIA refers to loss or deterioration of mental faculties and is characterized by confusion, lack of contact with reality, and apathy.

DEMENTIA PRAECOX, the old word, no longer used, for schizophrenia. *See* SCHIZOPHRENIA.

DEMULCENT, any gummy or oily substance which has a soothing effect on any part of the human body, especially on mucous membranes. The white of an egg, if it acts as a mollifying agent to the stomach, is also a demulcent. Among the best-known demulcents are glycerin, acacia, flax seed, Irish and Iceland mosses, licorice, sassafras, slippery elm, and starch paste.

DENGUE (deng′ ghee), an acute endemic and epidemic virus infection with severe symptoms which, however, rarely lasts longer than seven days, and from which recovery is almost always complete. The infection is transmitted by the same mosquito, the *Aëdes aegypti,* that spreads yellow fever. Hot weather and heavy rainfall provide ideal conditions for breeding both the mosquito and the virus, and epidemics of dengue are common in tropical areas. During World War II, outbreaks of dengue among soldiers stationed in the Pacific area were frequent. Epidemics have occurred in recent years in the southeastern and Gulf sections of the United States, in Australia, Egypt, Greece, and Vietnam. In some areas, epidemics take place at five-year intervals, and sometimes affect more than half the population. An attack of dengue ordinarily produces immunity for five years or more in most people.

About four to ten days after a person has been bitten by an infected mosquito, the symptoms begin suddenly, with severe headache, extreme exhaustion, and pain behind the eyes which is aggravated by any movement of the eyelids. Within a few hours, intense pain in the back and joints makes any movement difficult. Because of this characteristic pain, dengue is also called "breakbone fever." Temperature rises rapidly, sometimes reaching 106°F, the pulse is slowed, and the blood pressure drops. Often a pink, spotty rash appears, the face is flushed, the eyeballs congested, and some glands enlarged. After three or four days, the fever suddenly drops, there is profuse sweating, and the other symptoms disappear. This period of apparent improvement lasts about twenty-four hours, then temperature rises again and the symptoms return. A characteristic rash, resembling scarlet fever rash, appears over the knees, ankles, and elbows and sometimes spreads to the trunk, palms, and soles. The rash and symptoms continue until the fever drops again, usually within two days or on the sixth or seventh day of illness. Peeling of the skin frequently follows.

Convalescence is generally slow. Slow pulse, low blood pressure, and general loss of strength may persist for weeks. Bed rest and good nursing care are helpful. Physicians recommend large quantities of fluids, an ice cap on the head to reduce headache, and, if necessary, drugs to relieve the body aches and pains. To control the mosquitoes which spread the disease, repellents, DDT sprays, and screening should be used, and breeding places of mosquitoes detected and destroyed. Persons who are exposed to bites by the mosquito should wear protective clothing at all times and use repellents. Vaccines for immunization against dengue have been developed and may be effective in preventing the disease. *See also* AEDES AEGYPTI; YELLOW FEVER.

DENTAL CARIES, another name for *tooth decay,* a process in which bacteria form on the surface of the teeth and act upon carbohydrates to produce acids which gradually break down the enamel and dentine. Focal infection and ultimate decay and destruction of the teeth may result. To keep the teeth healthy, both preventive and corrective measures are necessary.

Prevention of tooth decay begins with proper diet. A balanced diet that includes meat, milk, eggs, fruit, and vegetables is essential for mouth health. Sweets, starches, and carbohydrates, such as candy, bread, and potatoes, which tend to cause acid formation should be limited. Regular brushing of the teeth and use of dental floss is important. The dentist can demonstrate the correct way to brush the teeth. Teeth cleaning is most effective when it follows eating. Experiments in adding fluorine to the water supply have resulted in a significant drop in the tooth decay of children. Another advance has been the discovery of a relationship between dental caries and vitamin C deficiency.

Regular visits to the dentist for x-rays, checkup, cleaning, and treatment should be a routine part of

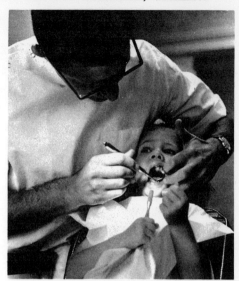

Dental Care—Three important factors in good dental care are: an adequate diet, including milk, fresh fruits, green and raw vegetables and eggs; regular brushing and care of teeth at home; and regular trips to the dentist, starting at about age three.

dental care. Children should be taken early for their first visit to the dentist with semiannual appointments thereafter. The dentist uses fillings as the best means of stopping decay in a cavity and also of preventing new cavities from forming. Fillings may be made of silver-mercury amalgams, cast gold inlays, or gold foil. By removing the decayed portion of the tooth and treating the tooth to receive the filling, the decaying process is stopped. The patient should, of course, follow whatever treatment the dentist recommends. *See also* DENTIFRICE; FLUORIDATION; TEETH; DENTAL RESEARCH, CURRENT.

DENTAL RESEARCH, CURRENT. Current research in dentistry promises great advances in dental prophylaxis in the foreseeable future. The National Institute of Dental Research in Washington, D.C. has reported experiments with hard new *ceramics* that can match the colors of original teeth, and with light but strong new *alloys*. These may be used for fillings in the future. Experiments have also been made with *plastic teeth* in animals with considerable success.

A *panoramic x-ray machine,* requiring only one exposure to photograph the whole mouth, will become standard equipment in dentists' offices in the near future. It was first developed for the United States armed forces.

Other experiments are being conducted with *anti-cavity vaccines*. Test animals have already been immunized against one type of cariogenic bacteria. Scientists hope to develop a vaccine which will extend immunity against all types of cariogenic organisms.

Research into *gum diseases* is expected to lead to developments in the treatment of related blood diseases, such as *leukemia. See also* DENTAL CARIES; TEETH.

DENTIFRICE, a powder, paste, or other substance used in cleaning the teeth. The effectiveness of a dentifrice in combatting tooth decay is one of the most debated subjects in modern dentistry and medicine. Many dentists believe that despite advertising claims a dentifrice does little more than help keep the teeth clean.

Some toothpastes, for example, are supposed to kill germs in the mouth. However, the first breath taken after brushing the teeth will introduce new germs which the previous brushing will not affect. Microorganisms exist throughout nature and a variety of them may be found in the mouth at all times. Other dentifrices claim to counteract mouth acidity by their alkaline content, although the value of mouth alkalinity is not even established. A variety of other claims exist, such as sterilization of the gums and digestion of food particles in the mouth.

The significant fact regarding all these preparations is that they are only in the mouth for a very short time, and therefore any effect they may have, apart from the actual cleaning, is temporary.

Normal teeth and gums do not need any special antiseptic. A rinse with plain water is as useful as any mouthwash. However, some people like the refreshing aftertaste of mouthwash. Most mouthwashes follow a fixed formula of the National Formulary, and are known as *liquor antisepticus* or *liquor antisepticus alkalinus*. Similar preparations are sold as LISTERINE® and GLYCOTHY-MALINE®.

When a serious infection, such as *trench mouth* or *Vincent's angina, canker sores* or *blisters,* exists in the mouth, the dentist applies substances, proven by use and experiment to be germicidal, to the infected areas. These include *hydrogen peroxide* and *sodium perborate*.

Research is being done to develop a control effective against tooth decay. Products containing *penicillin* or *chlorophyll* have been produced and sold, but the claims for them have not been scientifically established.

Fluorine in the form of *sodium fluoride* added to supplies of drinking water has been tested and found effective in reducing tooth decay in children, and increasing tests further corroborate this. Similarly sodium fluoride in a diluted solution can be directly applied to the teeth by the dentist.

Although there is still no certain means of preventing tooth decay, precautionary measures can be taken by everyone. Thorough brushing of the teeth morning and evening, and preferably also after heavy consumption of sugary things such as candy, is a deterrent to decay. A good balanced diet, containing adequate amounts of proteins, carbohydrates, minerals, and vitamins, particularly A, C, and D, and calcium is an important protective measure for the health of the teeth as well as of the entire body. According to studies cited by the *Journal of the American Dental Association,* reduction of sugar intake will decrease dental caries in about 90 per cent of the people. Although some carbohydrate is essential in the diet, most people can benefit by a reduction of sugar-containing foods. *See also* FLUORIDATION; VINCENT'S ANGINA.

DENTINE, the major portion of a tooth, the chalky part, found under the enamel and under the cement of the root. Specifically it resembles bone, except that it is harder and denser and differs in structure. Dentine contains numerous tiny tubelike passages which not only branch outward toward the surface of the tooth but also contain the same pulplike material which is found in the center of the tooth.

When exposed to the air, dentine may sometimes be sensitive, and occasionally it is defective in its lime content. This deficiency, which is inherited, gives the teeth a milky brown appearance. *See also* DENTAL CARIES; TEETH.

DENTURE, an artificial restoration of several teeth. If all the teeth of one jaw are replaced, the structure is known as *full denture,* and if fewer teeth are concerned, the substitute is called a *partial denture.*

DEPILATORY, an agent to remove hair. The hair-removing agent may be a chemical paste, a wax, razor, abrasive, or electric current. When a chemical-paste depilatory is used, the paste is placed on the skin for a short time and the hair comes off when the paste is removed. Care should be taken to leave the paste on for only the necessary time since it might be injurious to the skin if left on longer. The skin should be washed as soon as the paste has been removed, and a cold cream may be applied to soothe the skin. In the wax method, liquid wax is applied to the skin and allowed to harden. The hair comes off when the layer of wax is removed from the skin. Here the primary precaution is that the wax be applied at the proper temperature to avoid burning the skin. Electrolysis attacks the hair root, and if done by a skilled operator when the hair is still fine and thin the hair may be permanently destroyed, leaving no mark on the skin. *See also* COSMETICS; HAIR; SKIN.

DEPRESSION. *See* INVOLUTIONAL MELANCHOLIA; MANIC-DEPRESSIVE PSYCHOSIS; NEUROSIS.

DERCUM'S DISEASE. *See* ADIPOSIS.

DERMATITIS, the technical term for inflammation of the skin. *See also* ACNE; SKIN; CONTACT DERMATITIS. *See* MEDIGRAPHS pages 31, 339, 441, 681, 759, 763, 785, 879, 1043, 1171, 1195.

DERMATOMYOSITIS. *See* COLLAGEN DISEASES.

DERMOID CYST, a saclike growth found, for example, in the ovary or in the chest, and containing such startling elements as hair, skin, and teeth. This type of cyst, probably prenatal in origin, grows slowly and does not spread through the body. As the person grows older, however, the dermoid cyst may irritate parts of the body. Therefore its removal, by surgery, is usually recommended. Dermoid cysts do not tend to recur. *See also* CANCER; CYST; SKIN.

DESERT FEVER. *See* COCCIDIOIDOMYCOSIS.

DETECTING TWINS. A device known as a *phonocardiograph* is used in a technique for determining the presence of living twins in a pregnant woman's womb. This electric instrument can register the difference of frequency between the heart sounds of twins before birth.

DEVIL'S GRIP, also known as *pleurodynia* and *Bornholm disease,* an infection caused by the *coxahackie virus* which produces intense spasms of pain in the chest wall. Sometimes devil's grip occurs in epidemics throughout the United States, almost invariably during warm weather. The virus is present in discharges from the nose and throat and the infection is spread by contact. Children and young people are most often affected.

After an incubation period of from two to four days, sudden short but extremely sharp spasms of pain in the chest wall and lining of the chest (pleura) appear. The pain may vary from day to day from a dull pressure to an excruciating seizure. Coughing, sneezing, and even deep breathing aggravate the pain. Fever is generally present.

Although the pain is agonizing during the spasms, there are usually no serious complications. A chest binder or the application of heat is often helpful.

DEXTROSE, one of the sugars produced by the digestion of starches in the body. Made chemically, dextrose is widely used in medicine to supply energy to patients who cannot be fed by mouth. It is readily absorbed into the body and is usually fed intravenously. Dextrose is also useful in prevention of circulatory failure.

DHOBIE ITCH, a contact dermatitis common in India and caused by bhilawanol oil used in laundering. *See also* RINGWORM.

DIABETES, the ordinary designation for the condition in which the body cannot utilize sugar normally, causing unusually high sugar levels in blood and urine. Properly speaking, however, the medical term is *diabetes mellitus,* and is entirely unrelated to a completely different disease, *diabetes insipidus.*

The essential factor in *diabetes mellitus* is insufficiency of *insulin,* which is secreted by specialized cells in the *pancreas.* This lack has a profound effect on the body. Sugar is produced by the intestinal digestion of carbohydrate foods. It is then transported in the blood to the *liver* where it is converted into *glycogen* which can be stored in the liver and muscles and be readily converted to sugar for fuel when the muscles need it. When insulin is lacking, the body is unable to transform sugar into glycogen. Then the sugar remains in the blood, is excreted in the urine, and is unavailable to the tissues and organs that require it.

Diabetes insipidus is characterized by excessive overactivity of the kidneys and overexcretion of urine. Its source is uncertain, but it is believed to be related to some disorder in the central nervous system that involves the area of the brain with which the *pituitary gland* is associated.

Until the early 1920's, *diabetes mellitus* was an extremely serious

disease. All diabetics died young and a diabetic child had a short life expectancy. The discovery of insulin and its proper use in restoring order to the disrupted sugar metabolism of the diabetic has removed fear of this disease. Although diabetes requires constant attention and skillful management, even diabetic children grow up to live active lives, marry, and become parents. One physician who had treated diabetes for more than half a century and was one of the authorities in the field said his patients in 1900 averaged a lifespan

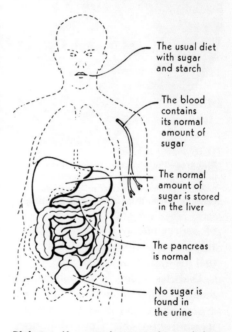

The usual diet with sugar and starch

The blood contains its normal amount of sugar

The normal amount of sugar is stored in the liver

The pancreas is normal

No sugar is found in the urine

Diabetes—If a normal amount of sugar is ingested in the diet and if the body is able to handle the sugar and perform the chemical changes (*metabolism*) necessary to convert the sugar to energy, then normal sugar conversion takes place as the above figure illustrates. However, should the liver not store sugar properly, or the pancreas not provide the substance (*insulin*) important for utilization of sugar by the body, there would be abnormal sugar levels in the blood and urine.

487

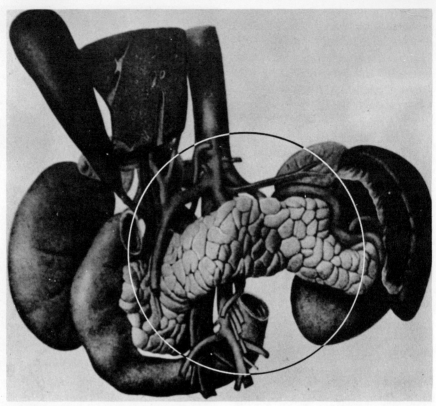

Diabetes—The *pancreas* (circled) is an organ in the abdomen. It produces *pancreatic juice* (utilized in the digestion of food) and the hormone *insulin* (important in the metaboliza- tion of sugar by the body). If the cells of the pancreas which produce insulin are damaged, blood sugar levels are not controlled and dia- betes may result.

of approximately five years. Today they can expect to live out their normal life expectancy.

Diabetes today is less menacing than a major infection. The discovery and use of insulin have made its control possible. But insulin does not cure the condition. It can only substitute for a critical deficiency. If this outside source is discontinued, the body will be in as dangerous a condition as before.

The basic concept of diabetes is that a disorder, such as an infection or a hereditary tendency, affects the pancreas or the insulin-producing parts of it. Excessive eating over a long time or emotional stress or mental shock can incite temporary attacks of diabetes. Studies now suggest that more may be involved than pancreatic disease alone. The pituitary and adrenal glands may be implicated and the whole diabetic process may be more complex than was formerly believed.

Without treatment, the diabetic, although eating and drinking in an endeavor to satisfy a perpetual hunger and thirst because of the sugar circulating in his blood, loses weight, becomes weak, and is susceptible to nervous complications. He is far more prone to infection than others, especially to *tuberculosis,* and is disposed to gangrene and skin damage. The characteristic terminal stage of the disease, when untreated, is a typical coma. Poisoned by *acidosis,* which results from disturbance of body chemistry, the diabetic person loses consciousness and dies without regaining it. Coma is also a threat to those treated. Therefore, careful regulation of the condition with insulin must be properly observed.

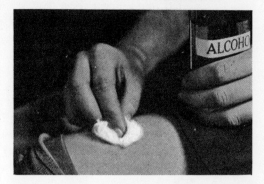

Diabetic coma results when the blood sugar level becomes high, and acid products of the incomplete breakdown of carbohydrates accumulate in the blood. It may occur when insulin dosage is missed or is inadequate to balance food intake, or under other circumstances, upsetting the necessary balance between the sugar and the insulin in the system.

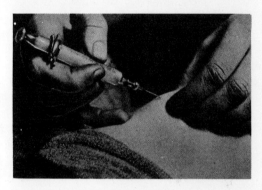

Diabetes—The proper technique for injecting insulin. The chosen spot of the skin is rubbed with alcohol. A different spot is selected each time, but the inner surfaces of the limbs should be avoided. A fold of skin is then pinched up, and the syringe is held by the barrel, not by the plunger. Since some spots feel the prick more than others, the needle should be moved a bit until a better spot is found. The needle is suddenly jabbed in the skin. The needle should land about midway between the tips of the thumb and finger, well beneath the skin but not into the solid muscle. The needle is directed straight ahead so as not to bend or break. Then the plunger is pushed in. After pulling the needle out, the cotton saturated with alcohol is held over the spot for a few seconds and the area of the skin is rubbed.

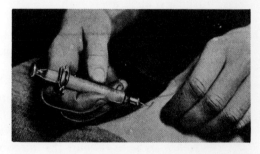

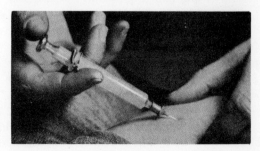

the disease and its causes   In a normal body, food sugar and starches are converted into a sugar form that is readily used as fuel by the muscles. In a diabetic, the pancreas does not produce enough insulin to turn food sugar and starches into this usable form. Instead of serving as fuel, they create a surplus of blood sugar that spills over into the urine. The proteins and fats consumed are not burned up as they should be, and the chemical balance of the body is affected.

Diabetes is common. It can occur at any age but affects the older group most—women slightly more often than men. It affects all races in varying degrees. The disease seems to run in families. And being overweight also seems to play a significant role.

The exact reason why the pancreas fails to function properly and produce the necessary amount of insulin is not known. But in addition to the influence of obesity and heredity, there appears to be a correlation with certain conditions increasing the body's need for insulin. Among these are infections and other hormonal disturbances.

symptoms   The onset may be slow or rapid. Children usually develop it suddenly and more severely. In adults the course is slower. There is a need to urinate frequently, and the patient complains of excessive thirst and hunger. There may be a slight loss of weight and strength. A clue may be repeated skin infections such as furuncles and carbuncles. A common complaint is itching of the external genitalia.

As the disease progresses there is marked weight loss. A frequent and characteristic symptom is a sweetish breath odor.

On examination, the urine reveals the presence of sugar, and the blood sugar is abnormally high.

complications   As shown in the Medi-Graph, complications are multiple and severe. Insulin shock can be a complication of concern to a patient who takes this drug.

The patient and his family should learn from their doctor to distinguish between *diabetic coma,* which results from uncontrolled diabetes brought about by a variety of factors such as insufficient insulin, infection, or perhaps prolonged vomiting or diarrhea; and *insulin shock,* which can follow by several hours the injection of insulin. Although in both cases the patient falls into a deep coma, the treatment is different and the life of the patient depends upon administering the correct treatment promptly.

prevention (or lessening of impact)   While a person can do very little to avoid getting diabetes, there are certain rules anyone can and should follow if he has a strong family history of this disease. He should have regular physical examinations with blood and urine checks. He should guard against overweight. He should have any infection promptly treated. And a patient who develops diabetes should minimize possible complications by strictly following the program of diet and medication prescribed by his doctor.

Diabetes

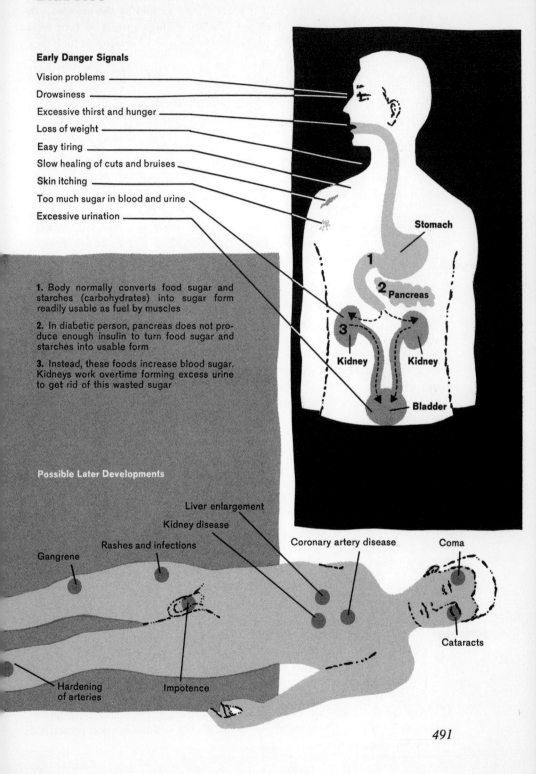

Early Danger Signals

Vision problems

Drowsiness

Excessive thirst and hunger

Loss of weight

Easy tiring

Slow healing of cuts and bruises

Skin itching

Too much sugar in blood and urine

Excessive urination

1. Body normally converts food sugar and starches (carbohydrates) into sugar form readily usable as fuel by muscles

2. In diabetic person, pancreas does not produce enough insulin to turn food sugar and starches into usable form

3. Instead, these foods increase blood sugar. Kidneys work overtime forming excess urine to get rid of this wasted sugar

Stomach

1

2 Pancreas

3

Kidney   Kidney

Bladder

Possible Later Developments

Liver enlargement

Kidney disease

Coronary artery disease

Coma

Rashes and infections

Gangrene

Cataracts

Hardening of arteries

Impotence

491

Diabetic coma is apt to be preceded by nausea and vomiting and, before these, by gradually increasing fatigue, weakness, and irritability. The physician should be consulted promptly on appearance of any of these symptoms. The patient should go to bed as a precaution against coma until the physician arrives.

Despite its slow onset, diabetic coma moves swiftly and may be critical. Once unconscious, the patient requires constant attendance by a doctor and, if possible, a nurse until he regains consciousness and during the following week or two of recuperation.

Diabetic patients need never suffer coma if they adhere to the prescribed diet, keep a check on their output of sugar, and maintain the schedule of insulin injections scrupulously. They should also know that extra insulin is needed to offset the effects of infection, which increases the severity of the condition.

During 1956, discoveries were announced of products which can be taken by mouth and which have an action like that of insulin in controlling metabolism of sugar. Extensive tests made in many countries have established the limitations of these products. They should never be used unless prescribed by a physician. In some cases, toxic side effects were observed. In the United States the two products now available are ORINASE® and DIABENASE®. The drugs work best in moderate cases of diabetes and in middle-aged persons.

Untreated diabetes in young persons strikes with greater force and results in death more quickly than in older persons. In the latter, it may be quite mild and exist for years without serious effect. Diabetes does not usually appear in younger people. Two-thirds of all cases start after the person has passed the age of forty.

Overweight is one of the most significant factors associated with the development of diabetes, and modern living, with more eating and less labor of the kind necessary to burn up what is consumed, makes that condition a constantly greater problem. People become overweight, and diabetes is a price that many of them pay.

Although a hereditary tendency for diabetes does exist, it is a recessive characteristic, which means that unless reinforced by the addition of new diabetes-prone members, a family will tend to breed it out. The marriage likeliest to produce diabetic children is that in which both parents are not only diabetic but also come from demonstrably diabetic precursors. All the children may well have the disorder. But the diabetic who marries a nondiabetic of nondiabetic stock has much less reason to fear that the children will be affected. In a marriage of two nondiabetics whose family records show a substantial number of cases, one of four children may manifest the tendency, though not inevitably.

Today control of the diet is an indispensible part of treatment. Unless it is coordinated with administration of insulin in the most rigorously careful manner, complications may occur. The phenomenon in-

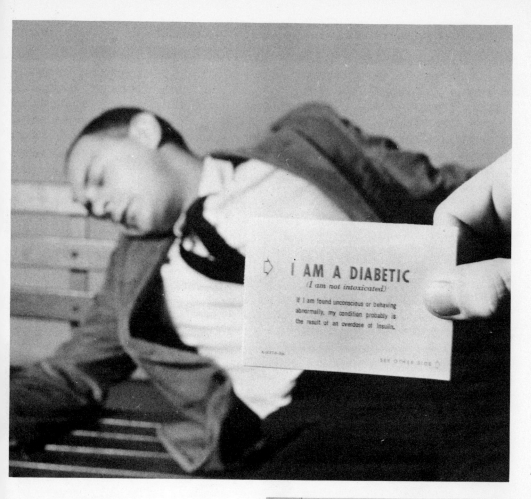

I AM A DIABETIC
(I am not intoxicated)

If I am found unconscious or behaving
abnormally, my condition probably is
the result of an overdose of insulin.

SEE OTHER SIDE

Diabetes is a serious chronic disease characterized by an inability of the body's chemistry to utilize glucose properly, due to an insufficiency in the production of insulin by the pancreas. The disease is frequently associated with obesity and is most common in individuals over 40. Arteriosclerosis may be an associated secondary disorder. To protect himself, the diabetic should join a local association of diabetics. The association can issue a card such as the one shown above identifying the diabetic and giving instructions to the reader in case of the victim's falling into a coma.

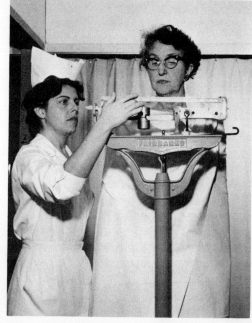

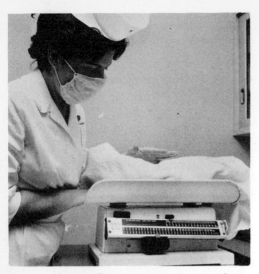

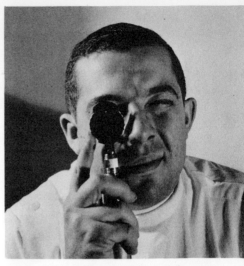

Abnormalities in pregnancy, eyesight, or the feet may indicate a diabetic condition. Abnormal concentration of sugar in the urine is a common symptom. Chemical tests and blood samples are used to confirm a diagnosis of diabetes. In severe cases, the blood glucose level is excessive due to faulty utilization.

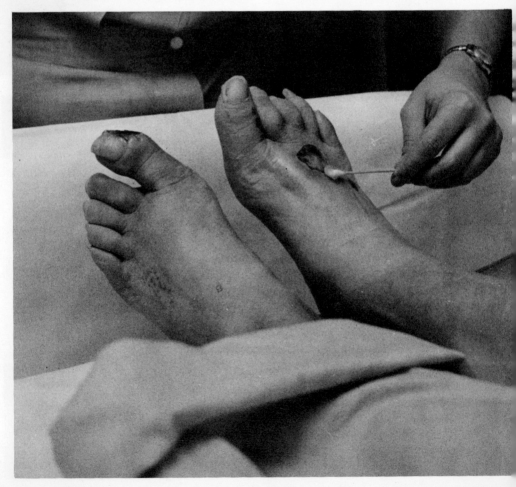

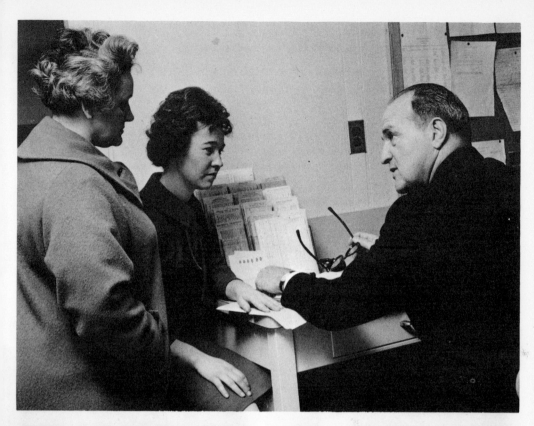

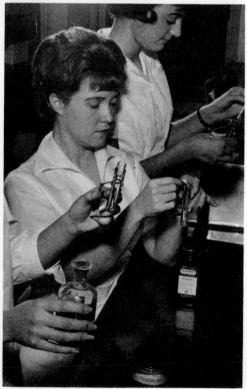

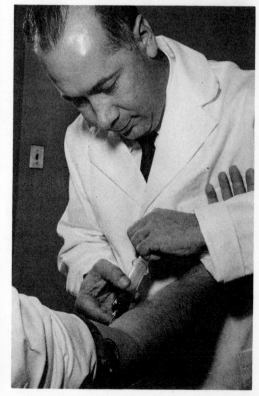

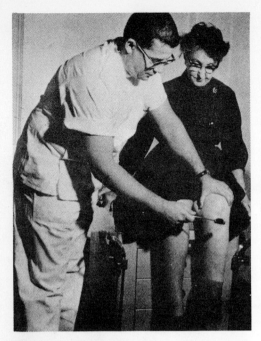

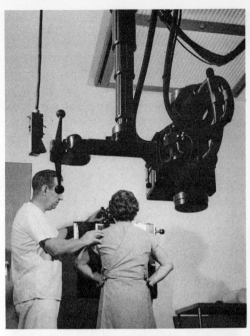

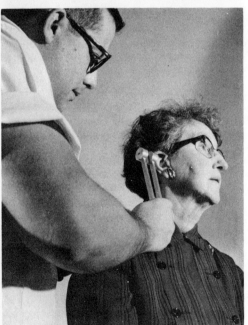

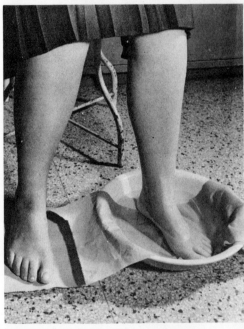

Regular thorough physical examinations should be scrupulously observed by all persons over the age of 40. Any diabetic condition will be revealed in the course of such an examination. Sometimes pain in the legs due to nerve involvement may be an early symptom of diabetes. Proper care of the feet is imperative for the diabetic. Although x-rays are not normally employed in identifying diabetes, they are useful in estimating the degree of arteriosclerosis that may be involved.

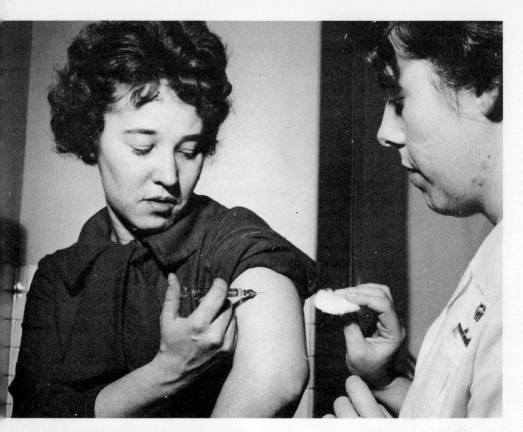

Under proper supervision, the diabetic can learn to administer insulin himself. Proper nutrition specified by a doctor or medical center can be instrumental in controlling a diabetic condition. The diabetic diet can be measured by regular household measures. The proper diet can be the difference between life and death.

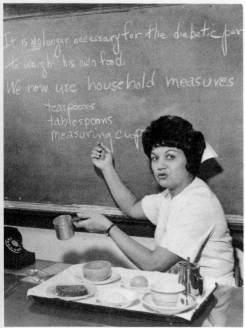

It is No longer necessary for the diabetic per to weigh his own food.

We now use household measures

teaspoons
tablespoons
measuring cup

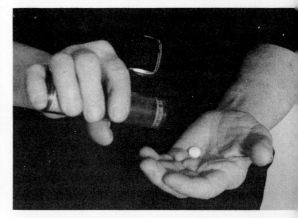

volved is not a single process and if one portion is disrupted, the whole network is disrupted.

The normal quantity of sugar in the blood ranges from 80 to 120 milligrams in each 100 cubic centimeters. The diabetic has much more. Thus, one basic element of diet modification is to reduce the intake of carbohydrates, sugars, and starches. This must be done with care, since fats are not properly metabolized in the total absence of carbohydrates, and acidosis may result. Acids resulting from incomplete breakdown of fats accumulate in the blood with the excess sugar, and coma may result.

Administration of insulin must be kept constantly in balance with the intake of food and the blood sugar levels in the body. The hormone is a potent substance which can cause shock and unconsciousness when an excess gets into the blood. This reaction is the basis of its use for *shock therapy* in mental illness, comparable to electric shock.

Diet control for the diabetic should provide the nourishment indispensable to health and growth, without overtaxing the body's diminishing capacity to metabolize sugars. The patient should keep his weight a little lower than average for his height, sex, and age. Insulin given to excessively obese people with mild diabetes is not very effective. Nevertheless, enough food should be consumed to satisfy hunger adequately. The diabetic diet should be calculated by a physician and dietician who estimate the patient's need in calories on a basis of his weight, age,

and occupation. The patient's capacity for disposing of sugar must be determined, and the doctor must decide to what extent diet may be relied on to relieve the basic condition and how much it must be supplemented by insulin.

In order to develop a diabetic's diet, his tolerance for sugar is established by beginning with an extremely simple intake and gradually increasing it until appearance of sugar in the urine begins to show that sugar capacity has been reached. At first, the patient will receive mostly vegetables with less than 5 per cent carbohydrates, such as cauliflower, celery, canned string beans, spinach, asparagus, lettuce, Brussels sprouts, artichokes, tomatoes, radishes, rhubarb, cabbage, and eggplant. The patient will receive from 150 to 200 grams of these and the bulk will relieve his hunger pangs without providing many calories. He should have a scale for weighing his meals.

In the absence of sugar in the excreted fluids, the diet is augmented on each successive day to include another five grams of carbohydrates, up to a total of twenty per day. Then the increase is slowed to the addition of five grams every other day. This is continued until either sugar appears in the urine or the patient is consuming three grams of carbohydrates for every thousand grams of body weight within each twenty-four hours.

Two or three days after the special diet has been started, vegetables containing 10 per cent carbohydrates may be included in the diet to pro-

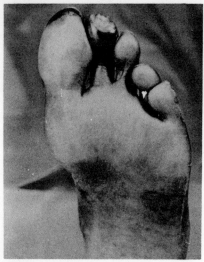

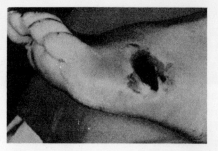

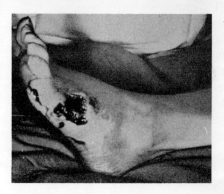

Diabetes—Patients with diabetes should be extremely careful to avoid damage or injury to the feet. Since circulation of blood in the feet is poor, infection can develop easily. Photograph (*top left*) showing skin damage wearing short shoes. The shoes rubbed against the toes, interfered with proper flow of blood in the tips of the toes and caused an infection. Photographs (*top right*) showing skin damage caused by poorly fitting shoes and improper foot hygiene. Foot lesions can be prevented if the feet are bathed daily and kept soft with applications of lanolin or oil. Diabetic patients should wear stockings and shoes which are a half inch longer than the feet to avoid binding the toes together. (*Below, right.*) What was a minor injury from walking barefooted developed into a serious infection for the person with diabetes. Shoes which fit properly should be worn at all times. Several pairs of shoes are necessary so they may be changed daily.

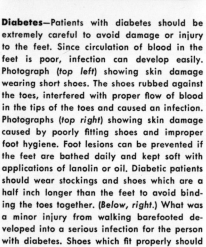

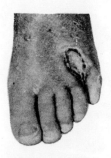

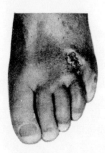

vide the added sugar intake desired. Such vegetables include canned peas, onions, beets, turnips, carrots, and squash. Later, vegetables of 15 per cent sugar content may be given, such as parsnips or canned lima beans, or even some with 20 per cent sugar content, such as succotash, beans, potatoes, and corn.

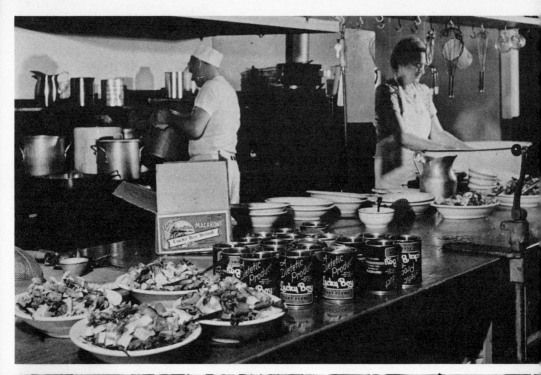
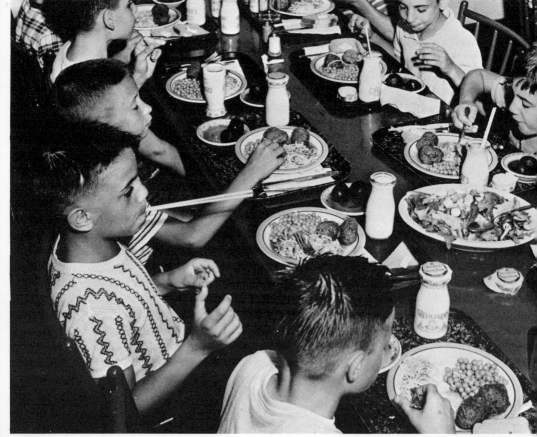

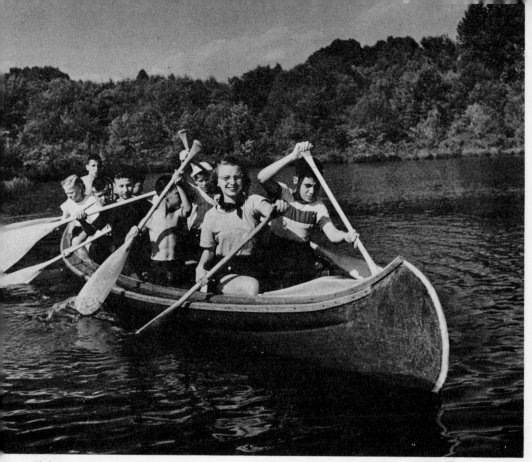

Diabetes—At a camp for diabetic children, every bit of food that goes into the making of meals is prepared with their special requirements in mind. Canned fruit is specially preserved without sugar. The amount of sugar in the diet must be rigorously supervised. The camp staff knows exactly how many units of sugar any child has in his system at any given time. A urine analysis is made on each child each day.

Diabetic children require plenty of food because they consume vast amounts of energy. Consequently, they eat six times a day—three full meals and three snacks between meals. At the camp, counsellors take the diabetic children for a supervised canoe ride across the lake. The amount of exercise is determined by the temperature and other weather conditions so as not to exhaust the limited facilities of the youngsters.

Vegetables should be cooked in a double boiler, so that all juices are retained.

Bread is usually omitted from a diabetic diet because of the large proportion of starch it contains. Special breads, however, made from gluten flour are available, and the label usually indicates the amount of carbohydrates and protein present.

The appearance of sugar in the patient's urine may demand fasting for a short time until the urine is clear again, or insulin may be needed. Insulin makes it possible for diabetics to eat a greater range of foods and diminishes or eliminates the need for fasting. Health and life expectancy are increased as a result.

Since diabetics are susceptible to certain health hazards, they must observe specific hygienic precautions. Eight to ten hours' sleep at night, as well as a daily rest after lunch, if possible, are advisable, along with plenty of fresh air and an adequate amount of sunshine. Sunburn should be avoided. The diabetic's skin is low in resistance and subject to serious infection if damaged. Diabetics should not let the skin become excessively dry. Strong soaps tend to dry the skin and increase the hazard of infection and should be avoided. Cold cream or lanolin cream are good lubricants.

Proper care of the feet is essential because foot difficulties may have serious consequences. The diabetic should take care to have proper shoes, to consult a chiropodist about calluses and corns, and to secure medical attention for even a minor bruise or wound. Iodine or other harsh applications should not be used. Tight garters should not be worn because they may create disturbances of circulation and may incite gangrene.

Exercise should be taken in moderation and be gauged to the age and condition of the person, the length of time he has been diabetic and his total intake of food and insulin. Exercise should be balanced against caloric consumption.

Excessively hot baths must be avoided because of danger of injury or destruction of the tissue from burning.

Any consumption of alcoholic beverages should be accompanied by exact knowledge of the quantity of calories taken, since a single gram of alcohol contains seven calories. Soft drinks, like ginger ale and other popular beverages, are too sugar-laden to be safe for the diabetic.

Dietetic soft drinks containing artificial sweeteners are now readily available.

Moderation should always be observed in smoking. Excessive smoking involves definite risk, both of increasing the sugar content of the blood and of disturbing the blood circulation, particularly in the legs.

The following group of simple rules is recommended for diabetics as a safeguard against the acidosis or coma which threatens them if the sugar levels rise unduly:

1. Be careful. Never permit yourself a careless attitude toward the disease.

2. Keep all your dietary rules and, especially, never overeat.

3. Never miss a scheduled insulin injection.

4. Protect yourself from infections; even a minor one may have serious results.

5. Inform those who should know of your condition, your surgeon, dentist, chiropodist, and barber, so that proper precautions can be taken.

6. Test the sugar content of your urine at least twice a week, and, if you have failed to observe the regulations, more frequently.

7. Keep the urine free of sugar as a good assurance against acidosis or coma.

8. Whenever you feel ill, take it seriously. Go to bed, avoid chill, call the doctor, and care for yourself until he comes.

See also ACETEST; CLINITEST; DIABETES INSIPIDUS; HYPOGLYCE-

MIA; INSULIN; ISLETS OF LANGER-HANS; PANCREAS. *See* MEDIGRAPHS pages 491, 1007, 1311.

DIABETES INSIPIDUS, a disorder of the urinary system in which large amounts of urine are excreted. The urine is itself normal and sugar is not present as in *diabetes mellitus.* The origin of *diabetes insipidus* is not yet definitely established. In a specific case damage to the pituitary gland, because of hemorrhage, infection, or a tumor, may be responsible. A disorder of the pituitary is probably accountable.

As much as four to ten quarts of urine may be excreted daily, as contrasted with 1½ to two quarts normally. One report describes the case of a sixteen-year-old boy who excreted thirty-three quarts of urine every twenty-four hours, and the equivalent of his own body weight in forty hours. Intense and practically uninterrupted thirst is another symptom, and sleep is disturbed frequently because of the urge to urinate. The abnormal excretions caused by the disease result in weakness and emaciation. If a tumor or serious abscess in the pituitary region is not present, the person may get along satisfactorily; but if one of these conditions is found, fatality usually ensues. Death then is the result of the original disorder and not of the *diabetes insipidus* caused by it.

Both the thirst and excessive flow of liquid can be controlled for as long as six hours by injection of an extract of the posterior part of the pituitary gland. This substance when inhaled as a dry powder has the same effect but is apparently ineffective when taken by mouth. In severe cases surgical removal of a tumor or of the pituitary gland has brought control of the serious symptoms. *See also* DIABETES; PITUITARY.

DIAMOX (*acetazoleamide*) is a drug used to treat congestive heart failure in which the patient is waterlogged from the accumulation of fluid in the tissues, and in other conditions in which elimination of fluids is inadequate. In some cases for which Diamox was used, the amount of urine increased 5 to 10 times the usual amount. Weight losses averaged 2.31 pounds during the first day the drug was taken, 1.93 pounds the second day, and a total of 10.75 pounds the first week. By regulating the acidity of the blood and of the body fluids through control of the action of an enzyme called carbonic anhydrase, Diamox forces powerful elimination of fluid from the body.

DIAPER RASH, a roughness and irritation of the skin in the area of the baby's diaper. Ordinarily infection is not involved and the rash is caused by the rubbing of the skin against a wet diaper. The irritation is aggravated if the diapers have been washed with a harsh soap, such as a soap with a high alkali content, and then carelessly rinsed. The rash is also intensified if a high degree of ammonia has been permitted to form in the diaper itself. This ammonia is produced when bacteria come in contact with urine which has soaked into the diaper.

A zinc ointment may be applied to relieve diaper rash. To prevent a recurrence of the rash, the diapers should be carefully washed with a mild soap and thoroughly rinsed. After laundering, the diapers may be soaked in a boric acid solution and hung in the sun. The presence of the boric acid will help prevent the formation of ammonia. These measures, plus careful attention to see that the baby's skin is kept dry and clean, ordinarily will bring good results. Protective lotions are available, such as silica preparations and DIAPERINE®. *See also* INTERTRIGO.

DIAPHRAGM, a wide muscle which separates the abdominal and chest cavities of the body, contracts and expands with breathing, and is significant both to the breathing process and to the circulatory system.

A disturbance of the action of the diaphragm due to injury to the nerves may have serious effects. Inflammation or infection of the diaphragm causes shortness of breath, soreness, and a sense of pressure in the lower chest region. Spasm of the diaphragm may be either *hiccups*—the more common form known as *clonic spasm*—or a constant tension of the muscle called *tonic spasm*. The tonic spasm is the more severe form and results from such diseases as tetanus, rabies, or epilepsy. Tonic spasm of long duration may cause exhaustion and, ultimately, death by asphyxiation. Sometimes vigorous rub-

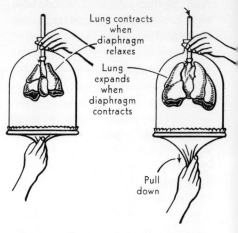

Diaphragm—This is a demonstration of the method by which the motion of the diaphragm expands the lungs. The diaphragm is a large muscle between the chest and the abdominal cavities. It is attached to the breastbone in the front, to the spine in the back and to the lower six ribs at the side of the body. With each expiration, the diaphragm moves upward and the lung contracts. On deep inspiration (drawing air in), the diaphragm moves downward against the abdominal cavity, the chest cavity is enlarged and the lungs expand.

bing around the chest walls, the back, and the region over the stomach will relieve the spasm.

Hernia or ruputure of the diaphragm may be caused by an injury, by a deformity before birth, or by a part of the stomach passing upward through the opening of the diaphragm at the esophagus. When a rupture occurs suddenly, symptoms of shock with severe pain in the lower part of the chest, hiccups, shortness of breath, and vomiting may be present. The most prominent symptoms of a hernia of long duration are shortness of breath and cyanosis. This is due to the possible displacement of the heart and to interference with the movement of the lungs. A child born with a large diaphragmatic hernia may also have what has been called an "upsidedown stomach." Unless this condition is detected promptly and corrected surgically, the infant may not survive.

Surgery of the diaphragm for control of rupture is usually successful. Special methods of study have been developed which include the introduction into the stomach and esophagus of specific substances which are opaque to x-rays. Thus the surgeon can determine the exact point at which the displaced organ has passed through the diaphragm before the actual operation. *See also* HICCUPS; HERNIA.

DIARRHEA, excessively frequent and moist or liquid evacuations from the bowels of the residual wastes from digestion; a symptom and not a disease. It may result from a tremendous range of different disorders, from indigestion to an acute infection or a cancer.

Diarrhea may be *transitory* and pass after a brief acute episode or it may be *chronic.* In simple *acute diarrhea* the frequent evacuations gradually change in character from soft to liquid. Intestinal pain and straining to evacuate still further are characteristic; and thirst, abdominal tenderness, and sometimes fever may be present. Frequently some toxic substance or food, such as green fruit, roughage, highly spiced foods, or alcoholic drinks, may be the cause. The diarrhea usually subsides after the elimination of the causative material, although the irritation accompanying it may prolong the condition.

When diarrhea is *chronic,* medical attention is imperative and failure to treat such a condition can result in serious weakness. The person will lose weight, strength, and appetite, develop anemia and become prey to various infections. *Chronic diarrhea has been classified under eight main headings and forty subheadings,* which suggests the variety of disease conditions with which it is associated. Some of these are a *stomach disorder* characterized by lack of a normal amount of acid, *ulcers, cancers, food deficiencies, Bright's disease, infections with different microorganisms and parasites,* the taking of *poisonous substances* such as *mercury* or *arsenic,* or of *cathartic drugs* or of *excessive alcohol,* various internal bodily disorders, special sensitivity to a certain food, and nervous and emotional disturbance. Various major infections which involve diarrhea are *amebiasis, typhoid fever, cholera,* and *bacillary dysentery.* It can also occur with *measles, pneumonia, smallpox* and *influenza.*

A thorough study of the person affected and of the evacuated material is essential to establish the specific cause of the diarrhea. The physician is interested not only in the patient's physical condition but also his emotional and mental state, the length of time the diarrhea has existed, the type and location of the pain, and the diet prior to the onset of the condition. The physician will try to establish the specific cause of the diarrhea and direct the treatment toward elimination of the cause rather than the symptom. *See also* CONSTIPATION, *and specific diseases. See* MEDIGRAPHS pages 77, 779.

DIET. *See* DIET, REDUCING; DIET, SPECIAL; NUTRITION; VITAMINS.

DIET IN DIGESTIVE DISOR-DERS. The primary purpose of diet for digestive disorders is to provide foods that do not cause chemical, mechanical, or thermal irritation to the digestive system. The foods selected for these diets should be easily digested, nourishing, and in a form (chopped, mashed, etc.) which requires the least amount of work for the digestive system. Foods and liquids should never be eaten too hot or too cold. A diet should be made of such foods as fresh milk and cream, cooked cereals, creamed soups or vegetable purées, cooked fruits and vegetables without skins and seeds, custards, junket, simple puddings, fresh soft-boiled eggs, toast made from stale bread, fresh butter, gelatin, plain ice cream, chopped beef patties, and jellies. Later, tender meats, broiled, stewed, or baked, and fresh fish may be served.

These foods contain proper quantities of proteins, carbohydrates, fats, and mineral salts. When the food is properly prepared and appetizingly served, such a diet should make digestion and absorption much easier.

When mashed or puréed, the food is more readily digested by the various digestive juices, the saliva in the mouth, the gastric juice in the stomach, and the bile, pancreatic, and intestinal juices in the intestine. Some people who have stomach or intestinal disturbances do not tolerate milk in its natural state; they must take such substitute fluids as sour milk, buttermilk, yogurt, acidophilus milk, or mullsoy.

Protein foods are chiefly meats, eggs, cheese, and fish. Carbohydrate foods are bread, cereals, vegetables, fruits, and sugars. Fat foods are butter, cream, lard, gravies, and oils. In these three groups are also present mineral salts and vitamins.

In arranging the diet for the treatment of digestive disorders, foods which will agree with the digestive system should be prescribed. The condition of the stomach, liver, gallbladder, pancreas, and intestine must be borne in mind.

When the stomach lacks acid and the proper ferments, intake of meats and other coarse foods must be reduced or stopped entirely, depending upon the degree of stomach weakness. Only liquid foods should be eaten for a time by a person with stomach or intestinal hemorrhage. If a patient has nausea or is vomiting all he eats, he may have to be fed intravenously, hypodermically, or rectally. Since symptoms vary considerably in different persons, the diet must be regulated accordingly. Some people with ulcer require one type of dietary regimen; others with symptoms of bleeding or profound spastic pain require other types. Since he knows just which foods are forbidden in a particular instance, the doctor's problem is to prescribe a diet consisting of the nonirritable rather than easily assimilable foods.

The average man or woman requires a diet furnishing from 2500 to 3000 calories a day and which should include all the vitamin factors essential to well-being. These vitamins are A, B-complex, C, D, K, and P. When a patient cannot assimilate food by mouth, vitamins may be added to the intravenous medication or given hypodermically. When bleeding is present and the blood examination reveals poor clotting, vitamin K in suitable doses is often administered.

Vitamin A is found in milk, egg yolk, cream, butter, cheese, lettuce, carrots, salmon, bananas, parsley, peaches, apricots, and cod liver oil. Vitamin B_1, with its associated complex factors is found in wheat germ, cereals, eggs, beef, liver, oysters, bread (particularly whole-wheat bread), salmon, prunes, oranges, carrots, lettuce, spinach, yeast, and tomatoes. Vitamin C is found in fruits and vegetables, such as lemons, oranges, limes, tomatoes, apples, bananas, apricots, peaches, leafy vegetables, carrots, parsley, peas, beets, asparagus, and in liver. Vitamin D is found in butter, cream, egg yolk, salmon, tuna fish, beef liver, and cod liver oil.

DIET, LOW SALT. Pure *sodium,* which is one of the two elements in *sodium chloride,* or common salt, is seldom found except in chemical laboratories. Many combinations of sodium with other elements are used in diet and in industry. Table salt is *sodium chloride*. Baking soda is *sodium bicarbonate*.

The average man takes in his diet about half an ounce of sodium chloride every day. It is easy, on a low salt diet, to reduce this to about one fifth as much. This is done particularly when excess of fluid accumulates in the tissues, as in *dropsy*. No one knows exactly the minimum or maximum of sodium chloride that any one person ought to have, but fortunately the human body is equipped with factors of safety, so that it can get rid of excesses of various substances. The average human body contains at all times about three ounces of sodium chloride. The use of salt by the body and its elimination by the kidney are apparently controlled by the cortex or outer layer of the adrenal gland.

Many vegetables contain another salt with an element similar to sodium, namely, *potassium*. A person who subsists on a vegetable diet craves salt, because vegetables contain less sodium than meat. The moment the salt in the human body falls below the amount necessary a craving is set up.

Salt is also important for supplying the *chlorine* element, since *hydrochloric acid* is secreted by the stomach regularly as an aid to digestion. *Pepsin* works as a digestive substance only in the presence of hydrochloric acid. However, hydrochloric acid should not be taken by the average person in that form except on the advice of a physician.

Various diets free from large amounts of sodium chloride have been developed. Most physicians are convinced that there is a definite relationship between salt in the diet and the occurrence of various conditions affecting the blood pressure and the kidneys. However, in the presence of unusual craving for salt, or, in fact, in any disease condition, it is well to be guided by competent advice.

DIET, REDUCING, a regimen of food and drink for the purpose of losing weight. In most cases of overweight or obesity, a reducing diet is the most desirable treatment. In addition to a wish to lose weight, the person should have a knowledge of the nutritional and caloric value of foods. The diet should include sufficient protein to prevent loss of body tissue protein. Carbohydrates should be limited and fat largely eliminated. To insure sufficient vitamin and mineral intake, supplementary multiple vitamin capsules should be taken daily. Losing weight involves a cutting down of regular everyday foods and does not necessitate specialized foods. Vegetables are to be cooked and eaten plain, without butter or sauces, and salads served without fatty dressings. Fruit should be fresh, or, if canned, without added sugar. Plentiful servings of low-calorie fruits and vegetables provide bulk and satisfy hunger. Only lean meats should be eaten. It is important to establish regular hours for eating meals. A simple bedtime snack, such as an apple or a glass of skim milk, will help prevent hunger in the early morning or the urge to eat during the night.

For an extremely obese person who is not active, a daily diet of 800 calories is possible. For moderate weight reduction, 1000 to 1200 calories can be taken daily provided the person is fairly sedentary, and 1400 to 1500 calories for persons requiring more energy for their daily activities.

To maintain health while reducing, certain foods are essential. The daily diet should include: 1 egg, 2 glasses of skim milk or buttermilk, 3 slices of bread, preferably whole wheat, 2 servings of lean meat, fish, fowl, or cottage cheese, 4 servings of raw or cooked vegetables, and 3 servings of fresh or unsweetened canned fruit. For the 800-calorie diet, the bread is omitted; for the 1200-calorie diet, an extra slice of bread and 3 teaspoons of butter are added, and the 1500-calorie diet can include 5 slices of bread, or 3 slices of bread and 2 small potatoes, and 3 teaspoons of butter. The bread can be the high-protein, low-calorie bread now sold commercially.

Following is a suggested day's menu for the 1000-calorie diet:

Breakfast
½ grapefruit
1 slice toast
1 egg
1 glass skim milk
Coffee or tea, without cream, milk, or sugar, may be taken any time.

Lunch
1 slice bread
1 cooked vegetable
3 oz. lean meat
vegetable salad
1 serving fruit

Dinner

Same as lunch; add 1 glass skim milk.

Bedtime snack: an apple or a glass of skim milk.

Following are lists of fruits and vegetables which may be selected:

Fruits

Apples	Peaches
Berries	Pears
Cantaloupe	Pineapple
Grapefruit	Plums
Grapes	Watermelon
Oranges	

Vegetables

Asparagus	Mushrooms
Broccoli	Okra
Brussels sprouts	Parsley
Cabbage	Peppers
Cauliflower	Radishes
Celery	Spinach
Cucumber	Squash
Eggplant	String beans
Greens	Tomatoes
Lettuce	Watercress

After the weight has been reduced to the desired level, it is essential to continue to watch carefully the diet and eating habits. The aim must be to maintain the new weight, and avoid the tendency to regain the pounds lost. *See also* OBESITY; WEIGHT, FACTORS WHICH INFLUENCE; WEIGHT-REGULATING MACHINERY OF THE BODY; DIET, SPECIAL.

DIET, ROUGHAGE IN THE. Most domestic animals are capable of eating and digesting roughage in considerable amounts. A horse and cow eat hay and get nourishment from it, but a human being cannot. The cellulose of hay cannot be digested properly by the human digestive tract, and the material is passed rapidly through the intestines.

Most vegetables and fruits and wholegrain cereals contain cellulose, which serves to give bulk to the material in the bowel and in that way to give the intestines something to work on.

Cellulose may be sufficiently tender to be partially digested, as, for example, in the form of lettuce, fruits, and cooked vegetables, but in general it is not digestible. Potatoes, beans, nuts, and olives have some cellulose, which may be utilized to a certain extent in the body, but in the majority of instances the cellulose is not properly utilized, except for roughage.

Cellulose is found in paper obtained from wood; cotton is practically pure cellulose, and the substance is also found in large amounts in bran. When water acts on cellulose it may swell it up somewhat, increasing its bulk still further.

Few people realize the danger of a diet containing too much cellulose. Such a diet interferes with digestion of the useful material, and it may irritate a sensitive intestinal tract to the extent of causing an erosion or inflammation.

The bran of rice and wheat contains vitamins which may be of great value to the human body. The bran contains about 22 per cent of the protein of the wheat kernel. Bran proteins are relatively rich in those nutritionally essential amino acids that are deficient in the endosperm of wheat. However, nature has seen to it that the vitamins are available in many forms, and it is not necessary to overload the intestines with roughage to secure a sufficient amount of any one vitamin.

The various Vitamin B components are found in the bran of cereals and in the embryo of cereals as well. The fiber of the green and yellow vegetables serves as a cleanser of the bowel and is not harsh enough to irritate. Too much bran, on the other hand, can easily irritate the bowel.

DIET, SMOOTH, FREE FROM ROUGHAGE. In the majority of cases of irritation of the colon and of associated constipation, the most important dietetic consideration is that the diets be free from unnecessary roughage or stimulation. Here are suggestions for a smooth diet:

Avoid sugar in concentrated form and take no candy or other food between meals. Hot cakes and waffles are permissible but should not be eaten with syrup. Fried foods are not bad if they are properly fried, that is, totally immersed in fat at the right temperature. Avoid eating when in a rush and when mentally upset.

The following are suggestions for breakfast: Orange juice, grapefruit (avoid the fiber in the compartments). Cantaloupe and melons are inadvisable. Coffee, if desired, is allowed in moderation, but it sometimes causes flatulence. If you are sensitive to caffeine try a caffeine-free coffee or a coffee substitute. Chocolate, cocoa, or tea; one or two eggs with ham or bacon (avoid the tougher part of the bacon); white bread, toast, or zwieback, with butter; any smooth mush such as farina, germea, Cream of Wheat, cornmeal, or rolled oats; puffed cereals and cornflakes are also allowed. Bran is harmful. Graham bread is permitted, but not the coarser whole-wheat bread.

Suggestions for lunch and dinner: In fruit cocktails avoid the fibrous pieces of orange and pineapple. Broths, bouillon, cream soups, and chowder are allowed; also meat, fish, chicken, squab, or game, except duck (avoid the fibrous parts and gristle). Veal may be tried; it is not digested well by many persons. Eat no smoked fish or pork. Crab and lobster had better be left alone. Oysters and sausage may be tried later.

Bread and butter are allowed, and hot biscuits if they are made small so as to consist mainly of crust. Rice, potatoes—mashed, creamed, or French-fried—are allowed; and later, sweet potatoes, hominy, stewed tomatoes (strained and thickened with cracker or bread crumbs), well-cooked cauliflower tops with cream sauce, asparagus tips, Brussels sprouts, squash, beets, turnips, creamed spinach, Italian pastes, noodles, macaroni, and spaghetti, all cooked soft, purées of peas, beans, lentils, lima beans, or artichoke hearts. All skins or fiber should be removed by passing the food through a ricer. Sweet corn may be used if passed through a colander. String beans are allowed if they are young and tender. Large, tender string beans, which can be used as a vegetable or salad, can now be obtained in cans.

No salad should be taken at first. Later you may try a little tender lettuce with apples or bananas, tomato jelly or boiled eggs. Mayonnaise and French dressing are allowed. Potato salad without much onion may be tried.

Suggested desserts are: simple puddings, custards, ice cream, gelatine, plain cake, and canned or stewed fruits, particularly pears and peaches. Cottage cheese is permissible; other cheeses often cause trouble. Apple, peach, apricot, custard, and lemon cream pie may be tried if only the filling is eaten.

Make no effort to drink excess water. Be guided by your thirst. Avoid excessive use of salt or other seasoning.

DIET, SPECIAL. In a number of specific diseases and bodily conditions, a special diet may be necessary —for example, in diabetes, heart disease, and in kidney, ulcer, and other infections. Such diets should be undertaken under the supervision of a physician. Conditions such as underweight and obesity, for safety and best results, should be properly supervised.

Some special diets may be self-administered. Among these are:

High-Caloric Diet: Add extra milk, cream, eggs, cheese, and dried fruits, such as raisins and dates, to the regular diet.

High-Protein Diet: Add extra meat, eggs, cheese, and fish.

Low-Protein Diet: Omit meat and all but one egg daily; add portions of vegetables and fruits.

High-Carbohydrate Diet: Omit meat and eggs, but add extra portions of vegetables and fruits, rice, pastas, and puddings.

Low-Carbohydrate Diet: Reduce intake of bread, potatoes, rice, and other starchy foods. Omit sugar, candy, cakes and pie altogether.

High-Fat Diet: Add extra butter, fats, fatty meats, oils, and cream to the regular diet.

Salt-Free Diet: Use only salt-free bread and sweet butter. Salt must not be added to food in cooking or at any other time.

See also DIET, REDUCING; OBESITY.

DIFFUSE LUPUS ERYTHEMA-TOSUS. *See* COLLAGEN DISEASES; LUPUS ERYTHEMATOSUS; ERYTHEMA.

DIGESTION, the complex chemical and physiological process by which food is converted into soluble form for absorption into the tissues and cells of the body.

In digestion, the food is first ground and chewed in the mouth, which prepares it for action by the saliva. Saliva contains an enzyme which acts on starch to convert it into sugar. Then the food passes through the esophagus into the stomach, where it is further disintegrated and acted upon by the stomach juices, which contain hydrochloric acid, pepsin, and other substances such as rennin (which coagulates milk). Protein is broken down by the action of pepsin and hydrochloric acid. The stomach usually requires about four hours of both mechanical and chemical action on food to complete its function. From the stomach the partly digested food passes into the small intestine, where both the mechanical and the chemical actions continue.

In the small intestine, bile secreted by the liver and pancreatic juice from the pancreas act on protein, starch, sugar, and fats. Intestinal juices from the lining of the intestines also act on sugars and proteins to complete the major part of the chemical process of digestion. All undigested food and debris pass, by muscular action, into the large intestine. Here water and glucose are absorbed, and finally the remainder passes into the rectum whence it is eliminated as feces.

The process by which the tissues utilize the food substances distributed to them by the blood is the secondary phase of digestion. In this process the living cells of every tissue and organ of the body absorb various food substances that they require and synthesize them into their own structure. *See also* STOMACH; INTESTINES.

DIGESTIVE DISTURBANCES. *See* INDIGESTION; CONSTIPATION; DIARRHEA.

DIGESTIVE SYSTEM. All the parts of the body concerned with intake, digestion, and elimination constitute the digestive system. The digestive tract is really a continuous tube whose parts are the mouth, pharynx, esophagus, stomach, small intestine, large intestine, and rectum. The linings of this intricate, con-

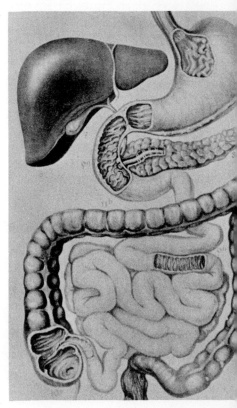

Digestive System—The digestive organs in the abdomen. Notice that the stomach is located high in the abdomen. The liver is the large, dark organ found to the right of the stomach and the upper part of the small intestine. The pancreas is depicted here as being below the stomach. The small bulb on the bottom of the liver is the gallbladder. Tubes from these three organs (liver, pancreas and gallbladder) lead into the small intestine. The small intestine takes up most of the space in the abdomen and empties into the large intestine. The large intestine frames the small intestine by ascending on the right side, crossing over and then descending on the left side to end as the rectum.

voluted tube perform chemical and mechanical actions on the food and absorb and transmit the resulting substances to the blood and lymph.

The principal glands and organs that open into the digestive system are the salivary glands of the mouth and the liver and pancreas which open into the small intestine. Mucous glands perform a lubricating function throughout the tract, which enables food and waste material to pass through.

Numerous disorders and diseases, both temporary and chronic, affect the digestive system.

DIGITALIS, a valuable drug derived from the dried leaves of the *purple foxglove*. It is a powerful stimulant for the heart, and may also be used to provoke the flow of urine in persons afflicted with *dropsy* (*edema*).

Digitalis can be dangerous and should never be used except in the dosage prescribed by the doctor. Even a slight excess over an extended period of time may cause the drug to accumulate in the system and act as a poison. The first symptom of poisoning may be palpitation of the heart, since digitalis slows the heartbeat. Often the lips tinge and at the same time the person may find it difficult to breathe. Whenever such an attack occurs, the person should be put to bed at once and a doctor called; sometimes the patient may receive a stimulant such as coffee. If his condition seems critical and the doctor is delayed, he may be given sips of tepid water to encourage vomiting. *See also* HEART.

DILANTIN, the trade name for *diphenylhydantoin sodium*. It is a white powder used as an anticonvulsant in the treatment of epilepsy, and is best taken with water at mealtimes, since it may be irritating if taken on an empty stomach. It should be taken only on the advice of a physician.

DIPHTHERIA, an infectious disease that may occur in nose or throat and is characterized by fever, sore throat, heart weakness and anemia. Formerly one of the most feared of childhood diseases, diphtheria is now comparatively infrequent and the death rate from the illness is almost at the vanishing point. Diphtheria can be diagnosed with complete accuracy. In conditions where it is suspected, a bacteriologist can determine from a culture of the infected area not only whether the disease-producing agents are the germs of diphtheria but also whether they represent any special type of that germ.

It has been found that diphtheria germs vary in their virulence in different epidemics. People may carry the germs of diphtheria in their throats without themselves being ill. There are germs which resemble the germ of diphtheria and which are nonvirulent. The diphtheria germ gets its effects in the body by producing a poison known as the *toxin of diphtheria*. When this poison or toxin is injected into animals, it kills them, provided the dose of the poison is sufficient. The virulence of the germ can be measured by the amount of poison necessary

513

the disease and its causes   Diphtheria is an acute (which is to say quick-developing), severe contagious illness caused by a specific type of bacteria. It involves mainly the respiratory system. The disease is spread by direct contact with an infected patient, with a carrier who may be perfectly healthy himself, or through contact with infected objects or from unpasteurized milk. It occurs mainly during the winter months, and usually affects children who have been ill with an infection of the nose or throat. Babies up to 6 months have some immunity. The disease has an incubation period of 2 to 5 days. The contagious period of the disease may last as long as from 2 to 4 weeks.

symptoms   The disease begins with temperatures in the 101° range, headache, and sore throat. The symptoms vary depending upon the severity of the case and the areas involved. The throat is usually covered with a grayish membrane which may extend to the roof of the mouth and even up into the nose. The mouth odor is foul, the voice becomes hoarse, and swallowing difficult. The glands of the neck become enlarged and painful. Nosebleeds may occur. Breathing may be difficult and noisy. The usual course is 7 to 14 days, and milder cases may improve even more quickly.

complications   In the 2nd to 4th weeks of this illness, severe complications can develop that involve the heart, lung, kidneys, and nervous systems. These include inflammation of the heart muscle, bronchopneumonia, nephritis, and paralysis affecting the muscles of speech, eye movements, arms and legs.

prevention (or lessening of impact)   A diphtheria vaccine is available which should be given to every child by the time he is ready for school. Booster injections are given until the age of 12 to maintain immunity. The Schick Test is used to reveal whether or not an individual is immune to the disease. Anyone who is not immune, or who has been exposed to the disease, should be immunized promptly with diphtheria toxoid or given booster shots of the vaccine. Antibiotic drugs are used in the treatment of the disease and in some of its complications.
Since the diphtheria germ attacks the body by producing a poison known as diphtheria toxin, an early diagnosis is very important. The longer the delay in administering the antitoxin or the toxoid, the more poison is absorbed by the body. Breathing can become difficult, and the patient may suffocate.
Diphtheria antitoxin is available for those not previously immunized with toxoid. In these patients it should be used early, and may be lifesaving.

Diphtheria

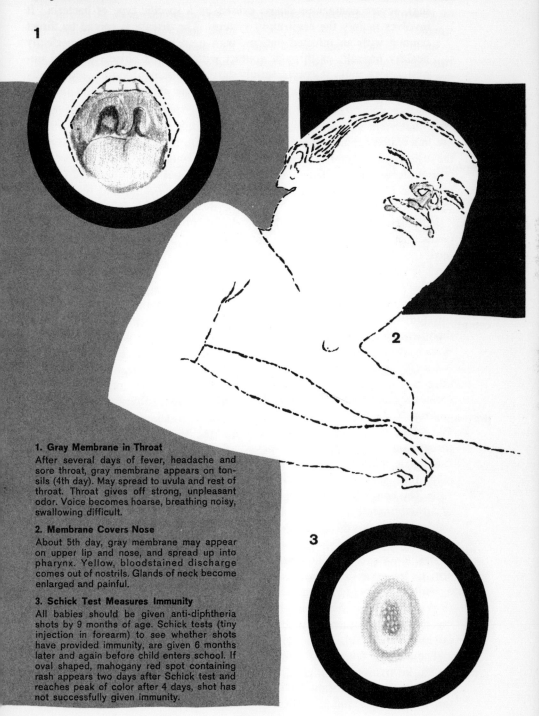

1. Gray Membrane in Throat
After several days of fever, headache and sore throat, gray membrane appears on tonsils (4th day). May spread to uvula and rest of throat. Throat gives off strong, unpleasant odor. Voice becomes hoarse, breathing noisy, swallowing difficult.

2. Membrane Covers Nose
About 5th day, gray membrane may appear on upper lip and nose, and spread up into pharynx. Yellow, bloodstained discharge comes out of nostrils. Glands of neck become enlarged and painful.

3. Schick Test Measures Immunity
All babies should be given anti-diphtheria shots by 9 months of age. Schick tests (tiny injection in forearm) to see whether shots have provided immunity, are given 6 months later and again before child enters school. If oval shaped, mahogany red spot containing rash appears two days after Schick test and reaches peak of color after 4 days, shot has not successfully given immunity.

to destroy an animal of standard weight.

In the United States more than two thirds of all the cases of diphtheria occur in children under five years of age and over 80 per cent in children under ten years of age. Now that great numbers of children are inoculated against diphtheria by the use of *diphtheria toxoid,* there is a tendency for the disease to occur more frequently in older rather than in younger children.

Diphtheria is spread by direct contact of a child who does not have the disease with one who does have it or with a carrier. Possibly there are indirect contacts. Before pasteurization of milk was adopted, infected milk sometimes spread diphtheria, but nowadays that source is no longer a menace.

Usually from two to five days after he has been exposed to the germs, a child who is infected will develop a slight fever, going up to 102 degrees Fahrenheit, a sore throat, general illness, and weakness such as is frequent with the beginning of almost any infectious disease. The congestion and the growth of a *membrane* begin usually in the upper part of the throat or *pharynx* and then spread downward into the *larynx,* or voice box, and perhaps also to the *nose.* The membrane is a thin, grayish film which then thickens. Associated with the swelling and redness there may be enlargement of the glands in the neck and increasing fever. The more the throat is involved, the greater the spread of the membrane in which the germs are found.

An early diagnosis is of the utmost importance in diphtheria. If the diagnosis not made promptly and antitoxin in sufficient amount not given quickly, the swelling in the throat becomes larger, hemorrhages begin, the voice becomes high-pitched and strangled, and there is a fetid odor from the throat. If the continuous absorption of the poisons goes on, drowsiness is followed by delirium, and the danger of death is great. When the membrane in the larynx grows in size, breathing becomes difficult and suffocation may ensue.

Before the discovery of antitoxin, 35 per cent of children with diphtheria died of the disease. In cases where the larynx, or voice box, was involved, 90 per cent died. Today the death rate has been reduced to nearly the disappearing point, due to the use of the antitoxin and the *Shick test.* The Schick test is important in determining susceptibility to the disease. *See also* CROUP; THROAT. *See* MEDIGRAPH page 515.

DISC, a plate of cartilage between the bones of the spine. When one of these discs is broken, the soft material which it contains may protrude in such a manner as to place pressure on the spinal nerves. The person so affected feels as if something has given way in his back, and will complain of a pain which seems to radiate downward along the side on which the break has occurred. This pain, constant and severe, will be intensified when he coughs, bends, or stands erect for a long time. Further symptoms may include muscle spasms, a disposition to protect certain nerve areas, a diminished skin sensitivity in the affected area, and a decrease in tendon reflexes. Sometimes the break is visible under x-rays.

If the injured person is permitted to walk, he will be required to wear a girdle or cast. Ordinarily, however, he will be put in a special type of bed, in which reinforcing boards have been placed under the mattress. Removal of the ruptured disc may be necessary and usually ends the difficulty. *See also* SLIPPED DISC; SPINAL CORD. *See* MEDIGRAPHS pages 947, 1211, 1221.

DISINFECTION, the destruction or removal of germs or articles which may be germ-bearing from a sickroom following recovery from an infectious disease. During the course of an illness, disinfection should be carried on constantly to prevent transmission of the disease. Discharged matter from the eyes, ears, nose, throat, skin, or other parts of the body should be destroyed by burning or other sure methods, after being collected in containers which can also be destroyed. Towels, bedclothes, and linens should be handled so that the infected side is turned inward, and those caring for these items should be careful to hold them by the noninfected portions.

The infectious material varies with different diseases. In chickenpox, the source of the infected discharges may be the mouth, nose, throat, or lesions of the skin; while in measles, meningitis, pneumonia, septic sore throat, and whooping cough it is usually from the mouth, nose, and throat. In typhoid, dysentery, and poliomyelitis, bowel discharge probably carries the infectious organisms. Moreover, in poliomyelitis the mouth, nose, and throat may also be the source. In scarlet fever and diphtheria, infectious matter comes from the eyes, mouth, nose, throat, and wounded skin surfaces.

After the patient has recovered, the sickroom and everything in it should be thoroughly disinfected. During the illness, upholstered furniture, carpet, curtains, and all extraneous ornaments should have been removed. At the end of the illness, beds, chairs, tables, floors, and woodwork must be completely scrubbed with soap and hot water, and linens and other washable fabrics boiled for at least fifteen minutes. Nonwashable materials can be exposed to direct sunlight out-of-doors for at least twenty-four hours; and rubber goods, such as sheets, hotwater bottles, and ice caps, can be washed with soap and water and placed out-of-doors to air and dry for at least two hours. Books, magazines, and toys which the patient has used should be burned.

Good disinfectants are *chloride of lime, creosol,* or *milk of lime* in solution. *Heat* is one of the best germ destroyers. Disinfection of the sickroom with *sulphur vapor* is a time-honored and effective method.

DISLOCATION, the displacement of a part of the body from its usual place. The term is used ordinarily in connection with a bone, such as the elbow, shoulder, or knee, moved partially or completely out of its normal position. Dislocations usually happen suddenly as the result of a blow, fall, or other accident, and recurrent dislocations are not uncommon, especially with athletes. Because of the danger of further injury, when any type of dislocation occurs, only a physician should reset the displaced joint. Until the doctor arrives, the person should be made as comfortable as possible and kept warm. Cold compresses applied at the point of injury may relieve pain and prevent swelling. *See also* JOINTS AND JOINT DISORDERS; FRACTURES. *See* MEDIGRAPHS pages 659, 1221.

DIURESIS. To release an accumulation of fluids in the blood, a physician may prescribe drugs known as *diuretics.* The excessive excretion of urine is *diuresis.* Urine contains both solids and water. Some diuretics increase the discharge of water and others increase the amount of solids released. Specific diuretics release various types of solids. Several drugs may be prescribed when a single drug to achieve the desired effect is not known. *Water* is a good diuretic, unless, of course, the body must get rid of an excessive amount of water. Diuretics which encourage the discharge of water are usually those which also stimulate circulation, such as *digitalis, Diamox, alcohol,* and *coffee.* Another group which includes *mercury combina-*

tions may be classed as the *mineral salt diuretics.* For this purpose, mineral salt is effective only in small amounts, since larger doses may act instead as a stimulant to the bowels. *See also* KIDNEYS; URINE.

DIVERTICULITIS. Pouches, or *diverticula,* which sometimes develop on the walls of the large intestines of adults, create *diverticulosis.* Inflammation or infection of these pouches is *diverticulitis.*

The severity of diverticulitis can be determined by a test, known as the *barium test,* in which the patient swallows a barium mixture and is then examined by a series of x-rays of the colon. Thus, the pouches and the bowel contractions can be seen clearly, and the x-ray film will also show whether or not a narrowing or obstruction of the bowel is present.

In acute diverticulitis, ulceration with consequent perforation of the wall of the bowel may result and cause massive hemorrhage which will require prompt surgery.

In older people, one of the dangers of diverticulitis is chronic irritation with a possibility of cancer. Treatment of inflamed diverticula includes rest and enemas to help cleanse the bowels when necessary. Sometimes mineral oil may be used to aid the passage hardened material. Persistent obstruction or constant inflammation and pain may also necessitate surgical treatment.

Persons with diverticulitis require a soft diet, similar to that for those with ulcer. Irritating spices and sharp foods must be avoided, as well as fibrous foods and those containing seeds or skins. *See also* INTESTINES; DIVERTICULUM.

DIVERTICULUM, a small pouch which sometimes develops on the smooth wall of the intestinal tract.

Meckel's diverticulum, named for its discoverer, is a congenital deformity or abnormality occurring near the middle of the small intestine. This pouch may collect partially digested food and become inflamed or infected and cause symptoms similar to those of *appendicitis;* also hemorrhage requiring surgical attention may result.

Diverticula may also form in the esophagus, stomach, duodenum, or jejunum, and a single diverticulum may occur in the cecum or elsewhere in the colon. Many diverticula do not cause symptoms and will not require treatment, but when they become inflamed surgery is recommended to correct the condition. *See also* DIVERTICULITIS.

DIZZINESS, sensation of swimming in the head; one of the commonest symptoms about which people complain. Like a cough, it may be a sign of something seriously wrong that demands prompt attention.

Dizziness follows recovery from all kinds of illnesses. It may result from poisoning by drugs, or sensitivity to certain foods. It is a symptom in high blood pressure, in menopause, migraine headaches, eyestrain, brain injury, punctured eardrum, malformation of the inner ear, syphilis, alcoholism, and many other diseases or disorders.

A common form of dizziness results from inflammation in that portion of the inner ear known as the *semicircular canals.* Anything that interferes with the delicate mechanism of these canals will produce attacks of dizziness.

If dizziness is temporary and the condition responds to treatment such as suitable attention to diet, correction of eyestrain, or regulation of kidney action, there is no cause for alarm. However, repeated and persistent dizziness calls for most careful diagnosis. There may be insufficient blood supply to the brain or weakened heart action. Recurrent dizzy spells sometimes signify the presence of a brain tumor. Dizziness in such cases is a distinct danger signal whose warning must be promptly heeded.

Dizziness caused by seasickness or airsickness, as well as by other forms of motion, is helped by the use of drugs like DRAMAMINE®, BONAMINE®,or MAREZINE®. *See also* MOTION SICKNESS; VERTIGO; EAR STUFFINESS.

DOG BITES. Because of the possibility of *rabies,* anyone bitten by a dog should receive the prompt attention of a physician. The wound may be carefully washed with soap and water, a weak solution of iodine applied, and the wound covered with a clean bandage. If possible, the dog should be confined and watched until it is determined whether or not it has rabies. The necessary information should be given at once to the city authorities. If the dog has rabies the person bitten is given the

Pasteur inoculations against rabies. The dog is killed and its brain examined for the presence of Negri bodies which are diagnostic of rabies. *See also* RABIES.

DOUBLE VISION. *See* EYE, *Diplopia.*

DOUCHE, a jet or current of water applied for cleansing purposes to any part, organ, or cavity of the body.

The danger of germs is always greater when washing an internal portion of the body. Water used for this purpose should, therefore, be boiled, then the temperature brought as close as possible to that of the blood, about 100° F. Cold water must not be used since it is harmful when applied internally.

Certain special equipment is necessary for the administration of a vaginal douche. First is the water container which may be made of tin, glass, rubber, or plastic. A length of rubber or plastic hosing is attached to the container with a vaginal tube of vulcanite or glass at the other end. Glass is more convenient for sterilizing purposes. This equipment must be kept absolutely clean at all times.

The container should be placed two or three feet above the point where the fluid is to emerge, in order that the force of the flow of water be satisfactory. If the container is placed too high, the force might be dangerous, and the liquid could reach unintended areas.

Before the tube is inserted, the fluid should be permitted to run through the entire hose so that all of the air is expelled. Petroleum jelly, if desired, may be smeared on the end of the tube, which should be thrust inward for a distance not exceeding three inches. Afterward the fluid may be ejected into any suitable receptacle. The vaginal douche is useful as an antiseptic, as a means of removing discharge, and also for controlling disagreeable odors. The solution employed will be chosen accordingly. *See also* ENEMA; NOSE; VAGINA.

DRAMAMINE, the trade name for *dimenhydrinate,* a compound with antihistaminic properties which has been found to be effective in the prevention and treatment of motion sickness.

DOWN'S SYNDROME is one of the more than 100 known causes of mental retardation. The old name, *mongolism,* derives from a superficial resemblance to the somewhat oriental appearance of the eyes.

Intelligence is limited in almost all cases but in very differing degrees. Walking and other motor development is often delayed, as is speech. As babies, most are quiet and easily managed; as children, they are especially friendly and affectionate. Most can learn usual daily care and can be trained to do routine jobs. Life expectancy may approach the normal. With appropriate training, many can lead satisfying lives at home, although some cases need institutional care.

There are three types of Down's Syndrome. In the most common type the condition has been found to be due to an additional chromosome, making a total of 47 instead of the normal 46. The incidence in the general population is said to be about 1 out of 600 births. Older women have a greater chance of having a child with this type of chromosomal disorder. The chance of having another such child is not much higher than in families with no previous history of such a condition.

The second type, which is far less common (1 in 12,000 births) but may run in families, has only 46 chromosomes because the additional small one is attached to another chromosome (*translocation*). In such cases the mother's chromosomes should be analyzed and if a similar translocation is found, the possibility of having additional children with Down's Syndrome is as high as 1 in 3. An extremely rare type of Down's Syndrome is *mosaicism,* where some cells are normal and some have the extra chromosome.

Chromosomal analysis from white blood cells of the Down's Syndrome child is available and establishes the type. A diagnosis also can be made before birth by examining the fluid surrounding the baby in uterus. *See also* FEEBLE-MINDEDNESS; CRETINISM; MYXEDEMA.

DRESSINGS, materials used to protect such injuries as burns, abrasions, and wounds. The most significant function of dressings is to protect the injured area from germs.

Since moisture encourages the growth of germs, a dry dressing is usually preferable. When the wound is inflamed or encrusted, however, a wet dressing may be more soothing and better for cleansing purposes.

Plain white dressings of lint, gauze, cotton, or wool, sterilized with heat and wrapped in antiseptic packages, may be purchased. These are useless, however if contaminated by unsterilized hands or brought into contact with any other unsterilized surface. Dressings may be stored in clean paper packages and kept in a suitable box, which is always tightly covered.

DROPSY. *See* NEPHROSIS.

DROWNING, suffocation in water or other liquid. A person removed from the water may be alive, even though he appears to be dead. Without delay his mouth should be cleared of any debris which he may have acquired in the struggle to breathe, and he should be placed on his stomach, the side of his head resting on his forearm. Artificial respiration should be given at once, for at least an hour, until the victim begins to breath naturally, or the effort is found futile.

As soon as the person regains consciousness, his blood circulation should be stimulated. He should be wrapped in dry blankets, warmed with hot-water bottles, if possible, and his limbs gently massaged. Stimulants, such as tea, coffee, brandy, or whiskey in water, may be given.

Although the victim might appear to have recovered, he should not be permitted to walk alone. Instead, if at all possible, a stretcher of some type should be used. Once the person has been placed in bed, he must be carefully watched for at least an hour, since his breathing might stop again, in which case it is essential to resume artificial respiration.

In cases of drowning, every effort should be made to secure the services of a physician promptly. *See also* ARTIFICIAL RESPIRATION; ASPHYXIA; RESUSCITATION.

DRUG ADDICTION. Traffic in drugs constitutes a major problem for the authorities and, because of the alarming increase in youthful addicts, for parents and teachers as well.

The loss of the power of self-control through drug addiction is not only harmful to the individual concerned, but also to society. A drug addict has such an overwhelming craving for the drug that he does not count the cost of getting it; crime, violence, and murder have been the price all too often. The addict develops a tolerance to the drug so that increasing doses are necessary in order to produce the desired effect. When not under the influence of the drug the addict tends more and more to manifest typical disturbances of the nervous system. If drugs are withdrawn from the addict, characteristic withdrawal symptoms appear, with acute physical pain in addition to such symptoms as severe cramps in the abdomen and legs, muscular twitching, vomiting, and diarrhea. The addict will be irritable, restless, and unable to relax, and will break out in sweat and "goose pimples." Rest and sleep are difficult or impossible to achieve.

The chief drugs used by addicts are opium and its derivatives, morphine and heroin; cocaine; hashish; and marijuana made from hemp. The widespread use of bromides and barbiturates, sedatives, and sleeping pills available to the general public, has also raised problems. The barbiturates fulfill all the requirements of habit-forming drugs. Overdose is often fatal. Therefore legal control of the sale of the drugs has been tightened.

Treatment for drug addiction is quite drastic and should be attempted only by qualified medical personnel with adequate facilities. The first step in treatment is withdrawal of the drug, abruptly, rapidly, or gradually, followed by a period of psychotherapy and rehabilitation. This final period should last at least four months, otherwise there is an even greater danger of relapse to the addiction among most patients. Information regarding treatment is available from the U. S. Public Health Service in Washington, D.C. *See also* MORPHINE AND OPIUM POISONING.

DRUG ALLERGY. The reactions, particularly to *penicillin,* have aroused a great deal of interest because of the widespread use of this antibiotic drug. Fatal cases have been reported. Apparently about five out of a hundred persons may have allergic reactions when injected with penicillin or when taking the substance by mouth. Fortunately, the *antihistamine drugs* are capable of controlling such reactions in most instances and this applies to treatment with ACTH and cortisone. *See also* ALLERGY.

DRUGS IN TUBERCULOSIS.
Sanatoriums for tuberculosis in the United States are finding themselves with vacant beds. The reason lies in the discovery of new drugs for controlling tuberculosis. The drugs principally responsible for this change include the antibiotic *streptomycin,* a product developed in Sweden known as *paraminosalicylic acid* and *isonicotinic acid hydrazines* better known as *isoniazid.* Added to these still more recently are *cycloserine* and such antibiotics as *viomycin* and *neomycin.*

The use of mass x-ray survey procedures has brought to light great numbers of cases of minimal tuberculosis defined as a tuberculosis lesion involving less lung area than that represented by the space above the first rib and without any evidence of destruction of lung tissue to the point of production of cavities. One attack on minimal tuberculosis has involved surgical removal of the small area of the lung which contains the nodules. Investigators have found that the combination of streptomycin and paraminosalicylic acid will prevent the development of resistant organisms and enable the destruction of the bacteria to be carried on for much longer periods than can be used when either drug is used alone.

The new drug isoniazid appears to have a direct effect on tubercle bacilli. Radioactive isotope study made with this drug shows that it actually invaded the bacteria and brought about their elimination. Strangely, physicians observe that when isoniazid was used for the control of tuberculosis it interfered in some way with the body's use of vitamin B_6 so that it was necessary to give extra vitamin B_6 to prevent complications.

As a result of these discoveries chemotherapy is now used as an outpatient or home treatment. The person with tuberculosis may be hospitalized for collapse of the lung or for surgery. With the drug methods, people are able to return home months earlier than under any previous method of treatment. *See also* TUBERCULOSIS.

DT stands for delirium tremens. *See* DELIRIUM TREMENS.

DUMDUM FEVER. *See* KALA AZAR.

DUODENAL ULCER. *See* PEPTIC ULCER. *See* MEDIGRAPH page 1297.

DUODENUM, the first portion of the small intestine, leading from the stomach. It contains the openings of the pancreatic and the common bile ducts. *See also* INTESTINES; PEPTIC ULCER. *See* MEDIGRAPH page 1297.

DUST, fine pulverized powder of dry earth or refuse, found all through the atmosphere except perhaps on mountaintops and out at sea. An atmosphere free of dust is far healthier than one which is not. Nature and industry produce dusts of various kinds, against which people cannot wholly protect themselves. In some instances, dust is disastrously harmful to humans.

Microscopic particles of pollen dust borne by wind come in contact with the mucous membranes of the eye and respiratory tract and produce symptoms of allergy such as seasonal *hay fever, hives,* and other disorders. Industrial dusts, produced by grinding of metals and in the manufacture of wood products, flour, sugar, textiles, leather, and feathers, also affect human beings.

Most dusts contain some carbon and other organic matter. Many people are sensitive to dusts and have skin reactions when the dusts come in contact with the skin. Other dusts, when inhaled, irritate the windpipe and bronchial tubes. Coal dust may get into the lungs causing pigmentation, and may stimulate the production of fibrous tissue. Inorganic dusts containing free silica incite *silicosis,* a special form of change in the lungs. In silicosis the silica acts to produce nodules throughout the lungs which can be detected by x-rays. Lungs damaged in this way are prone to secondary infections, including *tuberculosis.*

Organic dusts, like carbon, differ from inorganic dusts in that they do not cause the changes in the lungs such as produced by the action of silica. Organic dust particles do not penetrate lung tissue, but instead are absorbed into the tissues of the body.

Asbestosis is a special form of lung disorder in which the magnesium silicate contained in asbestos produces fibrous changes that are different from those caused by pure silica. However, asbestosis and silicosis are much alike, both being forms of the lung disorder *pneumoconiosis.*

To inhibit inhalation of dust, various forms of exhaust systems, air conditioning, and improved ventilation have been developed. Helmets and breathing devices worn by miners and workers employed in operations producing excessive dust have also been helpful.

Drought areas are great dust producers; but the immediate health hazard, aside from the relationship between dust storms and secondary pneumonia, is not serious. More harmful are the mental and economic hardships suffered by people living in the dust-bowl region. *See also* ASBESTOSIS; BRONCHITIS; INDUSTRIAL HEALTH; TUBERCULOSIS; INHALING OF DANGEROUS SUBSTANCES; RADIATION SICKNESS; OCCUPATIONAL HAZARDS IN INDUSTRY.

DWARFISM. *See* ACHONDROPLASIA.

DYSCHESIA. *See* CONSTIPATION.

DYSENTERY, inflammation of the colon. Its symptoms are pain and severe diarrhea and frequent passage of mucus and blood. *See also* AMEBIC DYSENTERY; BACILLARY DYSENTERY.

DYSMENORRHEA, pain at the time of menstruation. Discomfort in the lower abdomen or pains in the thighs and general feeling of pressure may occur. The causes vary from anatomic malformation, such as an undeveloped womb, to disturbances of hormone balance. If pain is constant or severe enough to cause nausea, vomiting, or headache, or to interfere with normal activity, the doctor should be consulted. Mental factors also may be responsible for unusual pain. Often the young girl has been prepared inadequately for womanhood. When the pain is not severe, the use of a mild sedative is helpful.

Strenuous exercise immediately before, during and after menstruation has been known to produce a period of pain later. Therefore, most physicians believe that violent exercise should be avoided.

While mild non-habit-forming drugs are helpful, the use of habit-forming drugs is dangerous. The relationship between the sex functions and the action of various glands studied by the physician permits him to prescribe endocrine or glandular products which are helpful in controlling dysmenorrhea. *See also* MENSTRUATION.

DYSPEPSIA. *See* INDIGESTION.

DYSPNEA, the medical term for difficult or labored breathing. This symptom occurs in attacks of asthma, acute laryngitis in children, cancer of the throat, weakness of the heart, and other conditions. *See also* ASPIRATION.

E

EAR, an organ which involves the sense of *hearing* and is also involved with the sense of *balance*. It consists of three parts: *external, middle,* and *internal.* The external ear comprises an outer section and the external *auditory canal.* It entraps sound and transmits the sound waves to the *eardrum,* a membrane that closes off the external ear. The middle ear, or *internal tympanic cavity,* contains bones and nerves for further transmission of sound, and connects with the *nasal passages* through the *Eustachian tube.* The internal ear is a bony labyrinth, containing the nerves that connect with the brain, and three semicircular canals which control equilibrium. The entire inner ear structure is encased by the *mastoid* region of the skull. Both ears, though related, function independently; and if the capacity of one is destroyed, that of the other is not necessarily impaired.

A number of disorders may affect the ear. *Earache* is caused by inflammation which, even though slight, should be cared for promptly by a physician, since neglect may lead to serious complications and even *mastoiditis.* The external ear, because of its position, is susceptible to many kinds of bruises and abrasions, as well as infection and invasion by fungi and insects. Swellings or boils on the external ear should be treated by the doctor. Bony growths on the external ear, known as *extosis,* are best treated by surgical removal. Congenital malformations are not infrequent and have been effectively treated by plastic surgery. Plastic surgery has also been successful on cauliflower ear, which results from repeated blows, as experienced by boxers, or from other injury.

The eardrum may also be subject to inflammation and is especially liable to puncture or rupture. A sharp instrument should never be used to remove wax or a foreign substance from the ear because of the danger of puncturing.

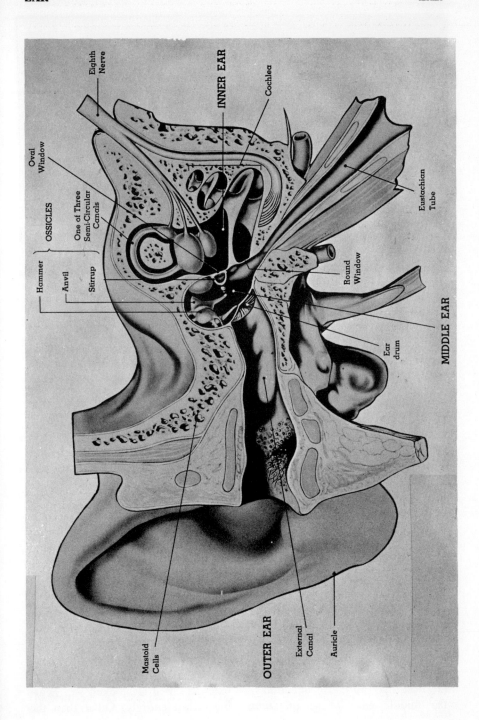

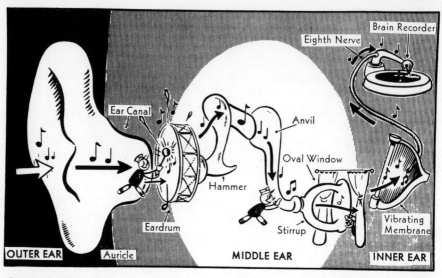

Ear—A simplified diagram of how we hear. Sound waves strike the *ear drum* which set off vibrations to the three smallest bones of the body, called the *ossicles*. These bones are also known as the *hammer, anvil* and *stirrup* because of their shape. The stirrup, in turn, vibrates the *oval window*—a thin membrane stretched across the entrance to the *inner ear*. Movement of the oval window is passed on to the *cochlea,* the organ of hearing which "feels" the mechanical movements caused by the sound waves. This vibrating membrane contains thousands of tiny, ciliated cells. It records the vibrations received and sends the results to the *brain* via the *eighth* or *hearing nerve* for analysis.

Rupture of the eardrum may be caused by extreme noise, such as an explosion, sharp descent from high altitude, diving into deep water, or even sneezing. Bleeding of the ear, dizziness, ringing sounds, and headache may be symptoms of ruptured or punctured eardrum. Careful diagnosis and patient treatment by an ear specialist generally corrects the condition.

The middle ear can be infected from without, through a ruptured or punctured eardrum, or from within through the Eustachian tube. Head cold, respiratory infection, diseased tonsils and adenoids, inadquate nasal hygiene, forcible blowing of the nose may all cause infection of the middle ear. These *infections* may be *acute, chronic,* or *temporary, draining* or *nondraining*. Symptoms are shooting pains in the ear, inflammation, ringing sounds, or impaired hearing. All the symptoms are danger signals and require immediate attention. Since many cases of deafness among adults are traceable to middle ear infection in children, it is obvious that the condition should be treated promptly. Children should be taught ear hygiene as a guard against ear infection.

Cases are on record in which living *insects* have entered the ear. They die and their bodies remain, gradually being surrounded by hardened wax, so that eventually the external canal is blocked and hearing is lost entirely. Other than the loss of hearing, no damage is likely to result. More damage comes from attempts to remove material from the ear than from the entrance of the material itself. It is not advisable for anyone to try to remove a foreign body from the outer ear if it cannot be washed out, unless he has had special training in this type of work.

Several instruments have been developed for removing objects. A bean or piece of chalk has been removed by the use of a probe with some adhesive material on the end. This becomes adherent to the bean or piece of chalk, which is then gradually withdrawn. Such performances are, however, best left to the experts.

A *pimple* or *boil* or any other infection in the tissue lining the external ear canal will cause intense pain, inflammation, swelling, and some fever and should have prompt medical attention.

Without special instruments and devices with electric light it is not possible for the average person to see the eardrum or to recognize trouble in the middle ear. The physician has devices, an *otoscope* and also an *ear speculum,* which permit him to see the lining of the canal and to throw light directly on the eardrum. When the eardrum is observed, it is possible to determine whether or not everything is normal, whether there is any obstruction in the external ear canal, and whether or not there is any infection.

It is also necessary in an examination of the ears to determine whether or not the Eustachian tubes are

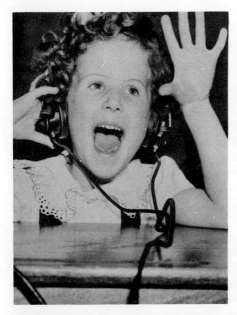 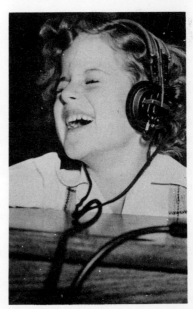

Ear—Photographs capturing the expressions of two girls as they hear their voices for the first time. Deaf since birth, they are enabled to hear by refined acoustical devices.

529

infected in any way, because infection or inflammation of these tubes will interfere seriously with hearing. The Eustachian tubes pass from the back of the nasal cavity to the middle ear. Frequently infection spreads from the tonsils and adenoids by way of the Eustachian tube to the ear canal.

Far better than the attempt to treat such conditions when they develop is the application of simple laws of hygiene that tend to prevent infections in the ear. Increased bathing and swimming have multiplied the number of cases of infection in the ear arising from that source. Children should not be permitted to swim more than fifteen or twenty minutes at a time. If they tend to have trouble with the ears they should not be permitted to dive. The child who complains of difficulties in hearing or of fullness in the head after swimming should give up this sport. This is nature's way of warning against trouble.

Unhealthy *tonsils* and *adenoids* may be the source of infections which extend into the ear. The vast majority of infections of the ear are secondary to *colds* in the head and *influenza*. About 10 per cent of children with *scarlet fever* and *measles* develop infections of the ear. About 5 per cent of those with *diphtheria* develop infections of the ear. Other cases develop after *mumps, typhoid fever, whooping cough,* and similar infections.

Prompt care of children with various infectious diseases will determine the presence of infection early, and immediate application of proper

treatment can prevent extension of the infection into the mastoid or inner ear.

Before the age of twelve children acquire infections of the ear more easily than do adults. Infections with virulent streptococci are more likely than others to cause infections of the ear. Removal of the tonsils and adenoids when repeatedly infected is important in preventing infections of the ear.

Most people nowadays know enough about personal hygiene to keep their ears clean. Boils and pimples still occur, and there are still cases in which the removal of hardened wax is necessary. The *cerumen,* or wax in the ear, when it becomes hardened is most easily removed by the use of the ear syringe filled with slightly warm water. Harm can be done by needles or too frequent syringing. The syringe should be sterilized by boiling before using, and water should be previously boiled and used warm but not hot.

The person whose ear is to be syringed should sit in a good light, a towel should be put around the neck and tucked inside the clothing so as to prevent soiling it, a pan is held at the edge of the ear so that the fluid which runs in will run into the basin and not down the patient's neck. The ear is pulled slightly upward and backward to straighten out the passage. With the ear held in this position, the nozzle of the syringe, which has been filled and has all the air expelled, is placed just inside the outer opening of the ear. The water is then permitted to flow along the back wall slowly and without too great pressure, so as to permit return of the excess flow of water as the water goes in.

Special instruments are usually needed for removing foreign objects. A probe with adhesive at the end may attach itself to a foreign object which can then be pulled out. Usually experts have the instruments and can do this performance easily.

A pimple or a boil or any other infection in the tissues lining the external ear will cause intense pain, inflammation, swelling and some fever. Prompt medical attention is required. With modern antibiotic drugs such infections are usually controlled.

Often the middle ear is infected because a child has not learned how to blow the nose properly. The worst technique is to hold both nostrils tightly when blowing, since this forces the infected material from back of the nose into the middle ear. The proper technique requires that only one nostril be held and that blowing be gentle. Preferably, the handkerchief or disposable tissue should be held quite loosely over the opening of the nostrils.

Middle ear infection may lead to some degree of deafness and rarely to permanent loss of hearing. Following an infection the child should be taken to a specialist—an *otorhinolaryngologist*—who will test the loss of hearing and do everything possible to stop the progress of infection and restore action to the damaged tissues of the ear.

Mastoiditis used to be frequent after infection of the ear, but now the total number of cases of mastoiditis has been greatly reduced by the antibiotic drugs. Pain and tenderness in the region behind the ear are the first symptoms of inflammation of the mastoid. The skin may be swollen so that the external ear seems to be pushed away from the head. Early treatment of infected ears will usually prevent this complication. Surgical treatment of mastoiditis involves an operation in which the infected area is opened and the infected material cleaned out. Unless controlled, a secondary inflammation of the coverings of the brain—*meningitis*—is possible. *See also* DEAFNESS; MASTOID; OTOSCLEROSIS.

EAR STUFFINESS. Ear stuffiness —one of the most common troubles of air travel—is suffered needlessly. By instructing the traveler in a simple procedure to keep the Eustachian tube (which passes from the back of the nose to the ear) open, pain can be prevented. The Eustachian tube functions in equalizing atmospheric pressure in the inner surface of the eardrum. When the tube is filled with mucus because of a cold or infection, changes in atmospheric pressure cause painful changes in the tension of the drum. If such an occlusion is complete, sharp changes in atmospheric pressure may cause rupture of the drum.

When ears become plugged, the procedure recommended is to clear the nose of accumulated secretions by a gentle blowing action and

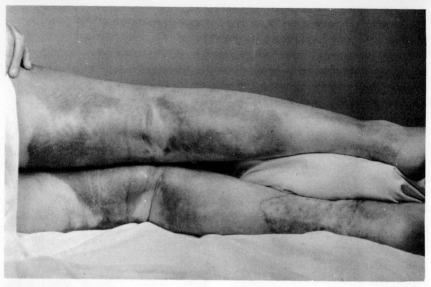

Ecchymosis—Ecchymosis seen in a case of scurvy. An ecchymosis is the black-and-blue spot in the skin which results from the escape of blood from the vessels to the tissues.

clearing of the throat; increase the negative pressure in this area by closing the mouth, pinching the nose and attempting to inhale vigorously. This procedure may release air which is trapped at a higher pressure in the middle ear.

If pain is not relieved, a one per cent solution of *ephedrine* combined with an antimicrobial agent is inserted through the nose so that the drops will fall on the Eustachian tube where it opens into the cavity of the nose and throat. If symptoms are not relieved by this procedure, the nose drops are "pumped" into the Eustachian tube by closing the mouth, pinching the nose and attempting to inhale and exhale vigorously. *See also* MOTION SICKNESS.

ECCHYMOSIS, the flow of blood into the surrounding tissues, after the rupture of a blood vessel. The term also applies to the discoloration of the skin caused by a hemorrhage under the skin, and to bruises which appear on the skin as the familiar black-and-blue spots after a blow and later turn brown, green, or yellow. *See also* BRUISES.

ECLAMPSIA, a serious convulsive condition occurring in pregnancy in women of any age. The cause is not definitely known. The prospective mother may suffer convulsions leading to unconsciousness. The first danger signal may be headache or failing vision. The blood pressure may rise sharply and albumin will appear in the urine. These early symptoms are pre-eclamptic. Scientific prenatal care includes constant guarding against this condition. Should any symptoms appear, precautions must be taken at once to prevent eclampsia, which is serious and in the past often resulted in stillbirth.

The woman should be hospitalized promptly. The intake of salt is restricted and a soft diet prescribed. Diuretic agents are given to induce sufficient elimination of urine, since in eclampsia the function of the kidneys is impaired and these organs must be relieved of any extra load. Anticonvulsant drugs are administered to control the tendency to convulsions.

Fortunately the warning symptoms usually develop slowly. However, cases do occur in which serious complications closely follow the first symptoms. Most doctors believe that pregnancy itself is responsible for the development of toxic substances in the body. This toxic reaction may affect certain organs more than others, thus inducing pre-eclampsia or eclampsia itself.

Improved methods of prenatal care in recent years have done much to prevent eclampsia and reduce the mortality rate from that cause. Frequent checking of blood pressure, periodic examination of the urine, and better weight control not only tend to improve the general condition of prospective mothers but make possible recognition of the pre-eclamptic state.

Nevertheless, physicians are always on guard against any eclamptic emergency that may arise. Extreme measures, including the use of oxygen, induction of labor, and even Cesarian section may be necessary in severe eclampsia. Even after a child is born, the mother must be just as carefully watched since pre-eclampsia and eclampsia occasionally occur immediately following childbirth. *See also* CHILDBIRTH AND PRENATAL CARE.

ECTOPIC PREGNANCY, an unusual form of pregnancy in which the fetus develops outside of the normal location, the uterus. It may occur, for instance, in the Fallopian tube. When ectopic gestation takes place the usual signs of pregnancy are present, though they may be overlooked. If a menstrual period is missed and slight bleedings begin to recur from the womb, a physician should be consulted. Prompt operation is the advisable treatment.

ECZEMA, a term which currently refers to a noncontagious skin rash for which a definite cause cannot be cited. Thus, a rash which is produced by a certain type of soap might be described as *dermatitis,* but not as eczema.

The possible causes of eczema, therefore, are always speculative. A change in the weather, in the temperature, or even in the intensity of light can be responsible. The cause may be found inside the body, perhaps in the contents of the blood, or possibly on the surface in the presence of warts or calluses, or in sensitized skin. Moreover, the area of the body may be significant. Eczema of the scalp can differ greatly from eczema of the face or groin. The skin may be sensitive to certain textiles or chemicals.

The symptoms of eczema are frequently associated with those of

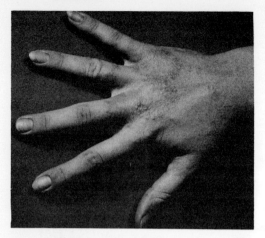

Eczema—Eczema of the hand prior to treatment. (*Below*) Photograph of the same hand three days following treatment with an ointment.

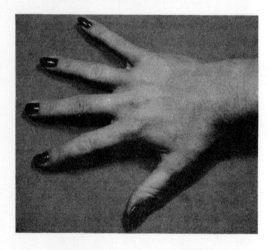

join to form larger ones. These rupture eventually and release a sticky substance. As this fluid dries it forms a yellow crust which drops off after several days, revealing a reddened and scaling area underneath. This scaling may continue for several days or weeks, after which the skin will recover its ordinary appearance. In the meantime, however, a relapse may occur and the entire sequence of blistering and healing will be repeated.

In children especially, the disease may spread and sometimes will cover the entire body. Often a high temperature is involved together with a disinclination to eat. The progress of the disease varies with the individual person; the blistering phase may predominate in one case, the dry and scaly phase in another, and the pimply stage in still another. Almost always, however, the person will suffer from severe itching. Heat may increase this itching so that it becomes almost unendurable. Eczema usually involves a thickening and breaking of the skin, and consequently the infected area is highly receptive to germs which may introduce complicating factors such as *boils* or *impetigo*.

asthma, and often attack alternately, or they can appear at the same time. Moreover, both may start suddenly, with the swallowing of certain food or the inhalation of a particular sensitizing substance. Both diseases may involve an inherited liability.

Often the first manifestation of eczema is on the face. The skin reddens, becomes swollen and hot, and small blisters appear which may

Since the possible causes are so numerous the treatment is often broad in scope. Although it may be impossible to identify the particular food which was responsible for the attack, nevertheless general dietary routine can be of considerable value. If the attack is acute, a strictly liquid diet may even be imposed. The free consumption of water is ordinarily advised but stimulating

534

beverages such as alcohol, tea, and coffee are seldom permitted. Medication is usually employed for special purposes only, for the relief of itching, or for the drying of open blisters. Radium, x-rays or ultraviolet rays may be used with good effect. Recently the use of cortisone ointments has permitted prompt control of this condition.

More than two-thirds of all skin diseases are classified as eczema. The symptoms and causes are so complex that successful treatment demands a qualified physician. *See also* SKIN; CONTACT DERMATITIS; IMPETIGO; INTERTRIGO; ERYTHEMA; ERYSIPELAS; LUPUS ERYTHEMATOSUS; PSORIASIS; HERPES ZOSTER; ACNE; RINGWORM; SPOROTRICHOSIS; ALLERGY; HIVES. *See* MEDIGRAPH page 441.

EDEMA. *See* NEPHROSIS.

EGGS of poultry are second only to milk in nutritive value, and many dietitians feel that every diet should include at least one egg a day. Eggs are rich in proteins, fats, phosphorus, iron, and in all the elements necessary for growth except calcium and vitamin C. They also contain cholesterol, a fatlike substance which may be involved in the growth of gallstones, cysts, and cancerous tissue. For this reason eggs in *large* amounts are not recommended for persons over forty years of age; however, anyone in this age range can safely have an egg a day unless specifically forbidden by a doctor. Ordinarily eggs are highly digestible; even a hard-boiled egg,

especially a minced hard-boiled egg, is only slightly less digestible than a soft-boiled egg. Eggs may induce constipation, discomfort, asthma, or eczema in some persons who presumably have become sensitized, perhaps only to the albumin. *See also* ALBUMIN; NUTRITION.

ELBOW, the joint at the middle of the arm where the large bone of the upper arm, the *humerus,* joins

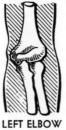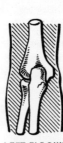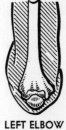

LEFT ELBOW
front view
joint extended

LEFT ELBOW
back view
joint extended

LEFT ELBOW
back view
joint flexed

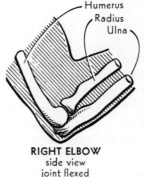

Humerus
Radius
Ulna

RIGHT ELBOW
side view
joint flexed

RIGHT ELBOW
side view
joint extended

Elbow—Drawings depicting the relationship of the bones in the elbow. The *radius* and *ulna* in the forearm meet the *humerus* (the single large bone in the upper arm) at the elbow. The large bone in the upper arm affords strength to the arm, while the two smaller bones in the forearm allow rotation. The ulna is the inner bone which extends beyond the elbow joint. The radius is thicker and shorter than the ulna.

the two smaller bones of the lower arm, the *radius* and *ulna*.

This joint can suffer any of the serious conditions that affect any other joint of the body. *Dislocation* is the most common disorder of the elbow and one of the most serious. Any dislocation should be examined immediately by x-ray and reset accordingly. If necessary, the elbow should be put in a splint or placed in a cast until it is completely healed. Such care must be given only by a doctor. *Ankylosis,* or locking in place of the joint, may result from inflammation or infection. This condition requires the attention of an orthopedic surgeon who will not only treat but prescribe subsequent manipulation, massage, and application of heat to restore free movement and avoid permanent crippling. So-called "tennis elbow" results from overactivity in playing tennis or other sports or even non-athletic motion involving lifting, sudden pulling, or extending of the elbow joint.

Besides injury involving the muscles and ligaments of the elbow joint, breaking or detachment of the small bones may cause pain and swelling. At the end of the elbow joint is the "funny bone," which is actually not a bone but a particularly sensitive nerve; a sudden blow or pressure on it may cause considerable pain.

In growing children, cartilage which controls growth of the bone at the elbow joint can also be damaged or dislocated. If damage does occur the cartilage must be replaced; if the cartilage is not replaced, the

arm will stop growing at the point where the *epyphisis* (cartilage) was damaged. *See also* DISLOCATION; FRACTURES; JOINTS AND JOINT DISORDERS.

ELECTRICAL INJURIES. Shock or injuries from electricity come from two major sources: accidental contact with electrical current and lightning strokes. Most of the fatal electrical accidents occur in industry, where electrical machinery and equipment are potential sources of accident to the worker. In the home, such accidents may result from faulty insulation or careless handling of lighting, heating, or refrigeration equipment.

A person suffering from electric shock must be immediately removed from contact with the source of the electric current. If a live wire must be cut, an axe with a wooden handle is the best tool to use. If the rescuer cannot cut off the current, he must be careful to handle the victim with the aid of some insulating material such as a dry rope, a wooden stick, or a leather belt. He must protect himself from receiving the shock which can be transmitted through the body of the victim. The doctor should be called immediately. If the person is unconscious or breathing has ceased, which is likely if the current has passed through the central nervous system and affected the respiratory center of the brain, artificial respiration should be given at once. Since artificial respiration may have to be continued for several hours, resuscitating equipment should be summoned if possible.

The clothing of the victim should be loosened to facilitate breathing and the victim allowed to rest several hours before he is moved to a hospital.

When struck by lightning, the person falls to the ground as if he had received a stunning blow on the head. After the shock, flashes of light seem to pass before his eyes and blindness or deafness can ensue. The nervous system may be dangerously affected with resulting symptoms of paralysis, pains in the limbs, and sometimes hemorrhage.

Dry skin offers a high resistance to electricity and therefore the local burns following electric shock are greater and the general effects on the body less. Moist skin lessens resistance and permits the current to have a greater internal effect with chances of death more likely, although the surface burns may be less severe. However, the attempt to sustain the life of the victim should, of course, have precedence over any treatment of skin injuries. *See also* RESUSCITATION; OCCUPATIONAL HAZARDS IN INDUSTRY.

ELECTRIC SHOCK TREATMENT. When electric shock therapy is given, two or more electrodes are placed on the sides of the head and a measured electric current passed through the brain. This type of treatment is used in mental disturbances. The application of electric shock to induce loss of consciousness has resulted in dramatic improvement for some persons, notably for those suffering severe depression, agitation, depression as-

sociated with menopause and catatonic states of schizophrenia. *See also* INSULIN SHOCK THERAPY.

ELECTROCARDIOGRAPH, an apparatus or instrument which records the electrical current created by the beating of the heart. Attached to the electrocardiograph are electrical conductors which are placed on each of the arms and the left leg. The currents of the heartbeat are conducted to the electrocardiograph where they are photographed. This resulting record of waves is the *electrocardiogram.* Several of these are made; one electrocardiogram is taken from the two arms, another from the left leg and right arm, and a third one from the left leg and left arm. Frequently a fourth picture is taken from the left leg and the top of the heart. The four photographs, altough not identical, resemble one another.

The electrocardiograph is exceedingly useful in diagnosis. It is invaluable in the study of the heart, and in many diseases such as rheumatic fever. It aids in diagnosing suspected cases of coronary thrombosis, a disease caused by clots of blood which block blood vessels leading to the heart and damage the muscle and induce rhythm breaks and other irregularities in the flow of the blood. *See also* CORONARY THROMBOSIS; HEART; RHEUMATIC FEVER.

ELECTROENCEPHALOGRAPHY, a method of recording the electrical activity of the brain, especially of the *cerebral cortex.* The

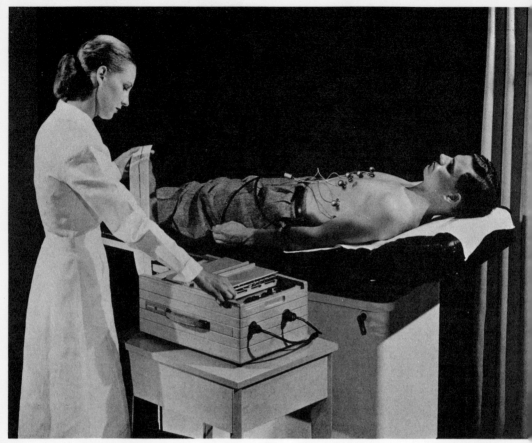

Electrocardiograph—This technician is preparing a record of a patient's heart action with an electrocardiograph. Small metal contacts, held in place on the patient's chest by means of a slight vacuum, pick up the electrical impulses from the heart. After being amplified, the impulses are used to deflect a stylus on the unit. This produces a wave pattern on a moving paper tape—visible evidence in the diagnosis and control of heart disease.

electrical impulses are detected by means of wires attached to the scalp and are recorded graphically in waves (EEG). Valuable information is gathered by this method in case of tumor, epilepsy, infections, and hemorrhages. The apparatus used is known as an *electroencephalograph*. It is also useful in locating a diseased portion of the brain, if not too deeply seated. *See also* BRAIN; BRAIN TUMOR.

ELECTRONIC MEDICAL AID.

A new electronic device able to translate metabolic functions—such as pulse rate, respiration rate, diastolic and systolic blood pressure, temperature, fluid loss, blood loss, and blood replacement—into electronic signals which are then recorded graphically has been developed.

Doctors are enabled by a glance at the graph compiled by the device

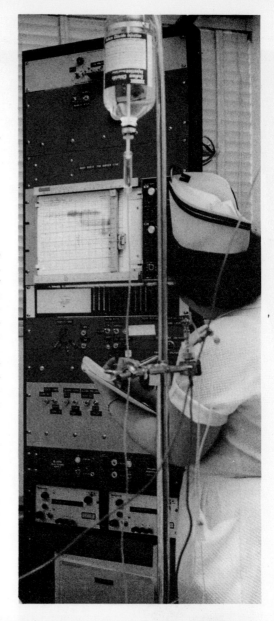

A patient-monitoring system now in use in several hospitals keeps an ultrasensitive, entirely electronic eye on various body functions. The findings are recorded on a graph, from which a nurse takes notes. The device measures and records blood pressure, both diastolic and systolic, including pulse rate, respiration, rate, temperature, fluid loss, blood loss, and blood replacement. The top photograph on the succeeding page shows the monitor's graph. The pen moves across one major division each hour. Up and down, a reading is plotted of each function every five seconds, and each reading is repeated every half minute—with the exception of blood loss and replacement, which are alternated and therefore measured once a minute. In the photograph at the lower left, the diastolic and systolic blood pressures are measured by a "strain" gauge which is connected with the patient's artery.

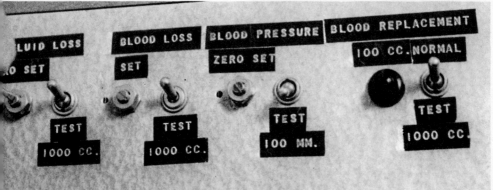

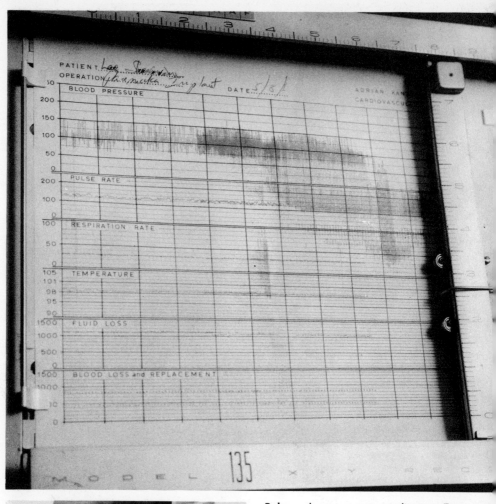

PATIENT *Leo Tureover*
OPERATION *fluid media Implant* DATE *5/8/*

ADRIAN KAN...
CARDIOVASCU...

BLOOD PRESSURE

PULSE RATE

RESPIRATION RATE

TEMPERATURE

FLUID LOSS

BLOOD LOSS and REPLACEMENT

MODEL 135 X-Y REC...

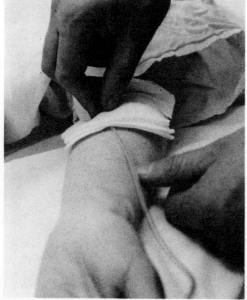

Below, the temperature indicators. Temperature is measured with a thermometer placed in rectum. In the lower photograph, opposite page, cables and wires relay information concerning loss of fluid and blood and rate of blood pressure.

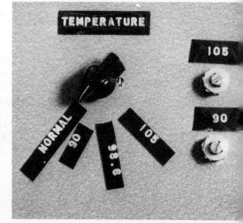

TEMPERATURE

105

90

NORMAL   90   98.6   105

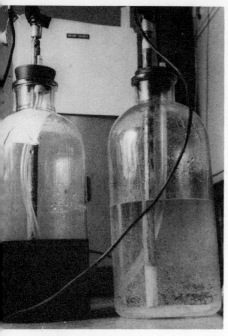

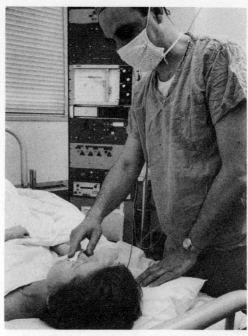

The bottles shown above left are used in measuring blood and fluid loss. One is collecting urine, the other blood from a chest opening. Inside each is a stick holding sensors having resistors. Rising fluid shorts out resistors in turn, depending on loss. Differing voltages thus generated create electrical signals recorded graphically.

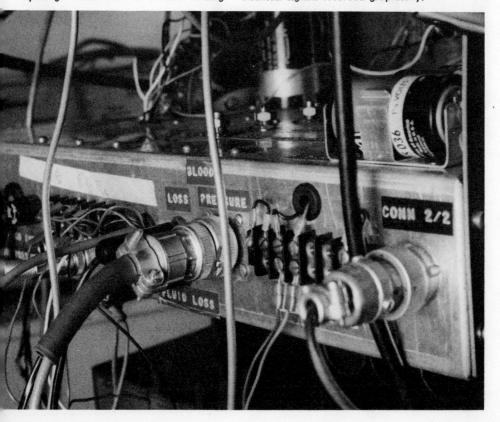

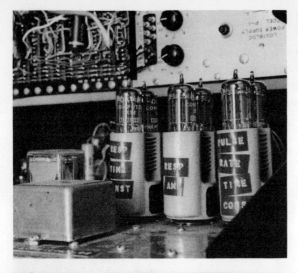

In top right photograph, preceding page, thermester tube monitors respiration rate. Left, a few of the many parts in the machine.

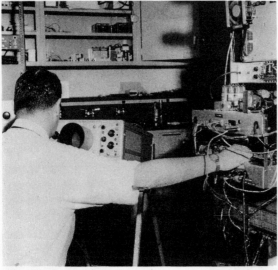

Left, the controls of the monitor. The device was originally developed at Maimonides Hospital, Brooklyn, N.Y.

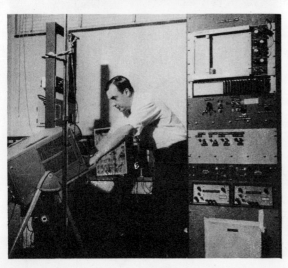

An overall view of the device. In the future, it will work as a console with several smaller sister machines connected to it.

to evaluate the status of the patient's condition, while nurses and other hospital personnel are liberated from routine functions for other responsibilities. *See also* ELECTROCARDIOGRAPH; ELECTROENCEPHALOGRAPHY; OXYGEN THERAPY, HIGH PRESSURE.

ELEPHANTIASIS, a chronic disease characterized by inflammation of the *lymphatic glands*. As the condition progresses, the skin becomes thickened, the tissues under the skin swell, and, in time, the parts of the body affected enlarge incredibly. The legs, for example, may resemble the legs of an elephant, whence the name, elephantiasis. Any part of the body may be affected, but enlargement of the arms, legs, or scrotum is most common. The breasts of women are less susceptible.

The disease occurs usually as a secondary effect of *filariasis*. The *filaria,* a parasite, gets into the lymph ducts and blocks them. However, blocking of the lymphatics by other means can also produce elephantiasis.

Elephantiasis, for the most part, is a disease of the tropics and a person may have it for many years. Tight bandaging and surgery can often reduce the deformities of the disease. Favorable results in the treatment of this disease have been obtained with *naphuride sodium* and *hetrazan. Sulfonamides* are used to combat secondary infections. Control of the mosquitoes that bear the parasite and of the worm responsible for the disease seem to be the best long-range methods of inhibiting elephantiasis. *See also* FILARIASIS.

EMACIATION, extreme thinness. Emaciation may have many causes, including a psychological basis. For example, a person suffering from depression may refuse to eat and waste away to the point of emaciation. Ordinarily the cause is basically physical, and is usually due to a degenerative disease of the muscles. Emaciation can also result from any degenerative disease of the spinal cord.

Diabetes, syphilis, or a growth in the gullet may cause emaciation. Persistent tuberculosis, in any part of the body will eventually cause extreme thinness. In addition, emaciation may also be produced by such diseases as cholera, extended diarrhea, disturbances of the thyroid glands, or even by extreme fever.

In the first six months of an infant's life, severe emaciation may seem to develop without any cause. The term *marasmus* is applied to this condition. Ordinarily the cause will be found in the baby's diet, and a change of diet will bring a cure.

Generally the treatment in cases of extreme emaciation varies greatly and depends on the source of the ailment. *See also* ATROPHY; MARASMUS; UNDERWEIGHT, HAZARDS OF.

EMBOLISM, obstruction of a blood vessel by a blood clot or by any foreign matter floating loose in the blood stream. An *embolus,* as the clot or particle is known, is dangerous because it may lodge in an im-

543

portant arterial blood vessel or vein and block the supply of blood to an organ or tissue on which life depends, such as the brain, heart, kidney, or lungs. If an embolus reaches a vital area of the brain, paralysis and even death may follow in a few hours. Embolism in the eye may cause blindness.

An air bubble may circulate through the blood and, if large enough, block a blood vessel. A bit of fat may get loose in the blood stream following fracture of a large bone. A collection of germs from an abscess may get into a small blood vessel, plug it, interrupt circulation, and produce a secondary abscess. Any of these disturbances is called an embolism.

In *endocarditis,* an inflammation of the lining of the heart, incrustations and growth may develop on the valves of the heart. These break off and get into the blood stream, and cause embolism. The two types of endocarditis are the *acute,* which arises suddenly and may cause death within a few days, and the *subacute,* which begins slowly and responds to early treatment.

The early symptoms of embolism are a slight rise in temperature and a rapid increase in the pulse beat. Within twenty-four hours, however, both the temperature and pulse rise rapidly, breathing becomes rapid, and the person has great mental anxiety and symptoms of shock. In postoperative embolus, the symptoms may be sudden pallor, rapid pulse, and collapse.

People past middle life are more prone to embolism than younger persons. Those who have had disturbances of the heart are affected frequently rather than those whose blood circulation has been normal.

Among the methods of treatment of embolism recently developed is an immediate surgical operation to release the blocked area, especially when the embolus occurs in the arms, legs, or in a region which can be reached. The development of such drugs as DICUMAROL, HEPARIN, and others which have the power to prevent blood clotting has been invaluable. Antibiotics have been useful also in the treatment of chronic bacterial endocarditis, thus lessening the danger of embolus. *See also* CO-AGULATION; CORONARY THROMBO-SIS. *See* MEDIGRAPHS pages 173, 231, 713, 731, 863, 1035, 1229.

EMBRYO, an organism in the earliest stage of development. In the human being, embryo refers to the individual during its first three months of life in the mother's womb. *See also* FETUS.

EMERGENCIES IN THE HOME. At least one person in every household should know the basic rules of emergency care.

Falls. Of the millions of serious accidents which occur in the home every day, almost fifty per cent are due to *falls.* The first rule to observe when a person has fallen is to estimate the extent of his injuries, whether or not he has suffered a broken bone, a hemorrhage, or just a bruise.

Usually, a *broken bone* can be recognized immediately by failure of the limb to function. A final diagnosis, however, can only be made by a doctor with the help of an x-ray machine. While awaiting the doctor, the injured limb can be placed in a homemade splint if there is someone present able to do it. The splint may be made by wrapping the limb in a large-sized magazine or equivalent which is then tied in place by means of handkerchiefs or strips of material.

A minor *hemorrhage* can be controlled by placing a piece of gauze against the wound. If the hemorrhage is more severe, pressure against the gauze may be necessary to control the bleeding. A tourniquet should be used with extreme caution. However, if one is absolutely necessary, it is applied in the following manner: A large handkerchief or towel is tied around the arm or leg above the hemorrhage. A small rod of any type, a clothespin or stick for example, is then inserted under the handkerchief. On the other side of the limb the handkerchief is tied in a knot and a larger rod is inserted

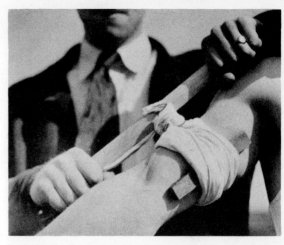

Emergency Treatment—Application of a tourniquet between the bleeding point and the body. A stick is placed in the knot so that when it is twisted the tourniquet will be tightened and the bleeding controlled. Pressure should be relieved at regular intervals to prevent gangrene.

through this knot in such a way that the tourniquet can be easily tightened, thus closing off the flow of blood.

A *bleeding tooth socket* can be controlled by filling the socket with antiseptic cotton. *Nosebleed* may ordinarily be halted by placing the victim face down and then stuffing the nostrils with gauze, or sometimes

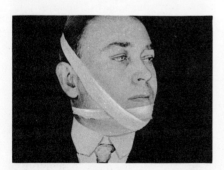

Emergencies in the Home—Some areas of the body are difficult to bandage. (On the left) the four-tailed bandage in place on the chin.

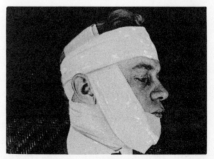

This is a good emergency bandage. (On the right) is the modified Barton bandage. It may be used with or without plaster.

545

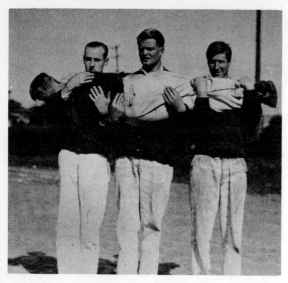

Emergency Treatment—Seriously injured persons should not be moved until medical assistance arrives. If it is imperative that the patient be moved, the method of carrying shown above should be used.

application of hot and cold packs will bring about the same result. If placing gauze on a *scalp wound* fails to stop the bleeding, a tight band wound all the way around the head may be successful. A real danger is unexpected *hemorrhage of the lung*. A doctor should be called and the person placed in bed and kept absolutely quiet.

A *bruise* is an injury caused by impact in which neither laceration or external bleeding occurs. The first symptom, pain, is usually followed by redness and swelling. Since blood under the surface has entered the tissue, the skin may become black and blue, and, later, brown and yellow. Though bruises do not ordinarily require treatment, ice packs will often lessen the pain. The pain and discolor of a black eye, which

is a type of bruise, will often diminish if iced compresses are applied. Later, when the blackness appears, hot compresses for half-hour intervals are more effective.

Foreign Bodies. Foreign bodies accidentally penetrating any orifice of the human body ordinarily should be extracted promptly. This must be done gently, however, since violence might do more harm than good.

An infant who has swallowed a foreign object should be laid face down, or held head down, so that he can cough up the object. If anything is caught in the nostril, blowing the nose or sneezing may help to extract it. Usually, however, the best solution is to call the doctor. When a foreign object lodges in the ear, an insect, for example, it may often be removed by filling the ear with warm oil. The insect cannot live in oil and when it dies it can be floated out with warm water.

Parents are justifiably frightened when a child swallows a broken piece of glass, a pin, or some foreign substance. If small, the object may pass from the body as part of a bowel movement.

A tiny particle in the eye may often be removed with the tip of a clean handkerchief. If it is under the lid, however, the most common method or removal is to turn the eyelid up over a small rod, such as a match.

These suggestions do not apply, however, to a speck which appears on the eyeball itself. When this happens, the wisest course is to place a pad of wet gauze over the entire eye, call a doctor promptly and keep the person quiet until he arrives. Such an accident is often extremely painful.

One should never attempt to pull a fishhook out the way it went in. Rather, it should be pushed all the way through and snipped off at the end. It may then be pulled out without damaging the flesh.

Wounds. A wound is an injury involving a break in the skin. Before caring for a wound, the person in charge should wash his hands thoroughly in soap and water, and perhaps also in alcohol. Any object applied to the wound should also be sterilized and cloth which is used as a bandage ought to be thoroughly boiled. Packages of sterilized bandages may be purchased at a drugstore or other shops.

After the wound has been washed in soap and water, or in some suitable mild solution, it should be treated with iodine or alcohol and then covered with a sterile dressing. If any pus appears in the wound, be sure to call a physician. If this is impossible, the pus should be removed before treating the wound, even if it is necessary to open the wound for this purpose.

Burns. Among the possible causes of burns are scalding water, hot irons, electricity and unexpected match blazes. Burns involving more than half the body are usually fatal. Any person who has been burned severely will suffer *shock* as well as physical damage and requires the immediate attention of a physician. Little can be done by the layman except to make the victim as comfortable as possible.

If a person has suffered lesser burns, however, the injured area may be covered at once with cold water or vinegar. Petroleum jelly can be used at a later stage. The wounds should never be covered with anything since these articles cannot be removed without doing serious damage to the tissues.

Burns caused by *nitric* or *sulphuric acid* should be washed at once to remove the acid. This may be done with a solution of *bicarbonate* of *soda*. If possible, the wound should then be permitted to soak in the same solution for as long as possible.

Injuries from fireworks, guns, cap pistols and similar toys are serious. Here the greatest danger is the pos-

Emergency Treatment—These men are demonstrating the basket method of carrying an injured person when it is necessary to transport him to another spot for treatment.

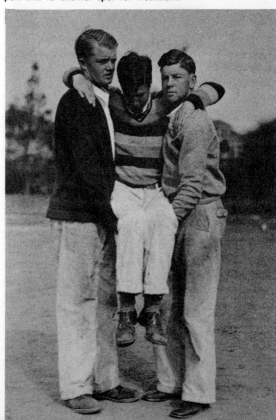

sibility of *lockjaw,* a disease in which germs, having entered a wound, are sealed in. A doctor is desirable because the wound must be cleansed, after which the victim may possibly need *lockjaw antitoxin.*

Resuscitation. Asphyxiation, suffocation due to deficiency of oxygen, is often caused by *drowning, electric shock* or by *carbon monoxide gas.* When a person has been under water for as long as five minutes artificial resuscitation is probably the quickest method of attempting to save his life. The most widely accepted method of artificial respiration, or resuscitation, is the direct *mouth-to-mouth-breathing,* using a special tube if available. This operation may usually be continued for at least an hour, or until the breathing has been restored. The person should be kept under close observation afterward, in case he should again cease to breathe.

If a person has suffered *electric shock,* the first step is always to remove the victim from the cause. Since every second counts and there is usually no time to turn off the current, the quickest solution is to throw a coat or similar article of clothing around the body of the victim and so pull him away from the current. Artifical respiration should then be administered until the doctor arrives.

Preventive action is the best method of avoiding death by *carbon monoxide gas.* Windows should always be kept open and an engine should never be permitted to run in a closed garage. Those who are especially sensitive to carbon mon-

oxide gas should avoid any occupation in which such gas occurs.

The first symptoms of monoxide poisoning are headache, faintness, nervousness and irritability. An apparent victim of carbon monoxide poisoning should be removed at once to fresh air and kept quiet and warm. If possible, while awaiting the doctor, the patient should be covered with hot-water bottles or blankets to prevent pneumonia. At the same time, artificial respiration should be administered.

Fainting. If a person has fainted, a physician should be called. While awaiting his arrival, the victim should be placed flat on his back in the coolest location possible. If the face is pale, the head should be brought as low as possible in relation to the rest of the body. If the face is red, however, the head may be moved to a position somewhat higher than that of the rest of the body. Cold water may be applied to the face or chest, and smelling salts or a teaspoonful of aromatic spirits of ammonia in a tumbler of water may be given.

Heat Stroke. Heat stroke may occur, not only in tropical weather, but in any area, a laundry or kitchen, for example, where the heat is intense. Persons working under such conditions should take salt tablets at regular intervals throughout the day.

The signs to watch for in heat stroke are *dizziness, drowsiness* and *fast breathing.* When the attack occurs, it is essential to transfer the victim at once to a cool place and then keep him flat on his back and absolutely quiet. Sponging with cool water will help to control the temperature, and the circulation may be stimulated with coffee or other drugs.

Some authorities advise that the victim of heat stroke be placed on a bed covered with a large rubber sheet, and his entire body then rubbed with ice until the temperature drops to 101°F. Then, the cold treatment is terminated and the patient is covered with blankets. If breathing stops, it is necessary to administer artificial respiration at once.

Bite Wounds. If a person has been stung by a *bee* or similar *insect,* the sting should be removed at once and a drop or two of diluted ammonia water placed on the wound. When a more serious bite has occurred, however, such as that of a *centipede, snake* or *scorpion,* bleeding should at first be encouraged as a means of removing the poison. Later, iodine may be applied, together with a cold pack to ease the pain. The sting of the *black widow spider* requires the additional attention of a physician who may employ a local anesthetic and also administer adrenalin to constrict the blood vessels so that the poison will not spread. Snakebite also requires urgent medical attention. The bite of certain species, such as the *cobra* or the *coral snake,* is usually fatal, but the bites of the more common North American species can usually be successfully overcome provided medical treatment is initiated without delay.

The treatment for a dog bite is the same as that which is given for any infected wound. If there is any likelihood of *rabies,* however, the wound should be cauterized by a doctor and the dog reported to the city authorities at once.

Hiccups. A hiccup is an involuntary spasm of the diaphragm, causing an inhalation which is suddenly stopped by the closing of the glottis. A characteristic sound is involved.

Popular cures for hiccups often involve the use of a ruse which is calculated to distract the victim's attention from his affliction. If the condition persists, a doctor must be consulted. *See* HICCUPS.

Migraine or Sick Headache. Migraine may have its source in sensitivity to food, in a disease of the stomach or brain, in hardening of the arteries, in disturbances of vision, in menstruation, or in mental problems. Sometimes the cause cannot be determined.

The headache will either come suddenly or its approach may be heralded by a feeling a depression, perhaps a disinclination to work or to carry on daily activities.

When the migraine headache actually strikes, the victim is usually required to lie down in a darkened room in absolute quiet. Often the patient is so uncomfortable that he rejects any assistance or attention. Drugs provide a satisfying relief for migraine and may become habitual unless their use is carefully supervised by a physician.

Food Poisoning. When a person appears to have eaten poisoned food, an attempt should be made at once to determine the nature of the poison. Evidence may be found in an empty bottle, a cup or spoon, perhaps on the table or floor, or possibly by smelling the patient's breath or inspecting his mouth.

While awaiting the doctor, the white of eggs, milk or strong tea can be given to the patient, all of which are antagonistic to certain poisons. Vomiting can be provoked by means of tickling the back of the throat or by giving the patient a cup of warm water mixed with salt. If there is any possibility that the person has taken an acid poison, vomiting should never be induced.

See ANIMAL BITES AND WOUNDS; ANTIDOTE; ARTIFICIAL RESPIRATION; BURNS; DISCOLORATION; EPILEPSY; ELECTRICAL INJURIES; FAINTING; FRACTURE; FIRST AID; FOOD POISONING; MIGRAINE; HEMORRHAGE; POISONING; SNAKEBITE.

EMERGENCIES, MEDICAL. A code alert—called "Code 99" at St. Vincent's Hospital, New York City, where it was first used—has been adopted in several leading hospitals for dealing with cases of critical cardiac arrest (heart failure). The announcement of the code over the hospital's address system alerts a specified group of doctors and nurses to immediate action.

New techniques in artificial respiration and circulation have made it possible to save many lives which formerly would have been lost, provided these remedial measures are administered within four minutes of heart stoppage. The announcement of the code number over the address system enables the medical team to assemble around the patient during these crucial four minutes. The requisite measures are implemented in order by those first arriving on the scene, supplemented by appropriate secondary procedures. See also RESUSCITATION; EMERGENCIES IN THE HOME.

EMETIC, a substance used to induce vomiting for various purposes —for example, to empty the stomach of poison. An emetic should never be used if the poison is an acid which might have a damaging effect on the lining of the stomach.

An emetic may also be used for persons suffering from bronchitis. This is indicated when the tubes which lead to the lungs are filled with a secretion which cannot be eructed except through vomiting. For old people, the emetic should be one which will not induce depression afterward. For these people, ten grains of ammonium carbonate, dissolved in water, is satisfactory.

One of the simplest emetics is a mixture of two tablespoons of salt with the minimum amount of water necessary to produce a liquid solution. Also effective is a mixture of one tablespoon of mustard in half a glass of water, or one tablespoon of alum in the same amount of water.

If an emetic is slow to act, vomiting can often be started by the old method of tickling the back of the throat with the tip of the finger, or with some object of similar shape. When regurgitation has finally begun, the process may be continued if the person drinks a large amount of lukewarm water at frequent intervals. This will also help to cleanse the stomach. See also VOMITING.

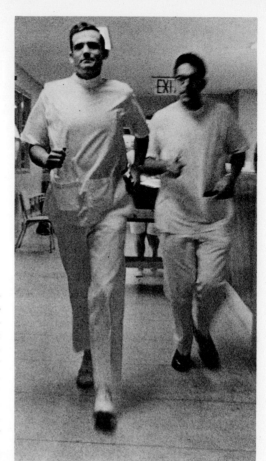

Several prominent hospitals have pioneered in the use of emergency teams to save the dying. The announcement of a predetermined code number over the public address system assembles a team of doctors and nurses in seconds to save a patient who has suffered a severe heart attack. Full breathing must be restored within a crucial four minutes if the patient's brain is not to suffer irreversible destruction. Right, doctors race for the necessary equipment upon hearing the code signal. Below, the full team in action shortly after the call.

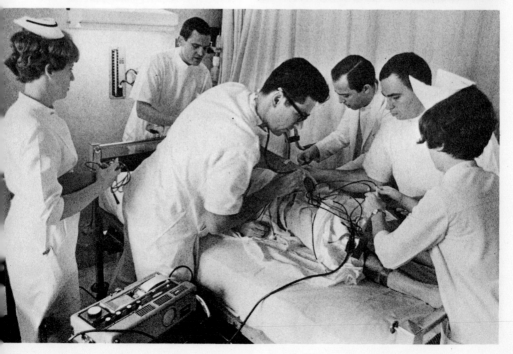

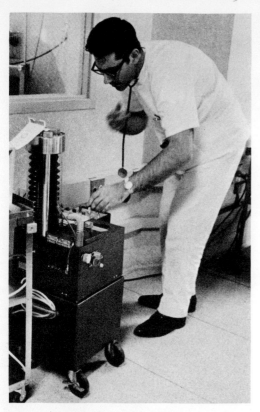

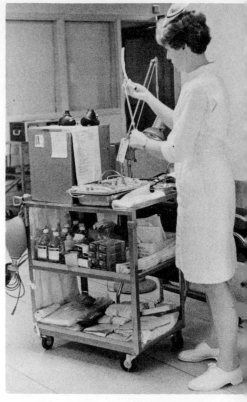

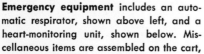

Emergency equipment includes an automatic respirator, shown above left, and a heart-monitoring unit, shown below. Miscellaneous items are assembled on the cart, above right. On opposite page, equipment is rushed to patient's bedside within seconds of alert. Patient is immediately positioned for emergency treatment.

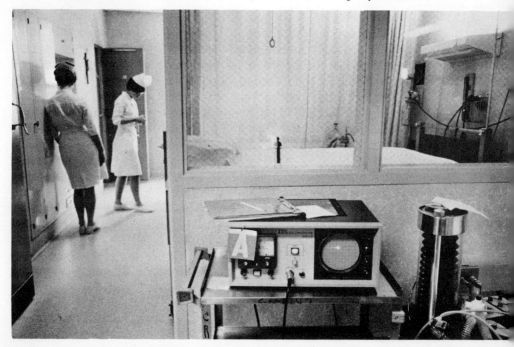

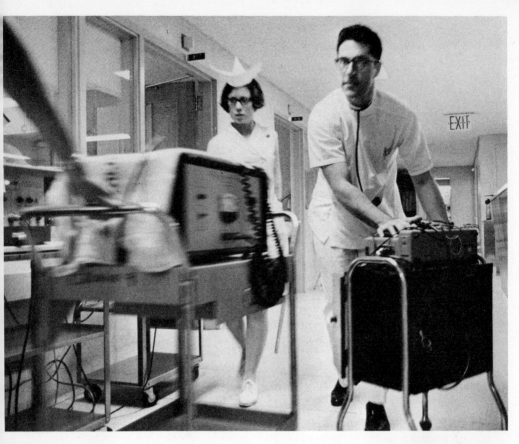
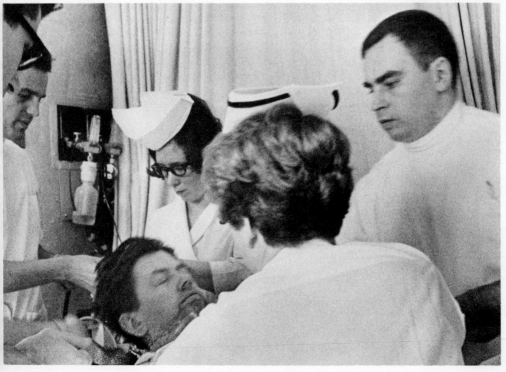

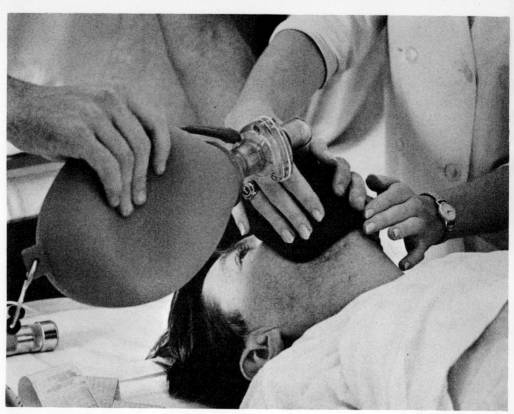

The most urgent task is to get air into the patient's lungs and hence blood into his brain. Above, the respirator forces air into the lungs. Below, a doctor begins external heart massage. On opposite page, the patient's breath is returning, and the doctor listens to determine if it is adequate. Massage continues. Patient is lifted so his lungs can be heard with stethoscope. Many lives can be saved by these procedures.

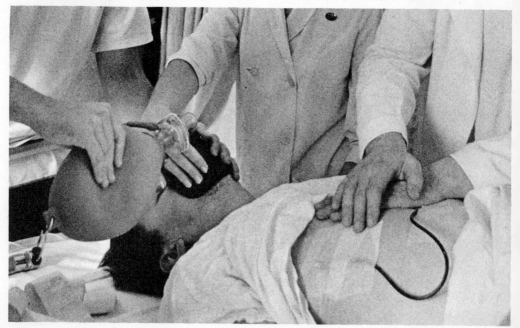

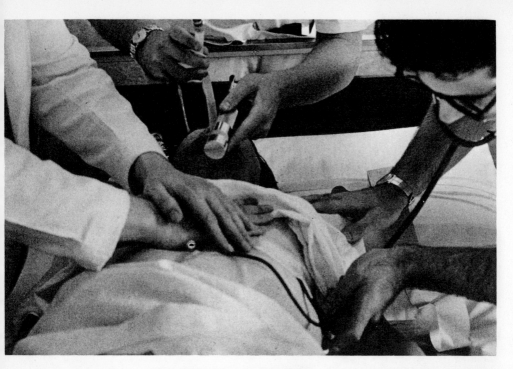

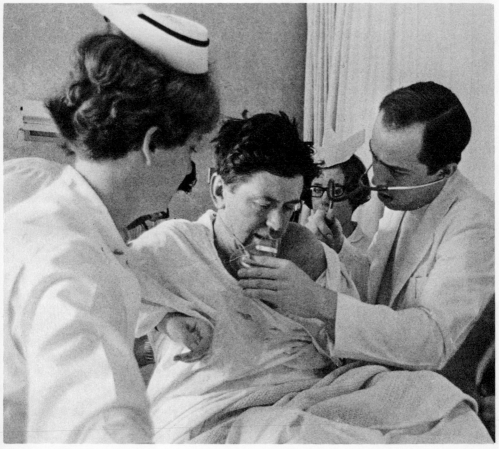

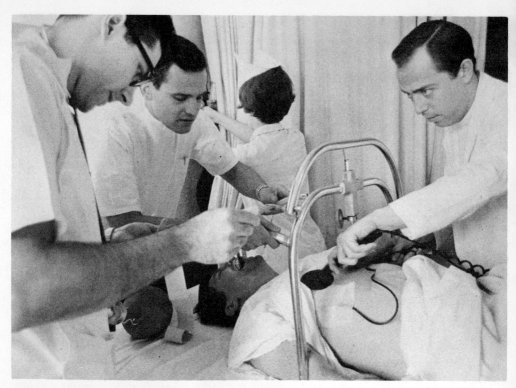

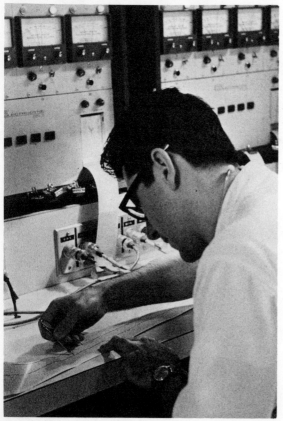

External cardiac massage apparatus, which shocks the heart back into action, is applied above. Nurse prepares injection of sodium bicarbonate to neutralize dangerous acids which otherwise accumulate when circulation is stopped. Left, the doctor interprets the electrocardiogram. On opposite page, the patient's heart activity has been restored and he breathes with aid of administered oxygen. Nurses follow the patient's progress as he begins to regain consciousness. They keep a constant vigil until he is back to normal.

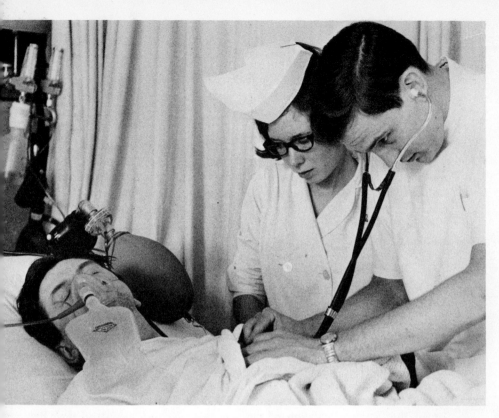

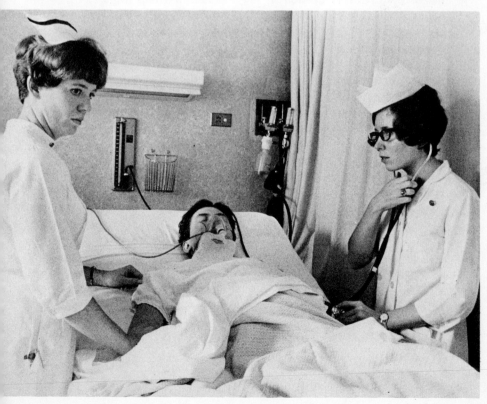

EMOTION, simply defined, an *expression of feeling.* In psychology it is a *response to stimuli,* involving certain physiological changes such as an increase in pulse rate, a rise in temperature, glandular activity, or a change in breathing rate. *Psychosomatic medicine* emphasizes the relationship of physical disorders to tension from unrelieved emotions.

In severe pain, fear, or anger, a person becomes pale because the blood vessels on the surface of the body contract. The skin feels cold and clammy, the mouth is dry because the saliva stops flowing and the tongue sticks to the roof of the mouth. Under such conditions, the heart beats rapidly and sometimes so strongly that the pulsation can be seen in the blood vessels of the neck. Other symptoms include wide opening of the eyes and dilation of the pupils. The tiny hairs of the body may actually stand on end and twitchings of the muscles may appear around the mouth and other parts of the body.

A rise in blood pressure or an increase in blood sugar may occur as a result of emotional strain due to excessive fear or to an accident involving severe emotional strain. The mere memory or association of some earlier incident later in life may provoke physiological reactions.

Continual worry is one of the significant causes of physical reactions and symptoms leading to various physical disorders. Violent emotions or prolonged minor emotional disturbances can affect the mental activity and the function of certain body processes. *See also* EMOTIONAL DISTURBANCES; NEUROSIS; PSYCHOSOMATIC DISORDERS; EMOTIONAL HEALTH; EMOTIONS AND ALLERGY.

EMOTIONAL DISTURBANCES.

Anxiety is an emotional state of fearfulness, apprehension, a feeling of impending disaster without reasonable explanation. It may reach highly distressing and disabling proportions and a person experiencing it may be completely overwhelmed. He cannot control his feelings and, at the same time, will agree that there is no logical reason for the magnitude of his feeling. He may not even be able to ascertain the cause of his anxiety. He may have a rapid pulse, dry mouth, difficulty in breathing, excessive perspiration, dizziness, and tremor. Probably most people will recognize at least some of these feelings as part of their life experience at some time. Anxiety reaches the level of an abnormal symptom, however, only when it is intense and frequent.

A *phobia* is an unreasonable fear of an innocuous object or an object that would not inspire a reaction of fear in an average person. Here again the standard is whether the response is appropriate or not. For example, a strong impulse to avoid contact with cats would not seem unreasonable if such contact produced asthma; otherwise an overwhelming fear of cats seems unreasonable. The term *phobia* is applied when there exists an extreme fear not objectively based on any danger involved. Fear of open spaces, fear of closed spaces, fear of infection, and fear of light are some of the many phobias that have been described in long technical terms. Sometimes these unreasonable fears seem related to early conditioning experiences.

Apathy. Whereas the forms of abnormal emotional response previously described have been too strong, another form exists in which there is too little emotional response. The emotions are dulled; nothing seems to matter to the person; he is completely indifferent to circumstances and events that to others have a strong emotional tenor. He is emotionally dull and does not have strong feelings of any type. At times of great physical fatigue or after prolonged severe illness, the normal person may know these feelings. But with returning physical vigor, the feelings disappear. Abnormal apathy, however, cannot adequately be explained by such physical factors.

Depression. Occasional moments of depression are part of normal experience but depression as an abnormal symptom has certain identifying features. It is prolonged, overwhelming, without sufficient cause, and may lead to suicidal attempts. A depressed person has a feeling of worthlessness and failure, is weighed down by sadness which he may or may not try to justify. He may say, "I don't know why I feel so sad and blue," or he may attribute his gloom to some trivial happening in the past. The feeling of hopelessness pervades all waking experience and he becomes retarded in activity and unresponsive to his immediate environment.

Furor. Exaggerated or even explosive outbursts of rage and anger are given the psychiatric label of *furor.* This symptom may occur in *schizophrenia, epilepsy, senility,* and in some other organic disorders. In such attacks, a person may be wildly destructive. Hospitalization and control by experts is imperative. Such behavior is, fortunately, rather rare as a symptom in the field of mental disturbance, although it was the basis of the stereotyped popular view in years past of the way people in mental hospitals act. This stereotype is, however, what people have in mind when they think that they are "going insane" or are worried and ashamed because some member of their family needs psychiatric care. Most people are surprised at the relatively peaceful and serene atmosphere of a psychiatric ward. *See also* ANXIETY; MENTAL DEPRESSION; NEUROSIS; SCHIZOPHRENIA; PARANOIA; INVOLUTIONAL MELANCHOLIA; MANIC-DEPRESSIVE PSYCHOSIS; EMOTIONAL HEALTH; STRESS; HYSTERIA.

EMOTIONAL HEALTH. A person's emotional health may be defined as the characteristic way in which he perceives, reacts to, and solves the main problems of life. The problems of life can be classified into three basic categories: (1) problems of biological and physical needs such as food, clothing, and shelter; (2) problems determined by cultural demands and prohibitions; (3) problems of internal psychological needs such as the need for security, love, belonging, self-esteem, independence, achievement, and adequacy.

Disturbances or conflicts in the manner of satisfying these needs may produce acute symptoms of mental or emotional illness or may become habitual modes of behavior called character disturbances. However, there is no fine dividing line between emotional health and emotional illness, or between normality and abnormality. Emotional health depends not only on the individual, but also on the particular situation in which he finds himself. Under extreme conditions of hardship, every individual can reach a point of emotional breakdown. Studies of prisoners of war have shown that conditions of extreme physical and mental stress can precipitate serious mental disturbances.

It is impossible to understand emotional health without reference to the cultural and social background of the individual. Certain societies—notably that of the United States—stress ambition, the accumulation of wealth and aggressive behavior as important. Other societies expect the individual to show no strong ambition, to refrain from aggressive behavior, and to cooperate with other members of the society.

Even within a particular society attitudes vary as to what is normal and abnormal behavior. Normality within a society is relative also to social status, age, and sex. For example, behavior that is harmless in the preadolescent of nine years of age may be unquestionably unhealthy in an individual of forty.

Although the difference between emotional health and emotional illness is often one of degree rather than kind, for practical reasons this distinction is very important. Many people have minor emotional disturbances that are not easily recognized, but because of their effects on the general health have medical significance. There are people in all walks of life who suffer from difficulties of adjustment to their environment. The anxieties, frustrations, and fears that stem from daily life experiences may induce headaches, ulcers of the stomach, asthma, or similar conditions. With the rapid advancement of medicine, the average lifespan today is much longer than was formerly common; as a result, cases of emotional disturbances at later age levels have greatly multiplied and have created a greater need for psychiatric services. *See also* ANXIETY; EMOTION; HYSTERIA; MENTAL DEPRESSION; PSYCHOSOMATIC DISORDERS; STRESS; MENTAL AND EMOTIONAL HEALTH.

EMOTIONS AND ALLERGY. Recently attention has been focused on the part that emotional or psychological factors play in allergic disease. At present, a complete answer has not been reached. To say that asthma, hives, and eczema, for example, are purely psychosomatic diseases is contrary to the experience and opinions of most allergists and psychiatrists. But to ignore emotional stresses also is unrealistic. Persons with allergic disease are ill, disturbed, uncomfortable, anxious, and apprehensive just as are those with other illnesses. Their symptoms may become more severe or may even be precipitated by situations of emotional stress.

Some persons subject to stress are allergic to begin with and their tolerance or reactivity is unbalanced by the state of stress or frustration. Allergic people can change their environment but they cannot run away from their allergic constitution. The same stress situation in nonallergic persons rarely if ever produces those diseases classified as allergic in nature.

Many nonspecific causes of flare-ups of allergic disease are recognized besides emotions. The physical effects of heat, cold, or barometric pressure may induce an asthmatic attack in an asthmatic person. Irritant smokes, dusts, fumes, or odors may have a similar effect. Commonly the onset of an infectious disease such as a common cold may irritate an allergic response of some nature.

There are many vagaries to allergic diseases. A person may not have any evidence of hay fever until late in life. Some with severe hay fever or asthma may suddenly or gradually lose their disease for reasons unknown. Some may have long periods of remission and then have their symptoms recur just as suddenly as they had disappeared. Women commonly have an increase in manifestations of allergic illnesses prior to their menstrual periods and many are completely relieved during pregnancy. One member of a family may be afflicted and others not, or different members of the same fam-

ily may have different forms of allergic disease. The same allergen may produce completely different types of disease in different persons. Allergy is a vital and provoking process. The condition still is in its early stages of recognition, implication, and understanding. A tremendous amount of knowledge has been acquired by biochemists, immunologists, pathologists, botanists, and clinicians and this knowledge has been utilized with success by practicing physicians. There are, however, many gaps in what we know about allergy. Many answers will need to be found before there is a final, satisfactory and completely successful control of allergic diseases. *See also* ALLERGY; PSYCHOSOMATIC DISORDERS.

EMPHYSEMA, the condition which exists when the normal air spaces in the lungs are dilated and the walls are overdistended. Various types of this disease are related to different causes. An obstruction of the breathing due to asthma or to chronic bronchitis or coughing produced by any one of a number of lung diseases may cause the walls of the small cells in the lungs to stretch and air to accumulate. The stretching occurs chiefly along the margins and upper edges of the lung where the muscular and bony framework of the lung less adequately support it. The stretching tends to destroy the elasticity of the breathing cells and causes distention of the lung.

Among the symptoms of emphysema are breathlessness on exertion and cough. The cough generally is due to chronic inflammation of the bronchial tubes. Cold air, dust, or exercise may start a coughing spell in the irritated tissues. A person with emphysema usually has a large barrel-shaped chest and prominent bones. The disease can be relieved by treatment of the asthma, bronchitis, or other chronic condition that causes it. Medical treatment of the cough which produces the distention is beneficial. Sometimes a properly fitted binder that sustains the chest walls without interfering with the movement of the ribs helps to control emphysema.

Emphysema is increasing in incidence, according to statistical evidence, and is now second only to heart disease as a cause of adult disability. Reports of deaths from emphysema have doubled every five years since 1945. Causation is believed to be related both to excessive cigarette smoking and to air pollution.

Pathologists have classified victims of emphysema into two types: PP (pink and puffing) and BB (blue and bloated). Advanced research into the intricate biochemistry of the lungs and the microanatomy of the lungs, bronchial tubes and cilia have expanded our knowledge of the disease but not yet demonstrated either the specific cause or a specific cure.

Mediastinal emphysema is caused by the introduction of air into the midchest region by a blow, strain, or coughing. It may result also from puncture wounds, or from incorrect use of machines for artificial respir-

ation. Symptoms include swelling of the neck and occasionally of the whole face and chest. If the condition interferes with breathing, the air can be withdrawn by an operation. However, if the amount of air in the tissues becomes so great as to interfere with the circulation to the heart and lungs, death may result.

In older people, chronic emphysema may exist because of inelasticity and weakness of the lung tissues. However, the cough generally is not as severe as in the case of younger people suffering from emphysema. A really effective treatment for emphysema associated with old age has not as yet been found. *See also* ASTHMA; BRONCHITIS; BRONCHOPNEUMONIA; LUNGS; TUBERCULOSIS. *See* MEDIGRAPHS pages 863, 1051.

EMPYEMA, a medical term signifying pus in a cavity or organ, especially in the chest cavity, the gallbladder, or in the pericardium which envelops the heart. Usually empyema is associated with infections of the lung and is called *suppurative pleurisy*.

Pleural empyema affects children more often than adults. Frequently it occurs in connection with pneumonia or influenza, particularly when the influenza virus is accompanied by a secondary infection of streptococci, staphylococci, or other pus-forming germs. Occasionally the tuberculosis germ may be present and fungi of various kinds may also be found. Empyema may also follow an injury or wound to the chest and lung.

Symptoms of empyema in influenza or pneumonia may be a sudden rise of fever, pain or interference with chest movement in breathing. If examination shows an accumulation of fluid, the doctor can confirm his diagnosis by tapping the chest wall with a needle. If the amount of fluid is so large as to cause pressure on the heart and lungs, prompt removal of the fluid is absolutely necessary. Most of the infectious material can be withdrawn with the needle and a cure affected by the re-injection of antiseptics or other substances to combat the infection. In extreme cases, however, surgical operation may be necessary. The prompt use of sulfa drugs and antibiotics has made surgery unnecessary when empyema is detected early. *See also* ABSCESS; INFECTIONS. *See* MEDIGRAPHS pages 1031, 1047.

ENCEPHALITIS, often called *sleeping sickness,* an inflammation of the brain which causes drowsiness and slowing down of mental and physical faculties. A number of distinct types of encephalitis are known, most of them caused by viruses. The condition sometimes occurs as a complication of another infectious disease, such as meningitis or measles, or may arise from poisoning or infection of a wound. *Virus encephalitis* should not be confused with *African sleeping sickness,* which is due to a parasite *trypanosoma* carried by the tsetse fly.

One type of encephalitis, *equine encephalomyelitis,* also affects horses, birds, mice, snakes, and possibly other animals. Since 1931, when it first occurred in California, the disease has appeared spasmodically in both human beings and horses and other animals. Sometimes it has reached epidemic proportions within a two-month period, and at other times has appeared in sporadic cases in a few scattered areas.

Another form of encephalitis appeared in a major epidemic in St. Louis during the summer of 1933 and has since been called *St. Louis encephalitis.* Still another form, *postinfection encephalitis,* occurs during the course of or follows an infectious disease such as measles or influenza. Sometimes it has appeared after vaccination against rabies, smallpox, or measles. Postinfection encephalitis, which is less common than the other types, attacks persons of all ages, although children are most susceptible. There is no evidence that this type is contagious.

Symptoms of encephalitis vary greatly, depending on the severity of the infection and the area of the brain and nervous system affected. The illness may be brief and mild or severe and lengthy. Acute forms usually begin with high fever and headache, dizziness, vomiting, and pain and stiffness of the neck and back. Drowsiness, stupor, and weakness of the eye muscles are common symptoms. In severe cases, delirium, convulsions and insomnia appear.

Damage to the nervous system is the greatest danger in encephalitis.

Parkinson's disease (shaking palsy or *paralysis agitans*) may follow an attack and sometimes a deterioration of mental faculties. Behavior disorders may develop in children who have had encephalitis.

In general, treatment consists in relieving pain and headache, reducing the fever, and making the patient as comfortable as possible. The physician may prescribe sedatives for restlessness and other drugs for insomnia or delirium. Special nursing care and regular supervision by the physician, even after the severe stage has subsided, are essential.

ENDARTERITIS, inflammation of the inner wall of an artery which occurs in certain types of endocarditis. *See also* ARTERIOSCLEROSIS; ENDOCARDITIS.

ENDOCARDITIS, inflammation of the lining of the heart. *See also* BACTERIAL ENDOCARDITIS; EMBOLISM; ENDOCARDITIS, MALIGNANT; HEART; RHEUMATIC FEVER. *See* MEDIGRAPHS pages 173, 1031.

ENDOCARDITIS, MALIGNANT. The proper name for this condition scientifically is *subacute bacterial endocarditis*. This disease used to be universally fatal as a complication of either rheumatic heart disease or similar conditions. By the use of the antibiotic drugs, the mortality has dropped drastically. Of course patients still die from heart failure or from breaking off of the bacterial clusters and their passing through the blood to important areas of the body or by the exten-

sion of the infection. Various germs can cause endocarditis but the one most frequently responsible is called the *streptococcus viridans*. The presence of the germ in the blood is detected by what are called *blood cultures*. Then vast amounts of *penicillin* may be given by injection into the muscles or even into the blood. In connection with the giving of the penicillin, a drug called *caronamide* inhibits the elimination of the penicillin from the body and permits the maintenance of large doses over a long period of time. Other antibiotics such as *streptomycin, aureomycin, terramycin* and *chloromycetin* are also used depending upon the extent to which the germ is found to be controlled by the antibiotics. *See also* ANEURYSM; BACTERIAL ENDOCARDITIS.

ENDOCARDIUM, the thin layer of tissue lining the inside of the heart.

ENDOCRINE GLANDS, any of the ductless glands, such as the adrenals, the thyroid, or the pituitary, whose secretions pass directly into the blood stream. *See also* GLANDS; HORMONES.

ENDOCRINOLOGY, the study of the endocrine glands and their secretions. *See* GLANDS; HORMONES.

ENDOMETRITIS, inflammation of the inner lining of the womb. It may follow normal birth or may occur as a result of abortion or infection. Malodorous discharge and fever are the two most common symptoms. This condition demands the attention of a physician. Treatment may require curettage or operation.

ENEMA, an injection of liquid into the lower bowel through the rectum. The purpose may be either to cleanse the intestines or to introduce drugs into the body.

An ordinary ear syringe, with a rubber tip, may be used to give an enema to an infant. A single bulbful of liquid is the maximum which may be safely introduced into the intestines of a baby at one time. The injection should be performed as slowly as possible.

For enemas of larger quantity, a douche bag with a capacity of at least a pint may be employed. The bag, or can, should be hung not more than two feet above the person's head. Placing it higher gives the stream excessive force. To this bag or can a length of rubber hosing is attached. At one end of the hose is a nozzle, made of bone or vulcanite, or the end of the hose itself, rounded off may be introduced into the rectum. A soft nozzle is preferable, since it is less likely to injure the fragile inner surface of the lower intestine.

To receive the enema, the person may kneel, or he can lie on his left side with his knees pulled up to his stomach. If he lies in bed, the bed should be protected with a rubber sheet. Before the nozzle is inserted into the rectum the fluid should be sent through the entire hose so that all the air is expelled. Petroleum jelly or paraffin should be applied to the nozzle, which may then be inserted for a distance of approximately one inch. Unless the liquid is inserted slowly, it will immediately emerge. If necessary, a folded cloth or towel may be held against the rectum to aid retention.

If the purpose of the enema is to empty the lower part of the bowels rather than to cleanse the intestines, the enema may be given with the patient sitting up instead of lying down, and the liquid, once it has entered, may be permitted to emerge at once.

The type of solution used will depend on the purpose of the enema. Some enemas are nutritional, and others are intended to fill the body with fluid. As a laxative, plain water may be satisfactory or a mild soap-and-water solution, although the latter type of enema is irritating to some people. Baking soda and water, glycerine and salt or soap-suds and salt solutions are also used. An enema containing a strong medicine should not be given except with the specific prescription of a physician. A barium enema is given before an x-ray or fluoroscopic examination of the lower intestines and organs of this region of the body. *See also* CONSTIPATION; DOUCHE; SYRINGE.

ENTERIC FEVER, the technical term for typhoid and paratyphoid fevers. *See* TYPHOID FEVER.

ENTERITIS, the medical term for any acute or chronic inflammation of the intestine due to any one of a variety of causes. Pain and diarrhea are among the symptoms.

ENURESIS, the scientific name for bed wetting, urinary incontinence in the absence of demonstrable organic causes, at an age when urethral sphincter control is normally expected; a habit disturbance. *See also* BED WETTING; CHILD CARE; INCONTINENCE IN WOMEN.

ENZYME, a complex chemical substance found largely in the digestive juices of the body which acts as a catalytic agent on other substances and causes them to split up. At least a dozen significant digestive enzymes are found in the secretions of the digestive system and aid in digesting fats, proteins, and carbohydrates. *See also* DIGESTION.

EPHEDRINE, a substance derived from a Chinese alkaloid called *ma-huang.* When injected or taken into the body it causes smooth muscle tissue to go into spasm. In hemorrhage it constricts blood vessels throughout the body, tending to keep the blood pressure normal. As an ingredient of nose drops it shrinks the lining of the nasal passages permitting more comfortable breathing during colds. It is also useful in asthma, by relaxing the smooth muscle lining of the bronchioles, permitting easier inflow of air into the lungs.

EPIDIDYMIS, (plural *epididymides*), that portion of the testicle lying like a hood over the upper end. When it becomes infected, as in *gonorrhea,* the condition is known as *gonorrheal epididymitis.* The epididymitis may also be associated with other infections. Treatment involves control of the source. The sulfa drugs and penicillin are most frequently and effectively used for these infections, but always on the advice of a physician. *See also* TESTICLES; VAS DEFERENS; REPRODUCTION SYSTEM.

EPIGLOTTIS, an elastic cartilage resembling a valve or lid, located behind and below the root of the tongue. It covers the *glottis,* the opening into the windpipe, during swallowing, thus preventing the entrance of food and drink into the larynx. Formerly it was assumed that the epiglottis was drawn down to cover the glottis. Actually, however, the glottis is drawn upward, to give protection.

EPILEPSY, a disorder of the central nervous system, perhaps among the most misunderstood of all human afflictions. Throughout recorded history, its victims have been at various times avoided, feared, scorned, ridiculed, flogged, and burned at the stake. They have been said to be possessed of the devil, and in some periods have been revered or even worshipped.

Epileptics are subject to seizures, temporary loss or alteration of consciousness, with or without convulsive movements. Five or more types of seizures are known, but only one, the *grand mal,* has the characteristics of the popular conception of a "fit" or convulsion. Even a violent *grand mal* seizure rarely lasts much longer than a minute, though it will probably seem much longer to an observer. After a seizure, the person may sleep for a few hours or resume normal activity within a few minutes.

Contrasted with the *grand mal* is the *petit mal* seizure, a momentary blackout, with or without a twitching of the eyelids or of other facial muscles. Its manifestations, however, are so slight that it may go unnoticed even in a crowd.

Little can be done while a person is having a seizure. At the beginning of an attack he may be lowered to the floor, well away from hard objects against which he might injure himself. Any tight collars or belts should be loosened, and a folded handkerchief inserted between the back teeth to prevent biting of the tongue. The patient should be turned on his side to permit saliva to flow from his mouth.

Science has made great progress in diagnosing and treating epilepsy through the use of an instrument, the electroencephalograph, which magnifies and records the electric impulses from the brain, much as an electrocardiograph checks the heart. An electroencephalogram, the written record, is unique for each person, like a fingerprint. This record is a significant clue to the type of medication most likely to be successful.

At present, approximately 0.5 per cent of the population of the United States is afflicted with epilepsy. Seizures begin prominently in early childhood and in adolescence, but many persons are subject to them after the age of twenty-one. The number of males and females who suffer from epilepsy is almost equal. The true cause of epilepsy is not as yet known. Epilepsy is known to be related to damaged brain tissue, or to a brain tumor in some cases, but it may be present when such conditions do not exist. Tension, although it does not cause seizures, may precipitate them. A well-adjusted person who is physically and mentally active will have fewer seizures.

The electric impulses of the brain of a normal person have been compared to a stream with a moderate flow, controlled by an adequate dam. In the case of a person with epilepsy, the level at times rises and spills over the dam and a seizure results. The level overflows when the predisposition to epilepsy combines with minor body or emotional disturbances which most people experience without ill effects.

The hereditary cause of epilepsy is more significant than the acquired one. Among near relatives of epileptics, the illness is about three times more frequent than among the population as a whole. Certain disorders which may bring about epilepsy are thus acquired causes. Among these are (1) congenital defects of the central nervous system—as, for example, degeneration of the nervous system, congenital mental defect, and scarring of nerve tissue; (2) changes in the development of the brain after birth—as, for example, various types of meningitis, multiple sclerosis, general paresis, tumors, hemorrhages, cerebral abscess, arteriosclerosis and senile degeneration; (3) general diseases such as uremia,

the disease and its causes Epilepsy is a disorder of the central nervous system which makes itself known intermittently. It is an extremely common disease, affecting people of all ages, and attacks can occur once in a lifetime or several times a day.

Epilepsy can occur as a symptom of other well-recognized diseases of the nervous system, such as brain tumor, brain injury, neurosyphilis, or stroke; or its specific cause may be unknown.

There are many theories about what causes epileptic convulsions. The one most generally accepted is that cerebral irritation stimulates some part of the brain. A reaction is triggered which sets up the seizure, and the patient experiences a disturbance of sensation, loss of consciousness, or convulsive movements. These can occur singly or in any combination.

symptoms There are three types of seizure in epilepsy: Grand Mal, or major attack; Petit Mal, or minor attack; and Psychomotor, or moderate attack (epileptic equivalent). In all of them there is loss of consciousness and loss of memory of the episode. In Grand Mal there are convulsions. The accompanying Medi-Graph illustrates clearly the characteristics of each type.

A patient suffering from one form of epilepsy can also present symptoms of another. Patients suffering frequent attacks may show some mental deterioration. Epilepsy in young children may be accompanied by feeble-mindedness.

complications As a rule, there are no serious complications in epilepsy, but patients can hurt their heads or severely lacerate themselves when they fall. Or else they can choke to death on food or saliva. In general, however, the life span of the epileptic is not affected.

prevention (or lessening of impact) The patient with any of the symptoms of epilepsy should undergo careful examination for signs of other diseases of the nervous system. Vascular disturbances within the brain, and even early brain tumors, often can be corrected if they are detected soon enough. A large group of medications are available for patients who have epilepsy from an unknown cause. These can lessen the frequency and even the severity of the attacks. The electroencephalogram or brain wave test has been most helpful in establishing the correct diagnosis.

Once an attack has begun, it is important to keep the patient from injuring himself. His clothing should be loosened, and a gag should be forced between his teeth to keep him from biting his tongue. No other treatment is necessary during an acute attack.

The frequency of attacks can be controlled somewhat if the patient stays on a wholesome, careful diet, avoids constipation, and takes no alcoholic beverages of any kind. His sleep habits should be regular and he should exercise moderately. He should not drive an automobile or operate dangerous machinery. Many communities have vocational rehabilitation centers where epileptics can learn to pursue a normal life.

Epilepsy A Disease of the Brain and Central Nervous System

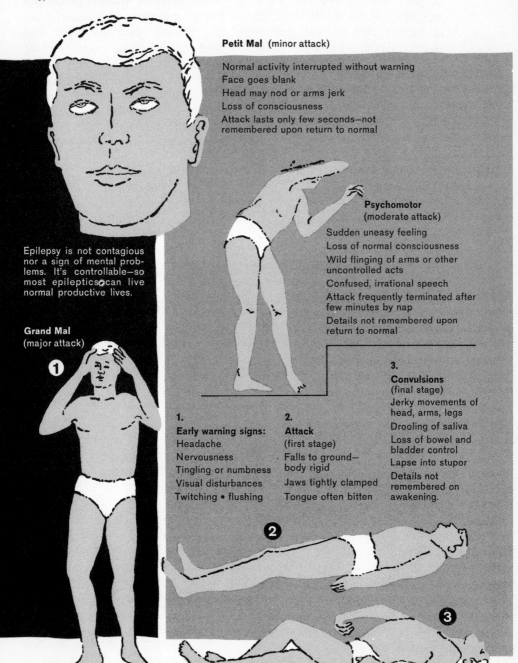

Petit Mal (minor attack)

Normal activity interrupted without warning
Face goes blank
Head may nod or arms jerk
Loss of consciousness
Attack lasts only few seconds—not
remembered upon return to normal

Epilepsy is not contagious
nor a sign of mental problems. It's controllable—so
most epileptics can live
normal productive lives.

Grand Mal
(major attack)

①

Psychomotor
(moderate attack)

Sudden uneasy feeling

Loss of normal consciousness

Wild flinging of arms or other
uncontrolled acts

Confused, irrational speech

Attack frequently terminated after
few minutes by nap

Details not remembered upon
return to normal

1.
Early warning signs:
Headache
Nervousness
Tingling or numbness
Visual disturbances
Twitching • flushing

2.
Attack
(first stage)
Falls to ground—
body rigid
Jaws tightly clamped
Tongue often bitten

3.
Convulsions
(final stage)
Jerky movements of
head, arms, legs
Drooling of saliva
Loss of bowel and
bladder control
Lapse into stupor
Details not
remembered on
awakening.

②

③

toxemia of pregnancy, fluid swelling of the brain, pernicious anemia, asphyxia, protein shock, acute fever in children, hypotension, insulin or electric shock; (4) effect of convulsant drugs—for example, camphor, caffeine, ergot, epinephrine, cocaine, magnesium sulfate, and sulfathiazole.

According to the Foundation to Combat Epilepsy, the incidence of epilepsy because of acquired causes is variable. The incidence related to convulsant drugs and brain tumor is not larger than 15 per cent, abnormalities at birth around 9 per cent, infections about 5 per cent, brain tumors about 1.5 per cent, cerebral circulatory defects about 1.2 per cent, and postnatal brain trauma about 6 per cent. In approximately 77 per cent of the patients, evidence of antecedent organic diseases of the brain does not exist.

A specific cure for epilepsy is not known, but medication can reduce the frequency of seizures or eliminate them completely in about 85 per cent of those affected. Many drugs and combinations of drugs are effective when taken under the guidance of a physician. Seizures can be completely controlled—that is, prevented from occurring—in about one-half of all persons with epilepsy. An additional 35 per cent under medication have the frequency of their seizures reduced by half or more, and the remaining 15 per cent of epileptic patients are not helped by medication.

A person with epilepsy should never try to treat himself, since the drugs and dosage needed vary from person to person and only a physician, specially trained, is competent to prescribe. Mail-order remedies should never be used. For most persons with *grand mal* or psychomotor seizures, the doctor employs among other drugs *phenytoin sodium* or DILANTIN®; and, if this drug is not fully effective, *phenobarbital* may be added. Another drug, MESANTOIN®, can be tolerated in larger amounts by some patients than others. These drugs can be obtained only by prescription and changes and directions in dosage must be supervised properly to be effective. For convulsions, the physician may employ first *phenobarbital* or MEBARAL®. *Bromides,* although now replaced by newer drugs, are still useful in some circumstances. In cases of *petit mal, tridione, paradione,* MILONTIN®, and *phenurone* have been successfully used in many cases.

The person subject to epilepsy must take his medicines regularly, avoid alcohol, emotional upsets, and fatigue and live as regular a life as possible. He should not be overprotected by his family, but should be encouraged to lead a full life. Children should not be kept out of public school and should play with their friends as usual. The epileptic must never be put into a position of feeling that he is "different."

In prevention of epilepsy as regards marriage and having children, each patient must receive individual consideration. Only the predisposition to epilepsy is inherited, not the disease itself. The chances that a child of epileptic parents will have epilepsy are about 1 to 40; and that a child will have more than one convulsion during childhood about 1 to 70. If an acquired cause is responsible for epilepsy in parents, these chances are greatly reduced.

If the number of cases of infectious diseases that involve the brain were reduced, a great step toward controlling acquired epilepsy would be made. Many of these diseases are the result of traffic accidents, occupational accidents, and war injuries. Concentrated efforts to reduce asphyxia and injuries at birth should be made.

Psychologically the illness may have a great effect. Approximately 80 per cent of all victims of epilepsy are capable of leading normal lives; those persons about them should recognize that epilepsy is not communicable and not a sign of insanity. Unfortunately, through misunderstanding of the disease, a person with epilepsy may find himself shunned by other people and discriminated against in employment. Concealment of the disease may deny many epileptics the advantages of education and marriage. Not only must the public be educated about epilepsy but the epileptic himself must learn to have self-confidence and courage.

Many people with epilepsy have achieved great heights of accomplishment. An organization, Epilepsy: Self-Help, sponsored and financed by the Variety Club Foundation to Combat Epilepsy, has been organized for people with epilepsy to meet for mutual association, understanding, and encouragement. The self-confidence of the epileptic can be strengthened when he has an opportunity to discuss his problems with persons who understand them. For information about epilepsy, write to the National Epilepsy League, 130 North Wells Street, Chicago, Illinois. *See* MEDIGRAPH page 569.

EPINEPHRINE, one of the chief hormones of the inner portion of the adrenal glands. Its trade name is *adrenalin*. It has the power to constrict blood vessels and is employed in medicine as an astringent to stop the flow of blood and to increase the blood pressure in anesthesia. *See* ADRENALIN.

EPISTAXIS refers to the common *nosebleed*. Nosebleed may be due to many factors. In children, it is usually the result of picking the nose and breaking small blood vessels. In adults with high-blood pressure, nosebleed may occur, which tends to relieve the blood pressure. Nosebleeds may result from frequent blowing of the nose, from a cold, foreign bodies in the nasal passages, or during the menstrual period. Fleshy growths in the nose—such as polyps—vitamin deficiency, food allergy, or even leukemia may all produce a nosebleed. Chronic nosebleeds can lead to general weakness.

Treatment at home should include having the victim lie down, applying ice-cold compresses about his lips and nose, and inserting small wads of cotton into the nasal passages. If this does not stop the bleeding, the doctor should be called. *See also* NOSE.

EPITHELIOMA, any cancer or tumor of the skin or other epithelial tissues. *See also* CANCER.

EPITHELIUM, tissue composed of contiguous cells with little intercellular substance. It forms the *epidermis,* lines all the hollow organs and passages of the respiratory, digestive, and genitourinary systems of the body. The hair, nails, and enamel of the teeth are modified epithelial cells. *See also* SKIN.

EPSOM SALT, a bitter white or colorless crystalline salt of *magnesium sulphate heptahydrate*. It acts as a cathartic and also as an antidote in lead or carbolic acid poisoning.

EQUILIBRIUM, physically the sense of balance, and mentally a well-balanced condition of mind or feeling. Physically it is controlled by information from the inner ear and elsewhere sent to the brain and transferred to the necessary muscles.

If the head is rotated rapidly and then suddenly stopped, the fluid in the semicircular canals of the inner ear continues to move. The result may be a giddiness so pronounced that the person may not be able to stand. The same sensation will be experienced if pressure is brought on the inner ear by means of a syringe, or if blood should enter the semicircular canals. Likewise the victim of *locomotor ataxia* may possess such a faulty sense of balance that he cannot walk without watching his feet.

Finally, if the cerebellum is itself diseased, the sense of balance is destroyed, and the victim may walk as if he were suffering from alcoholic intoxication. *See also* EAR.

ERGOT, a fungus that grows on grains and cereals. It is used to aid the uterus to contract after childbirth, to prevent blood loss. It does not affect normal pregnancy. Any form of this drug must be used only under the supervision of a doctor, since it may have adverse effects on the blood pressure as well as the blood vessels themselves.

ERGOTISM, a disease caused by overuse of ergot-containing food or drugs; it is characterized by gangrene of the fingertips and toes.

ERYSIPELAS, also known as *St. Anthony's fire* because the skin becomes a bright red as the inflammation spreads, a skin disease due to streptococcal infection. It manifests itself in headache, vomiting, chills, and fever, pain in the joints and prostration. The poison emitted by the streptococcus transmits the inflammation which spreads rapidly. The infection appears on the face, but may affect any part of the skin. It usually starts in a wound, fissure, or minute abrasion of the skin.

Erysipelas occurs more often in cold weather when the cracking of the skin due to exposure predisposes persons to its attack. The condition begins as an irregular round or oval patch. As it spreads, the patches become livid red, slightly swollen, hot and tender. The disease may be fatal, particularly to young children or old and infirm people, and it is essential that a doctor be called at once.

The development of sulfa compounds and antibiotics in recent years has rendered all other forms of treatment of erysipelas obsolete. These drugs reduce the fever, check the spread of inflammation, and bring the condition under control. People with erysipelas should be given plenty of fluids, at least ten glasses of water a day, and nourishing food, since the disease devastates the blood and weakens the patient. Erysipelas frequently reoccurs and therefore particular care should be taken to avoid scratching or irritating the skin.

ERYTHEMA, a redness of the skin, in uneven patches, caused externally by sunlight, ultraviolet rays, x-rays, heat, cold, friction, or by chemical irritants. Also erythema may result from the action of internal poisons, as in scarlet fever and other infectious diseases.

This condition may be caused by drugs or by poisons generated in the bowels or in other parts of the body. Sometimes it is accompanied by fever, sore throat, and pain in the joints. This type of erythema affects young people, especially girls, and may last for several weeks. Another species may occur as lesions of the skin, surrounded with red rings. The treatment includes rest in bed, a light diet, and the application of a soothing powder or lotion.

In the nodular form of erythema, round or oval nodular patches appear on the legs below the knees, and on the lower arms. The patches are tender and discolored, resembling bruises. Treatment is somewhat similar to that for the patchy type of erythema. Antihistaminic drugs, ACTH and several related drugs are sometimes effective in controlling these cases.

Another form of erythema, known as *erythromelalgia,* is of nervous origin and appears suddenly on the hands and feet. A more serious variety of erythema affecting the internal organs is *lupus erythematosus* in acute form. *See also* CHAFING; ECZEMA; INTERTRIGO; LUPUS ERYTHEMATOSUS; COLLAGEN DISEASES. *See* MEDIGRAPH page 869.

ERYTHROBLASTOSIS FOETALIS. When a mother is Rh negative and the embryo is Rh positive, antibodies are developed before birth which may cause the newborn child to suffer from jaundice and anemia. This condition is known, medically, as *erythroblastosis foetalis,* which means destruction of red blood cells in the fetus. It is also called *hemolytic anemia. See also* BLOOD TYPES; RED BLOOD CELLS, DISEASES OF.

ERYTHROCYTES, the scientific term for red blood cells. For conditions affecting the red blood cells, *see also* ANEMIA; BLOOD; RED BLOOD CELLS, DISEASES OF.

ESOPHAGUS, the tube, also known as the *gullet,* which connects the mouth with the stomach.

The modern physician possesses a special instrument by which he can actually examine the walls of the esophagus, where food will some-

the disease and its causes DIVERTICULUM Diverticula are pouches that form off the wall of the esophagus, which is the passage between the throat and the stomach. A patient may have been born with a weakness in the wall of the esophagus, causing it to balloon outward in pouches; or pouches may be the result of an inflammatory disease in the region of the esophagus, which has weakened the wall. These pouches tend to grow larger as time goes on.

CANCER OF THE ESOPHAGUS Cancer of the upper end, middle, and lower end of the esophagus is not uncommon, occurring in about 5% of all patients with cancer. Men over 40 are affected most frequently. The cause is unknown.

symptoms DIVERTICULUM The most noticeable symptoms in diverticulum are difficulty in swallowing, and vomiting undigested food several hours after eating. Pain is not an important factor, although occasionally there may be some pain under the breastbone. The patient often has a feeling of fullness beneath the breastbone and is relieved only after vomiting.

CANCER OF THE ESOPHAGUS As the cancer grows, it obstructs the food passage, and so the first symptom is difficulty in swallowing, progressing to vomiting. This may begin with solids, extend to soft foods, and eventually even liquids are brought up. Occasionally the matter brought up is bloody. Pain is a rare symptom. The diagnosis is usually made by X ray.

complications DIVERTICULUM A patient with diverticulum can live for years without any real difficulties unless the vomiting is so severe that he is unable to tolerate food and suffers from malnutrition. Rupture of the pouches is a rare but serious complication. Ulceration and hemorrhage can also develop.

CANCER OF THE ESOPHAGUS The progressive obstruction of the food passage can result in actual starvation. Sometimes the cancer can rupture into the windpipe and allow food to pass into the lungs at the site of the rupture and cause pneumonia. Complications from the spread of the cancer to other parts of the body inevitably result in death.

prevention (or lessening of impact) DIVERTICULUM There is no way a condition such as this can be prevented. The only treatment when the diagnosis has been established would be one of surgical correction. The need for this type of surgery would be as a life-saving measure only.

CANCER OF THE ESOPHAGUS There is no way the cancer can be prevented. When it becomes a matter of saving the patient's life, surgical correction is attempted. This is resorted to only if the obstruction becomes so large that it effectively prevents the digestion of food.

Diseases of the Esophagus

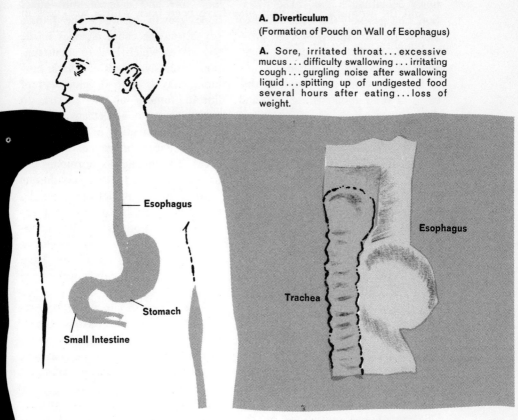

Esophagus

Stomach

Small Intestine

A. Diverticulum
(Formation of Pouch on Wall of Esophagus)

A. Sore, irritated throat...excessive mucus...difficulty swallowing...irritating cough...gurgling noise after swallowing liquid...spitting up of undigested food several hours after eating...loss of weight.

Esophagus

Trachea

B. Cancer of the Esophagus

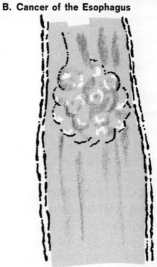

B. Difficulty swallowing...spitting up of undigested food...excessive saliva...feeling of fullness, pressure or pain high in chest...eventual obstruction.

times accumulate and cause irritation. Occasionally the walls will then adhere to each other, or even grow together, so that the doctor must surgically reopen the organ.

The two chief symptoms of diseases of the esophagus are pain and difficulty in swallowing. The principal disorders, besides foreign objects and irritation by food, include congenital abnormalities, inflammation, ulcers, spasm, tumors, rupture, and dilated or twisted veins. Cancer may occur in the esophagus, usually in the lower or middle portions of the tube.

Psychological problems may also be reflected in the esophagus. People have starved to death because they could not emotionally undertake the task of swallowing, a condition known as *hysterical dysphagia.* However, starvation from this cause is rare, because food can be introduced into the body by means other than through the esophagus. Dilation of and operations on the walls of the esophagus are performed with a high degree of success. *See also* STOMACH. *See* MEDIGRAPH page 575.

ESTROGENS, the female sex hormones, are produced primarily in the ovaries. However, they also occur in the afterbirth, the adrenals and other glands. Estrogens are responsible for the development of female physical characteristics. They cause the breasts to enlarge, the deposition of fat around the hips, and development of the female reproductive glands. They make the voice relatively high-pitched, the skin and

hair soft and delicate, and affect bone growth as well. The female sex hormones cause changes inside the uterus which lead to menstruation. Excessive levels of female hormone may lead to development of fibroid tumors of the uterus, to ovarian cysts, bone defects and possibly to aggravation of tendency to breast cancer or cancer in other areas. The female sex hormones are used medicinally for many conditions —for instance, to help regulate the menstrual periods, to lessen the severity of symptoms of the menopause, and to hasten development of female characteristics. They have been used in men with cancer of the prostate, to lessen the progress of the disease. They should never be employed without the constant supervision of the physician. Production of the female sex hormone ceases at the menopause. *See also* OVARIES.

ETHER, a thin, colorless, volatile, and highly inflammable liquid whose chief use is as an anesthetic in operations and as a solvent.

EUCALYPTUS OIL, an oil developed from the leaves of the eucalyptus tree, useful as a stimulant, antiseptic, and astringent.

EUNUCH, a male deprived of his testicles. *See also* CASTRATION.

EUSTACHIAN TUBE, or *auditory tube,* the canal connecting the nasopharynx with the middle ear. Its function is to equalize the pressure between the middle and external ears. *See also* DEAFNESS; EAR.

EXANTHEM, any eruption on the skin. Any acute disease, like measles, scarlet fever, or chickenpox, in which there is an eruption of the skin is called an *acute exanthematous disease*.

EXCRETION, the discharge from the body of waste products, including feces, sweat, and urine. The greater part of this function is performed by the kidneys. *See also* BOWEL; CONSTIPATION; DIARRHEA; URINATION.

EXERCISE. Many people believe that the road to health lies in exercise. This has led to the development of innumerable systems of exercise, as well as to the sale of all sorts of extraordinary springs, bicycles, walking machines, dumbbells, and similar apparatus alleged to lead the user directly into vim, vigor, and vitality.

Actually, exercise is merely a means of stimulating the action of the muscles, improving the coordination of nerve and muscle, and improving the circulation of the blood. The chief value of exercise is to stimulate the general chemistry and physiology of the body through its effect on the circulation and on elimination.

Various authorities have suggested the proper amounts of muscular activity for persons at various ages. One suggestion is that there be four hours of muscular activity daily at the age of five years, five hours daily from the age of seven to nine, six hours from nine to eleven, five hours from eleven to thirteen, four hours from thirteen to sixteen, three hours from sixteen to eighteen and two hours from eighteen to twenty. Another authority has said that one hour should be given daily to activities involving the use of the large muscles of the body after twenty years of age and that anything less will result in physical deterioration.

However, man does not live for his muscles alone. Certainly there is not the slightest evidence that big muscles are necessarily associated with good health. However, everyone should have sufficient strength of muscle to carry on the ordinary activities of life and to permit some exceptional use in time of emergency. For young people exercise has the value of stimulating body growth. Competitive sports of a vigorous kind, such as running, tennis, handball, football, and baseball, are available and useful up to the age of thirty. Serious overactivity after that age may do more damage than good.

The use of calisthenics, setting-up exercises, so-called "daily dozens," and similar performances is valuable within limitations. Such systems are not, however, to be considered as the single road to good general health. It is the regular use of exercise in moderate amounts that maintains health, rather than the occasional overindulgence to the point of muscle strain and exhaustion. Among muscular activities suitable to people of all ages are swimming, walking, golf, horseback riding, fishing, and gardening.

People who do not exercise do not have positive health. They do

577

not seem to have the vigor, vim, and vitality of those who take a reasonable amount of exercise. The muscles of our chests and hearts and of our bodies generally need a certain amount of activity in order to give them a factor that is called *tone*. Tone denotes the ability of a muscle to respond when called on.

The chief purpose of exercise is to obtain a normal development of tissues, so that they will be capable of performing their ordinary functions. The muscles of the trunk and of the back must be well-developed to maintain good posture. The muscles of the back, legs, and feet are needed to make walking, running, and jumping easy and graceful.

Exercise increases the circulation of the blood and thus aids nourishment of the individual cells of the body. Improved circulation also helps to remove waste material from the body. The proper circulation of the blood is related to the regulation of the heat of the body.

Exercise also increases the depth and rate of breathing, thus giving the red blood cells more oxygen to carry, and helps to eliminate the waste carbon dioxide from the body.

Following a reasonable amount of exercise in the open air the body feels refreshed and not exhausted. With such refreshment comes the relaxation that is exceedingly important for rest and good mental hygiene.

Finally, there is a psychological sense of satisfaction associated with being able to swing a golf club, a tennis racket, or an ax as well as the next man or in being able to row a boat or to swim when such an activity may be required.

There is apparently no absolute evidence that physical training produces a condition which helps to protect the body against disease. The chief value of exercise it that it increases the competence of the body to do physical work, improves fatigue and endurance, and produces perfection of movement.

The virtue of exercise does not lie in any increase of muscular strength but in its maintenance of the normal activities of the tissues. When a muscle contracts it uses up a substance called *glycogen,* which is present in muscles in large amounts. A waste product, *lactic acid,* accumulates. The blood takes up *carbon dioxide,* which develops from waste material, and carries it to the lungs, where it is eliminated from the body.

If carbonic acid and lactic acid accumulate, the muscles become acid in their reaction. If lactic acid accumulates in considerable amounts, the movement of the muscles will stop. Oxygen is required to aid continuous movement of the muscles.

Exercise—The charts on the succeeding pages depict some of the more common and useful exercises employed in maintaining good muscular tone and development. While these exercises are recommended for adults, it is also advisable for parents and physical education instructors to train children in their practice. Both adults and children benefit from regular systematized exercises such as those shown here.

1. THE STRETCHER

(Minimum 4; Maximum 10)

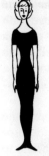

Starting position
standing erect

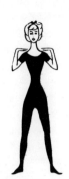

1. Right foot sideward,
hands at shoulders
(pull elbows
down)

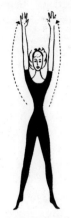

2. Hands upward,
rise on toes
(stretch)

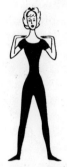

3. Hands at shoulders,
heels normal
(pull elbows
down)

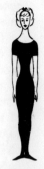

4. Right foot
normal, hands
normal

2. THE KICKER

(Minimum 6; Maximum 12)

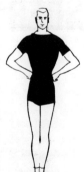

Start. pos.—
standing erect,
hands on hips

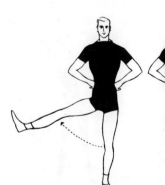

1. R. foot raised
sideward (kick
high)

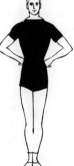

2. R. foot normal

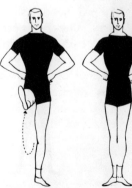

3. R. foot raised
forward (kick
high)

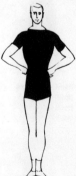

4. R. foot normal

579

3. THE TWISTER

(Minimum 6; Maximum 15)

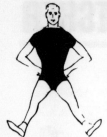

Start. pos.—
sitting on floor,
hands on hips,
feet apart (chest
high)

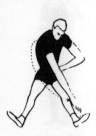

1. Trunk turned
L., R. hand on
L. toe

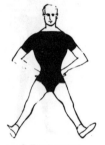

2. Trunk normal
R. hand on hip
(chest up)

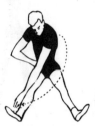

3. Trunk turned
R., L. hand on
R. toe

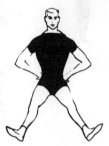

4. Trunk normal,
R. hand on hip
(chest high)

4. THE SIDE BENDER

(Minimum 6; Maximum 15)

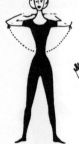

Start. pos.—feet
apart, hands at
neck (elbows
back)

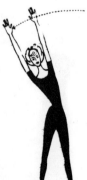

1. Trunk bent R.,
hands upward
(stretch)

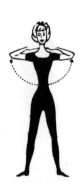

2. Trunk normal,
hands at neck
(elbows back)

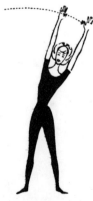

3. Trunk bent L.,
hands upward
(stretch)

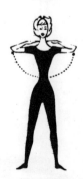

4. Trunk normal,
hands at neck
(elbows back)

580

5.THE NECK PRESSER

(Minimum 6; Maximum 15)

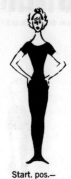

Start. pos.—
hands on hips

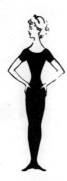

1. Head turned
R. and drawn
backward

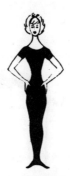

2. Head normal
(don't let head
sag)

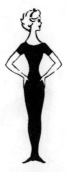

3. Head turned
L. and drawn
backward

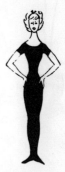

4. Head normal
(don't slump)

6. THE LEG LIFTER

(Minimum 6; Maximum 15)

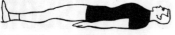

Start. pos.—back
on floor

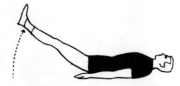

1. Feet half
upward (knees
kept straight)

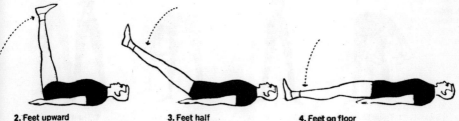

2. Feet upward
(keep hips on
floor)

3. Feet half
upward (same
as count one)

4. Feet on floor

581

7. THE SQUATTER

(Minimum 6; Maximum 15)

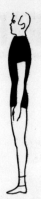

Start. pos.—
standing erect

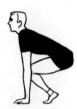

1. Squat on floor
(hands near
feet)

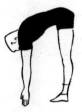

2. Knees straight
(keep hands
on floor)

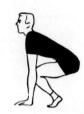

3. Squat on floor
(same as
count one)

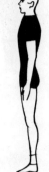

4. Stand erect

8. THE COMPRESSOR

(Minimum 6; Maximum 15)

Start. pos.—feet
straddle hands
sideward

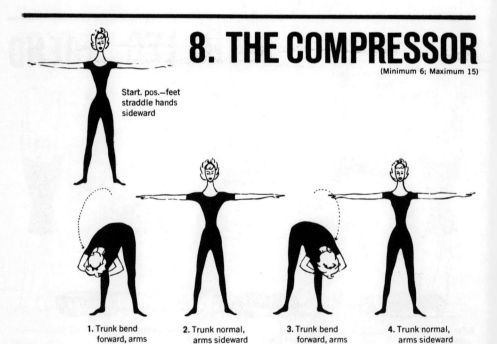

1. Trunk bend
forward, arms
about right
knee

2. Trunk normal,
arms sideward

3. Trunk bend
forward, arms
about left
knee

4. Trunk normal,
arms sideward

582

9. THE DIPPER

(Minimum 6; Maximum 15)

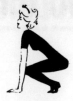 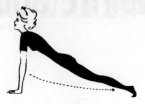

Start. pos.—squat on floor (hands near feet)

1. Feet backward (trunk and legs straight)

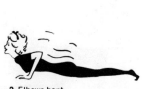 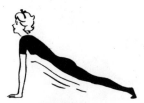 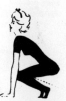

2. Elbows bent (only hands and toes touch floor)

3. Elbows straight (same as count one)

4. Squat on floor (same as starting position)

10. THE TURN AND BEND

(Minimum 6; Maximum 15)

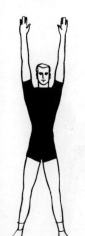 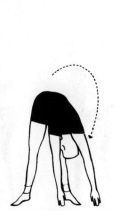 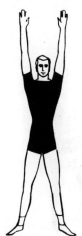 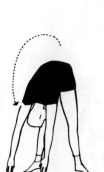 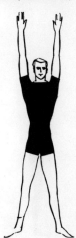

Start. pos.—feet apart, hands upward

1. Trunk bent L., drawn downward (stretch)

2. Trunk normal (keep chest high)

3. Trunk bent R., drawn downward (stretch)

4. Trunk normal, arms overhead

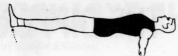

11. THE LEG CIRCLER

(Minimum 6; Maximum 15)

Start. pos.—back on floor, feet raised one foot

1. Legs to L., knees straight (keep legs together)

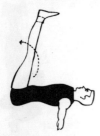

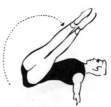

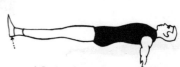

2. Legs in front of chest (arms stay outstretched)

3. Legs to R., knees straight (keep legs together)

4. Back on floor, feet raised one foot

12. THE HIGH STEPPER

(Minimum 10 steps; Maximum 20 steps)

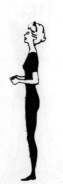
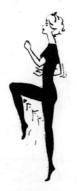
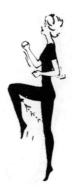
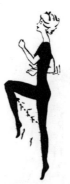
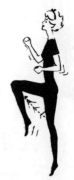

Start. pos.—standing erect, fists clenched

Run in place. (raise arms and knees vigorously)

Left

Right

Left

13. THE EXPANDER
(Minimum 5; Maximum 10)

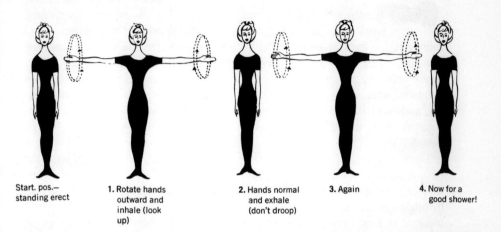

Start. pos.—
standing erect

1. Rotate hands
outward and
inhale (look
up)

2. Hands normal
and exhale
(don't droop)

3. Again

4. Now for a
good shower!

14. THE ROWER
(Minimum 6; Maximum 15)

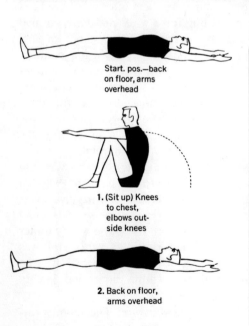

Start. pos.—back
on floor, arms
overhead

1. (Sit up) Knees
to chest,
elbows out-
side knees

2. Back on floor,
arms overhead

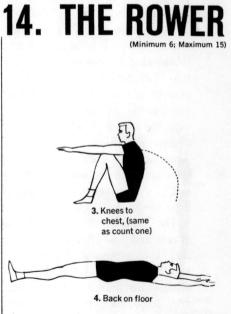

3. Knees to
chest, (same
as count one)

4. Back on floor

When oxygen comes in, the lactic acid disappears, the glycogen accumulates again, and the muscles become alkaline rather than acid. Large amounts of oxygen are necessary for continuous work by the muscles.

Thus, a person who is doing hard muscular work requires ten times more oxygen than he needs when he is resting. The extra oxygen, which is provided by speeding up the circulation, increases the rate of breathing and sometimes raises the pressure of the blood in the blood vessels.

During exercise the pulse rate becomes more rapid, the blood pressure rises, and more blood goes through the tissues. The amount of increase depends on the rapidity and continuity with which, and the length of time during which, the muscles are being used.

In addition to the value of exercise for improving the general health is its value in improving the condition of tissues that have been weakened by disease. Therefore, restricted exercise is prescribed for people who have such conditions as heart disease or high blood pressure. These exercises must be controlled by trained attendants, so that the sick person never becomes fatigued, exhausted, or overexercised.

The balance between beneficial effects and bad effects is so delicate that it is impossible for anyone to regulate the exercise in relation to disease for himself. Even doctors who have such conditions cannot regulate for themselves the amount of effort they may put forth.

Serious harm, at times even death, has resulted from having a doctor tell such patients casually that they need exercise, without specifically prescribing the character and the amount. In determining physical fitness the doctor studies the pulse the blood pressure, the breathing, and the condition of the blood.

Pulse. Everyone should know how to measure the rate of the pulse. The rate is much faster in children than in adults. It varies from just over 100 beats a minute for a three-year-old to eighty-one for a boy of twelve; sixty-eight or seventy for a youth of eighteen, and sixty-eight for a man of sixty. The rate for women is five to nine beats higher in each age group.

Here is how the pulse gauge works in relation to exercise. Count your pulse beat after you have been sitting for a while and have not had any exercise. Then stand up and simulate running for a few minutes. Running of this type for five minutes will speed the heart and pulse more than the same exercise for three minutes. The longer the exercise, the longer time required for the rate to return to normal.

Among a group of boys who ran the 100-yard dash there was an average increase of forty-five beats per minute in the pulse at the end of the race. The pulse of a sprinter who had run 400 yards still was sixteen beats above normal after he had rested one hour and twenty minutes.

Blood pressure. The blood pressure averages from 110 to 120 above the age of twenty years and up to the age of forty. From ten years to twenty years it averages about 100.

Exercises of strength, such as weightlifting, will raise the blood pressure. Exercises of speed, such as tennis or speed swimming, will cause the blood pressure to rise somewhat less rapidly and to return to normal more slowly.

When the blood pressure of a woman who had run up three flights of stairs in forty-five seconds was measured it was found to have risen forty points. In exercises of endurance, such as thirty-six holes of golf, a long hike across the country, or a slow bicycle tour, the blood pressure will not rise as high as it does in speed exercise. At the end of the trip it may actually be lower than ordinary.

Breathing. Breathing also varies according to the nature of the exercise. Training in breathing makes the difference between winning and losing an athletic event. In the short dashes the racer breathes normally through the time when the starter says, "On your mark." At the order "Get set" the sprinter will take a breath and hold it until the gun indicates the start. He will retain this breath until he is underway. Better sprinters hold their breath longer than those who are untrained.

Swimmers mostly shorten the time when the breath is taken in and given out and increase the rate of breathing with the rate of the stroke.

Expert golf players take a deep breath before the drive and hold it during the swing of the club. This serves to stiffen the chest muscles and aids in control of the arms.

After the drive the golfer lets out the air and breathes normally. During the putting the breathing should be quiet and shallow.

The average person breathes from seventeen to twenty times per minute. Women breathe a bit more rapidly than do men. All of us breathe more rapidly when standing than sitting. The amount of air taken in a single breath averages three quarts for a grown man; two quarts for a grown women.

Superstitions about exercise. Big muscles are not necessarily a sign of strength or a guarantee of long life. Overdeveloped muscles may be a liability rather than an asset.

The length of life depends on the general physical condition of the body as a whole and a great deal on the nature of the body that one has inherited from one's ancestors. People who live long tend to have children who live long.

Many peculiar devices have been developed for producing expansion or development of various portions of the body. Some contend that breathing exercises, which will greatly increase the expansion of the chest, are beneficial to health and long life. Actually the evidence shows that most such exercises are more harmful than beneficial.

Most of the important functions of the body related to health are automatic, including the work of the heart, the lungs, and the kidneys. This natural automaticity regulates the rate and depth of breathing in relation to the functions of the body of the person concerned.

Increased work brings increased need for oxygen and more and deeper breathing. Young people who participate regularly in a certain amount of wholesome physical activity, including ordinary games and competition, swimming, tennis, walking, rowing, and bicycle riding, will not worry about their rate of breathing.

Large lungs and vital capacity developed beyond the usual needs of the body mean that much of the tissue concerned will not be called on enough of the time to be helpful. Unused tissue tends to become infiltrated with fat and to become weak. This happens to the man who develops tremendous muscles and an enlarged heart by exercising during youth and then giving up all exercise as he gets older.

Young people need more exercise than do older ones, because their bodies are growing. They, therefore, take in more oxygen and give out more waste matter than does the ordinary adult.

Training improves an athlete and the quality of his performance. Training helps to coordinate the muscles, so that they give a better performance without using up as much energy as might otherwise be required. The danger of exertion may be overcome if boys and girls will be careful to warm up slowly before any activity, exactly as athletes do before football games or track meets. The warming-up process enables the body to reach its maximum requirement and prevents the short breath and discomfort which usually precede what athletes call the coming of the second wind.

Training increases the vital capacity—that is, the amount of air that can be handled by the lungs. The average athlete has a capacity of four to five quarts of air in contrast to three quarts for the non-athlete. The increase in endurance resulting from good physical training is shown by the fact that the onset of fatigue is delayed. Most important in training is practice in using the correct form. *See also* PHYSICAL THERAPY.

EXHAUSTION, a condition produced by loss of vital power from fatigue or protracted disease. Extreme exhaustion is known as *nervous prostration* or *psychasthenia,* sometimes referred to as *neurocirculatory asthenia* or *weakness.* The symptoms of exhaustion often include insomnia, loss of memory and appetite, listlessness, palpitations of the heart, and vitamin deficiency. Psychasthenia is rarely fatal, but it may render the person useless to himself, his family, and society. Corrective measures require a thorough examination, both mental and physical, of the person. Ordinarily a complete rest is imperative and possibly a radical revision of diet or even a change of occupation. *See also* ANEMIA; ASTHENIA; FATIGUE; HEAT SICKNESS.

EXHIBITIONISM, a variety of sexual deviation, seen most frequently in men, in which there is a compulsion to display the sexual organs, usually without desire for sexual union. Organized *nudism* is a related form of exhibitionism. The adult exhibitionist is typically an immature person, usually beset by feelings of inadequacy. Often he is conscientious in his daily work, and the tendency is not suspected by friends. Exhibitionists act from an uncontrollable inner tension and afterward experience depression and intense remorse. Psychiatrists believe that the disorder is the result of a subdued intense rage of some sort, a feeling of arrogance or hatred toward women and a desire to shock. Inner feelings of cruelty and sadism exist as well. The exhibitionist usually does not desire to inflict any physical harm. Treatment demands intensive psychiatric study; seldom can the person cure himself. *See also* HOMOSEXUALITY; NARCISSISM.

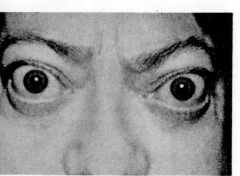

Exophthalmos—Protrusion of the eyeballs which occurs with enlargement of the thyroid gland. There is a great increase in appetite, and the patient is nervous and irritable. In severe conditions the eyeballs may protrude from the eye-sockets to such a degree that the eyelids cannot be closed. Repair of the thyroid gland and medical treatment can control the disease but the eyes do not return to their normal position in the sockets.

EXOPHTHALMIC GOITER, also known as *Graves' disease,* a disease caused chiefly by overproduction of the thyroid hormone with consequent enlarging of the thyroid gland. It is characterized by goiter, rapid heart action, protruding eyeballs, nervous excitability, fine involuntary tremor, loss of weight, muscular weakness, and a tendency to intense, acute exacerbations called *thyroid crises. See also* GLANDS; GOITER. *See* MEDIGRAPH page 769.

EXOPHTHALMOS, bulging or forward displacement of the eyes. Usually it is caused by an increase of pressure within the eye or by changes in the muscles of the eye. This condition is seen most often in cases of *exophthalmic goiter*.

EXPECTORATION, ejection of material from the mouth by coughing or spitting. Fluid or semifluid matter may be expelled from the lungs or air passages, or merely saliva. The matter expectorated, called *sputum,* may contain disease microbes, and spitting on floors and streets and public places is not only unesthetic but also unhealthful. Expectoration should be done into a handkerchief, or in places where it cannot do harm.

EYE, the organ of sight. Constructed like a camera, the eye is intricate and efficient. Most living species ordinarily have two eyes. The eyes of many other species surpass the human eye in certain respects. Many insects, for example,

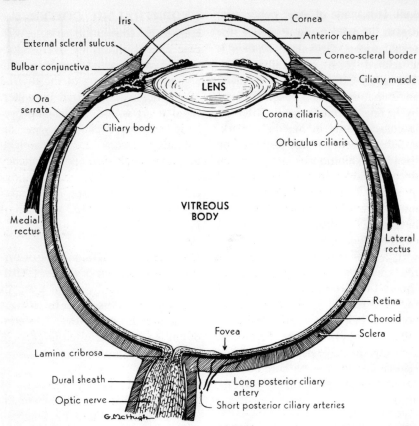

Iris
Cornea
External scleral sulcus
Anterior chamber
Corneo-scleral border
Bulbar conjunctiva
Ciliary muscle
Ora serrata
LENS
Corona ciliaris
Ciliary body
Orbiculus ciliaris
VITREOUS BODY
Medial rectus
Lateral rectus
Retina
Choroid
Fovea
Sclera
Lamina cribrosa
Dural sheath
Long posterior ciliary artery
Optic nerve
Short posterior ciliary arteries
G.McHugh

Eye—A vertical section of the eyeball, organ of vision. The eyeball is held in its socket by strong muscles. The *cornea* is the transparent external layer which protects the eye. If a portion of the cornea is defective and loss of sight is threatened, it is possible to remove the diseased area and transplant a piece of healthy cornea from another person's eye. Corneal transplantation does not restore sight in every case, despite the modern techniques developed, because other parts of the eye as well as the cornea may be unhealthy. The *lens* which focuses the image is held in place by the *suspensory ligament*. The *retina* receives the image and the *optic nerve* transmits it to the *brain*. The *iris* controls the amount of light entering the eye. It is like a colored curtain with a hole, the *pupil*. When one is looking at the eye, the iris appears doughnut-shaped, and the color may be brown, blue, green or gray, depending on hereditary factors. (Brown is by far the most common color in the world as a whole.) In strong or bright light, the pupil in the iris becomes smaller; in dim light, the pupil becomes larger. The *vitreous humor* is a clear, gelatinous substance behind the lens.

and some animals have eyes which are far more acute and efficient than those of human beings.

The eye in man is relatively small in relation to the total size of his body. If his eye were comparatively of the same size that the eye as- sumes in certain birds, an average- size man would have an eye weigh- ing five pounds.

Structure and mechanism of vision. The eye is nearly a perfect sphere and occupies the anterior part of the frontal cavity of the skull. It is made of three concentric layers: the *cornea,* the *iris,* and the *retina.* The cornea is transparent and fits into a white membrane called the *sclerotic coat.* The iris connects with the *choroid layer* by means of the *ciliary body.* The iris itself is a colored, circular membrane with a central perforation, the *pupil.* The retina, the innermost of the three layers, is a delicate transparent membrane containing the ends of the *optic nerve.* The *vitreous body,* a firm transparent jelly, constitutes about four-fifths of the eyeball. In front of the vitreous body is the *crystalline lens,* slightly yellow, disc-like in shape, transparent, and curving out on each side. The space between the lens and cornea is divided by the iris into two parts, the *anterior* and *posterior chambers,* which contain the *aqueous humor,* a transparent fluid. In front the eye is covered by the *conjunctiva,* a mucous membrane, and posteriorly by a *fibrous capsule.* The entire eyeball is moved by a group of muscles attached on the outer surface. The curvature of the lens is changed by the *ciliary muscle,* while the pupil is dilated by the action of the *dilator* and *constrictor fibers* in the iris.

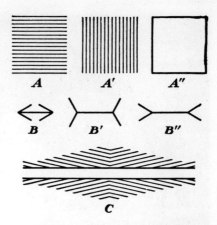

Eye—While the eye is one of the most precise instruments known, it is subject to optical illusions. Figures A, A', and A'' are of exactly the same size but appear to be of different sizes because the horizontal and vertical lines create a misleading impression. The lines shown in B, B', and B'' are of exactly the same length, but the diagonals induce a distorted interpretation. The two center lines shown in C are exactly parallel, but the diagonals again distort the image, making the parallels appear to diverge at the center.

To understand the mechanism of vision, some knowledge of the construction of the eye, as has been outlined above, is helpful. Actually *we do not see with the eye but with the brain and nervous system.* The chief factors involved in seeing are the *optic nerve* and the *brain's center for vision.* The retina, part of the

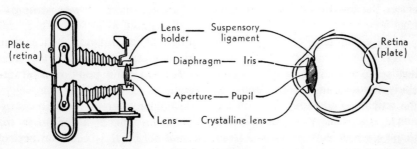

Eye—The eye is, in effect, a natural camera. Here are shown a camera with its principal components and the portions of the eye that correspond.

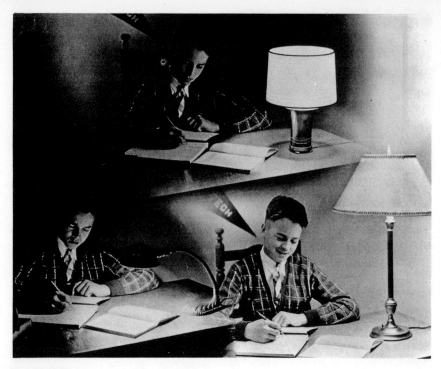

Eye—Eyesight can often be preserved if proper lighting is used at all times. Inade- quate light places strain on the eyes and makes work much more difficult.

nervous system, serves to convey images to the optic nerve. The lens is truly a lens, and serves to focus images on the retina, while the muscles control the size and shape of the lens in its focusing. Accessory muscles move the eyeball. The iris controls the amount of light which enters the eye by dilating and contracting.

Ideally the lens of the eye receives light from the outside and bends it so that the image is precisely focused on a small point of the retina. To maintain focus on the retina, the lens must change its shape when objects are viewed from different distances. This is called *accommodation*. When the eye is

unable to accommodate properly, *nearsightedness* or *farsightedness* may result.

Nearsightedness—*myopia*—is the condition in which one is unable to see objects clearly at a distance. It may be hereditary and frequently is not discovered for some time.

Farsightedness—*hypermetropia*— is the condition in which one sees things at a distance better than things close up because the light is focused at a point beyond the retina.

Another common condition is *astigmatism*. This is a change in the curvature of the outer surface of the eye, and the use of a proper lens 'will correct this curvature in most

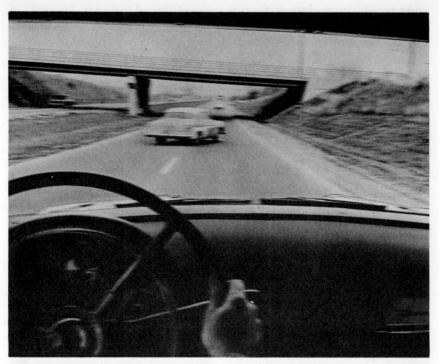

Astigmatism—Here, a representation of the effect produced by astigmatism is presented. In this case, horizontal lines are sharp but vertical lines are unsharp.

cases. In some cases, however, the curvature may be so irregular that lenses cannot be adapted to the curve.

When the muscles of the eye are unbalanced to such a degree that the action of the two eyes is dissociated and one eye tends to deviate away from the point at which vision will be correct, a number of possibilities exist for correction. One method is, of course, training to improve the strength of one muscle or another. Another method is operation on the muscles, shortening them or lengthening them to make conditions more balanced. A third possibility is the use of correct lenses to overcome the imbalance of the muscles.

The eye in its normal functioning has the ability to adapt itself to various conditions of light. Overuse will exhaust this ability, and proper lighting is necessary to prevent the eye from becoming strained or fatigued.

A newborn baby is farsighted and for that reason pays little attention to objects close to him. By two months, he is able to use his eye muscles to bring his eyes into range for what he wishes to see. The baby does not see small objects clearly until he is at least six months old. Because the eye of a baby is so delicate, it should be protected against strong light, injuries and irritants.

As people grow older, their eyes change. The most significant changes are those in which the lens becomes clouded, resulting in *cataract*. The muscles connected with change of shape of the lens to accommodate seeing at various distances do not respond as well as formerly. People past forty may require glasses when previously they had not needed them. Moreover, all the tissues concerned with the nutrition of the eye change as age increases, and the eye becomes functionally a less competent organ.

Except for time spent in sleeping, the eye is used almost constantly from the moment of birth until death. Overwork of the eyes results in earlier exhaustion, just as with any other organ. Therefore, vision should be facilitated in every possible way. The eye needs regular rest periods. To reduce strain, it is essential that suitable working conditions be given the eye.

The eye may be used for measuring the general state of health. Conversely the body may reflect trouble with the eyes. If the doctor finds the eyes clear and bright he will feel less concern about any immediate danger to general health. When a severe cold, fever or weakness from any cause is present, the eye will reflect this condition by lack of luster, heavy eyelids, and sluggish movement. In jaundice, the white of the eye becomes yellowish.

The eye may also reflect general disturbances of the body, such as hardening of the arteries, anemia, and diseases of the kidney and nervous system. A tumor in the brain is sometimes discovered because of difficulty with eyesight. Frequently double vision—*diplopia*—is the first symptom of inflammation of the brain. The pupils of the eye may be constantly contracted, dilated, or even unequal in size because of the effects of drugs on the body.

The dominant eye. Each eye transmits an image; these are fused by a higher center in the brain. Eyes may differ, one from the other. When a person sees everything with one eye and depends on the image from one eye only, he is called a *monocular*. If he sees with both eyes and the images are properly fused, he has *binocular* vision. A person may be right-eyed or left-eyed, just as he may be right-handed or left-handed, and the eye on which he depends is called the *dominant eye*. When anything happens to the dominant eye, the other must then dominate. Little difficulty occurs if the eye that had not been dominant previously works satisfactorily. However, if that eye cannot assume dominance, a variety of symptoms may result, such as stuttering, fatigue, or various types of hysterical attacks in addition to symptoms related to vision.

Many animals are organized on a one-sided basis, so that the eye, the hand, and the foot on the same side work together in order to achieve the best possible results. Obviously throwing the eye out of function on that side will interfere with the activities involving the foot and hand as well.

Various tests have been devised to determine which eye is dominant.

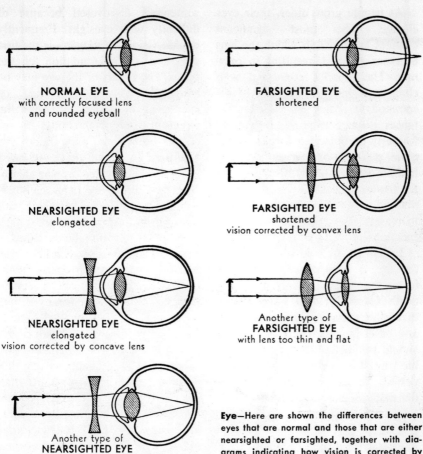

NORMAL EYE
with correctly focused lens
and rounded eyeball

NEARSIGHTED EYE
elongated

NEARSIGHTED EYE
elongated
vision corrected by concave lens

Another type of
NEARSIGHTED EYE
caused by the lens of the eye being
too thick and too greatly curved

FARSIGHTED EYE
shortened

FARSIGHTED EYE
shortened
vision corrected by convex lens

Another type of
FARSIGHTED EYE
with lens too thin and flat

Eye—Here are shown the differences between eyes that are normal and those that are either nearsighted or farsighted, together with diagrams indicating how vision is corrected by wearing suitably curved lenses.

One test is merely to ask the person concerned to look through a cylinder-like roll of paper. The eye that he uses for this purpose is the sighting eye. He uses the sighting eye when shooting. Another test is to ask the person concerned to look through a hole in the middle of an 8 × 10 inch piece of cardboard. He will look through the hole with one or the other eye and that will be the dominant eye.

If the person is found to be using the left eye for most such purposes and the right hand for other functions, the question of harmony between these activities needs investigation. Thus, a right-handed person with a dominant left eye may represent a problem. If a person's natural left-handedness has been changed so that the hands no longer work in harmony with the dominant eye, many difficulties will be understandable.

Color blindness. Color blindness is more common among men than among women. Difficulty in distin-

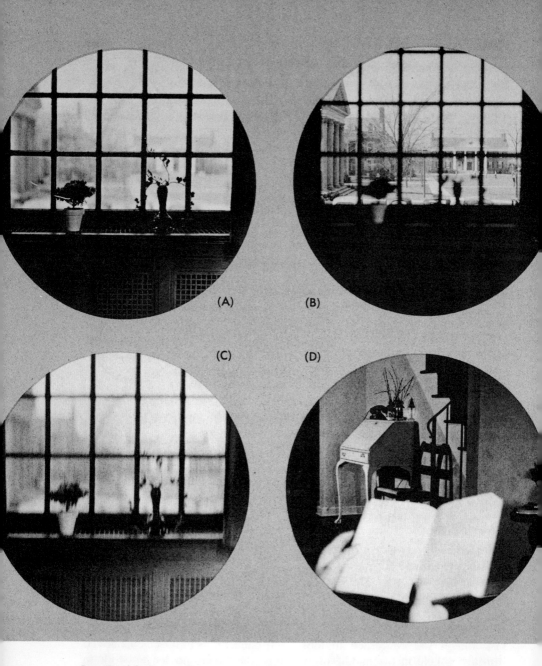

(A)

(B)

(C)

(D)

Eye—(*Top left*) The *myopic* eye sees near objects sharp and distant objects unsharp. (*Top right*) The *hyperopic* eye has sharp distant vision but unsharp near vision. (*Bottom left*) The *anastigmatic* eye sees lines in different directions with varying degrees of sharpness. In this photograph, the vertical lines are sharper than the horizontal. (*Bottom right*) The presbyopic eye, like the hyperopic, results in unsharp near vision, although distant vision may be satisfactorily sharp. However, the cause is entirely different from that of hyperopia. Presbyopia is caused by the loss of the accommodative function of the lens; it loses its elasticity so that it can no longer focus near and sharp with equal ease.

guishing between red and green is the most common form of color blindness. The blue-yellow dilemma is much rarer. Color-blind persons see objects as lighter or darker, but are unable to distinguish the shades. Sometimes they may distinguish between red and green lights on roadways by their difference in brightness.

Everyone who drives a car or works in an occupation in which color detection is significant should have a test to determine whether or not he is color blind. A test for color blindness may consist of sorting and matching color samples. Traffic signals are most frequently red, green, and yellow and occasionally blue, colors most frequently concerned in color blindness. Therefore, a color-blind person should not drive a car.

A specific cure for color blindness is not possible, since the defect is one of structure of the eye. However, color vision may be developed or substitutions found.

In certain branches of the armed services, like the navy and air force, color blindness is a bar to admission.

Vision of the child. When a child reaches one year of age, parents can, with a simple test, determine whether or not his vision is perfect. A bandage may be tied over one eye. Then a block, a ball, or any toy that the child uses may be placed near him. If the vision of the child is normal, he will pick up the object when either eye is bandaged, indicating that each eye functions properly by itself. If, however, the child is slow to detect the toy or unable to recognize it, an eye specialist should be consulted.

The next significant time for testing vision is when the child begins to read. Difficulties of vision may be present if the child holds the book too close to his eyes, too far away, or at an unusual angle. Such peculiarities call for immediate testing of the child's vision.

Certain other elementary symptoms are quickly apparent. A child with a pronounced degree of *astigmatism* may frown as he reads; he may have an aversion to reading because he associates it with headaches and discomfort. Sometimes one eye alone may be farsighted and the child will be able to get along by using just the good eye.

Unfortunately the child who is nearsighted has few readily detected symptoms. He sees things that are close and is not concerned about objects at a distance. The difficulty may first become apparent when the child plays a game, such as baseball or basketball, or is taken to a motion picture.

Cross-eyes. Any straining of the eye or imbalance of the muscles may result in cross eyes or squint (*strabismus*). Children may be born with one or both eyes crossed. A squint or walleye may develop from excessive strains placed on the external muscle of the eye by the extra effort which is required to see when there is an extreme degree of nearsightedness.

Children rarely outgrow cross-eyes. The sight of the crossed eye may never develop and, in many instances, the squint or crossed eye

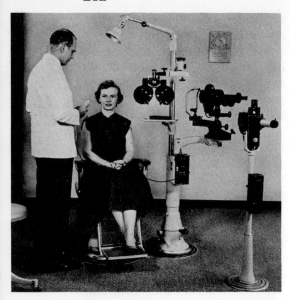

Eye—By the use of this modern refracting unit, the doctor has within easy reach all the instruments he needs for a complete visual analysis.

becomes worse. Early diagnosis and treatment are essential for the best results. As soon as one notices that a child is cross-eyed, an eye specialist should be consulted. Sometimes good results are obtained merely with proper eyeglasses, which tend to hold the two eyes in position. Children have been found able to tolerate eyeglasses at the age of fifteen months.

The weak eye may be exercised by various training devices to correct the habit of suppressing the image of one eye. In certain disorders, when the deficiency is slight, this *orthoptic training* is successful. The most favorable age for such therapy is between three and six years. After the age of seven the results are less satisfactory.

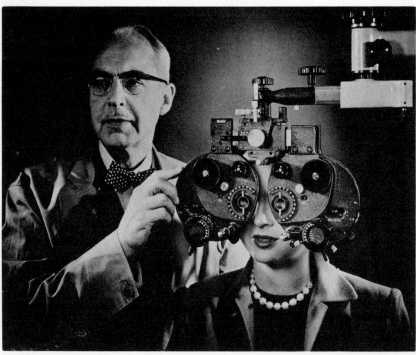

Eye—With this instrument, the doctor is measuring the *refractive error* of the eye.

The surgical procedure for overcoming cross-eyes is the most certain method of correction. Proper placement of the eye muscles by the surgeon tends to bring the eye back into proper relationship to the other eye and permit binocular vision. The operation is not a guarantee that vision will be improved, but it will prevent the vision from being eventually lost from failure to use the eye successfully. In addition, the correction of cross-eyes is essential in establishing a proper mental attitude in the child. Children with cross-eyes may be so sensitive to ridicule that they become shy, withdrawn, introverted personalities and their lives affected as a consequence.

Color of the eyes. The color of the eyes is apparently governed by heredity. When a blue-eyed person marries a brown-eyed person and there are four children, one probably will have blue eyes, one brown eyes, and two may have blue eyes with traces of brown. Brown-eyed parents may produce not only children with brown eyes but also blue-eyed children. The color of the eye is helpful in determining paternity but is hardly conclusive.

Colored rings. When one looks at bright light at night—for example, street lamps—they may seem to be surrounded by areas of color or colored rings, blue on the inside and red on the outside. This is not a disturbance of the eye, for these colors are due to the tissues and cornea of the eye. The tissues are not seen in ordinary light.

Specks before the eyes; muscae volantes. Because of the structure of the eyes, several disturbances of vision may develop which are not actual defects but merely tricks of eye function. If a person suddenly looks up at the sky or at a white ceiling after the eyes have been closed, he will probably notice a number of minute specks that move in front of the eyes. These specks are blood corpuscles moving in the smallest blood vessels at the back of the eyes. If the heart beats faster because of exercise, the blood corpuscles will move faster and the specks will also seem to move faster.

Eyestrain. Eyestrain is common. Unsuspected eyestrain may be associated with twitching of the eyelids and face. Nausea and vomiting may appear, with headache, loss of appetite, and many other similar con-

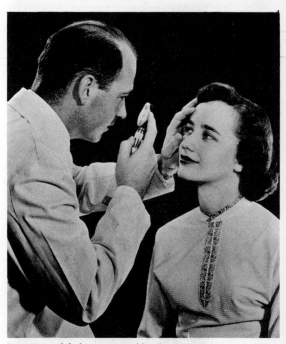

Eye—The *ophthalmoscope* enables the eye specialist to examine the retina of the eye.

599

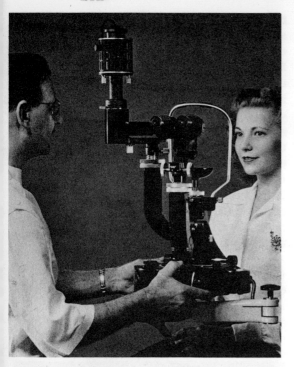

Eye—The *biomicroscope*, consisting of a stereo-scopic microscope and special light source, makes it possible for the doctor to study and observe the anterior portion of the eye (the conjunctiva, cornea, lens, and vitreous area).

lighted, and long periods of viewing may produce an uncomfortable condition.

Conjunctivitis. The tissue which lines the eyelids and runs out over the eyeball is called the *conjunctiva*. Inflammation of this tissue is known as *conjunctivitis* or *pinkeye*. Its symptoms are smarting and burning of the eyelids, formation of pus, and reddened eyelids. The inflamed eye becomes exceedingly sensitive to light, and tears flood it constantly. After sleep, the eyelids may be crusted together. This ordinary disorder of the eye demands care by a qualified doctor. Treatment is based on the severity of the infection and the character of the particular germ.

Styes. Styes involve infection of the glands of the eyelid by one of the common pus-forming germs, usually near a hair follicle, and often appear in crops. In some instances they are associated with uncorrected errors of vision. Under such circumstances the eye does not resist invasion by outside organisms as well as the normally functioning eye.

A stye behaves like a pimple or small boil. After a day or two it softens and bursts, the infectious material is discharged, and recovery usually follows. Before the stye has softened, its progress can sometimes be stopped by pulling out the hair that runs through it, and by treating the spot with an antiseptic that is not dangerous to the eye itself. Usually it is helpful to apply hot compresses to styes, to hasten the development of the inflammation. When a yellow spot appears, the infectious material should be released at once.

ditions. The only conclusive way to determine whether or not eyestrain actually exists is to test the ability of the eyes to see, and then to overcome the condition by rest or with eyeglasses.

Glare or bright light places stress on the eyes. Special care should be taken to insure proper lighting in the home, schools, offices, and factories. Although motion pictures and television may provoke eyestrain and fatigue, under normal conditions they do not cause serious eyestrain. However, the wrong type of lighting in the theater or home, films that are jerky, spotted, or badly

In the case of repeated formation of styes, physicians collect the germs causing them, make a vaccine from them, and reinject this vaccine into the patient. This may help the patient to develop specific resistance against the germs responsible for the styes.

Glaucoma. Glaucoma causes 15 per cent of all blindness in the United States, and about one-half of the blindness in adults. In this condition, pressure within the eyeball brings about loss of sight. Interference occurs with the circulation of the fluid that comes into the eye. The accumulation of this fluid causes pressure, and as the pressure increases there is pain, the eye becomes hard and reddened and the pupil gray and cloudy. This describes the acute form of glaucoma.

In a second and more serious form of glaucoma, gradual obstruction of the drainage system occurs so that the pressure increases slowly and the loss of sight is gradual.

The physician can determine the extent and effect of the pressure with the *ophthalmoscope* and the *tonometer*. Drugs have been developed which eliminate fluid and lower pressure within the eye.

As the glaucoma develops, the person finds that he can see straight ahead as well as he ever could, but not so well to the sides. Gradually the vision in front also becomes narrowed until finally there is complete loss of sight.

Eye—With the *retinal camera*, actual photographs of the retina can be taken in black and white or in color to record its condition exactly and permanently.

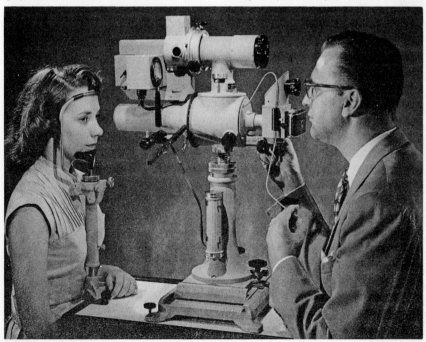

In the treatment of early glaucoma, drugs, such as DIAMOX®, may be sufficient. In later stages, drugs prepare the tissues of the eye so that an operation to relieve the pressure, known as an *iridectomy* because part of the iris is cut out, may be more easily and successfully performed.

An instrument useful in measuring the width of the field of vision is the *perimeter*. If the field is steadily narrowing, glaucoma is present. A correct diagnosis early in the development of glaucoma is invaluable in preventing pain and pressure and in saving sight.

Older women should be particularly watchful of their eyes, as they are more likely to suffer from glaucoma than men.

Excitement is often a factor in producing glaucoma, because of the increased flow of blood to the eyes during excitement, with consequent rise in pressure. Early symptoms may include headache, blurred vision, eye pain, and nausea. Prompt attention should be paid and an ophthalmologist consulted.

Tumors. Tumors may arise in the lids, the eye socket, or within the eyeball, and may interfere with vision and cause irritation of the eyeball. They should be removed, even though they are generally benign tumors. Malignant tumors sometimes occur, which can spread and may require removal of the eye. The most common malignant tumor of the eye, *retinoblastoma,* usually occurs in children under ten years of age, and may even occur at birth. *Malignant melanoma,* a sometimes fatal form of eye tumor, occurs most commonly in adults, arising inside the eye and spreading throughout the body if not checked in time and removed.

Fatigue. An eye which is fatigued and unable to work satisfactorily becomes easily irritated. Moreover, it is more apt to be invaded by foreign bodies, like cinders and dust, simply because the tissues do not react to rid the eye of such foreign material. Persons with bad eyesight frequently have red rims on the eyes, swollen eyelids and constant watering, and the eyelids may be crusted together in the morning. The appearance of any of these signs should be an indication that the eye needs medical care.

Iritis. The iris is the colored portion of the eye. It becomes infected and inflamed due to various causes. When it is infected it becomes swollen, dull, and discolored. The pupil gets small, gray, and sluggish. There is pain, which is worse at night, radiating to the forehead and to the temple, and there is much disturbance of vision. In most infections of the eye the person who has an inflammation of the iris cannot stand to look at the light, and there is constant watering of the eye.

One of the most common causes of this condition is *syphilis*. However, the iris may also become infected by other germs and may be involved in rheumatic conditions. It is of the utmost importance to take care of this condition immediately because the inflammation and infection may result in scarring which will either block the pupil entirely or bind the iris down in such a manner as to prevent its motion. Obviously this will cause a permanent disturbance of vision.

When a doctor takes care of this condition, he applies drugs which relieve the congestion and put the part at rest. Dilatation of the pupil will prevent the scarring and tend to break up the small scars that have already formed. Various preparations of *atropine* are useful for this purpose. There are other drugs which are anesthetic in character and which prevent pain. The doctor may prescribe also moist, hot compresses for several hours, which will tend to diminish the pain and the inflammation.

Of particular importance, however, is the treatment of this, as of other conditions, through the body as a whole. Syphilis affecting the eye means syphilis elsewhere in the body and demands the kind of consistent and persistent treatment that is necessary for this condition. The rheumatic condition with which iritis is sometimes associated must be treated for the general rheumatic disturbance, with the detection, if possible, of the focus of infection of the body and with the elimination of that focus when it is found. Other types of septic infection must also be controlled. When there is *diabetes,* the treatment of the condition by diet and insulin so as to control the diabetes throughout the body generally is even more important than the treatment of the condition as it affects the eyes.

Once the condition is healed, surgical operations of various kinds, in-

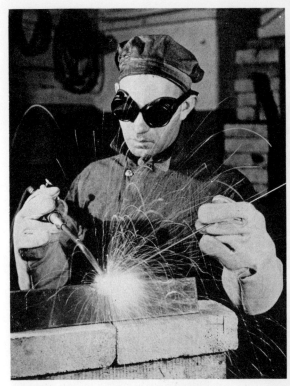

Eye—Many jobs in industry are hazardous. This man is dressed properly for arc welding. Note the large goggles which protect his eyes.

cluding plastic operations, may be necessary to bring about normal restoration of the iris and thus aid vision.

Trachoma. This is a serious infection affecting the eyelids. These infections may spread to the cornea, causing large ulcers, with partial or complete loss of eyesight. It may be necessary to use treatment that is practically constant day and night, to save the eyesight. Indeed, most physicians recommend that the patient be put in the hospital. Sulfadiazine and other drugs and streptomycin have also been found useful in controlling trachoma.

Ulcer on eye. The most dangerous infection of the eye is ulcer on the eyeball. This may be due to any kind of infection, but the worst forms are those due to the germ that causes pneumonia, the *pneumococcus,* and the one that causes gonorrhea, the *gonococcus.* In both of these types there is rapid destruction of the tissue of the eyeball. If there is penetration or perforation due to such destruction, the interior of the eyeball is also infected, and then there is complete loss of vision.

There is another type of infection of the cornea or covering of the eyeball which occurs most frequently in young children who are undernourished and have frequent colds, and particularly in those who have *tuberculosis.* In such cases there is an excessive flow of tears and a great aversion to light. This symptom is called *photophobia.* Because of the aversion to light, which produces blinking and pain, the person is likely to keep the eyelid shut on the inflamed eye. If the eye is studied, it will be found full of little flecks of material deposited by the inflammation. Syphilis is also sometimes responsible for inflammation of the cornea.

It must be remembered that there are various ways in which germs can attack the eye. They may come in from the outside or from the inside. The same germs that cause inflammation in the joints or in the nervous system, coming from infection in the tonsils, or the teeth, or the throat, may also be carried by the blood to the eyes and bring about serious infection there. Under the

circumstances, the mere healing of the condition in the eye is not sufficient. It is necessary to find the systemic cause responsible and to take care of that as well.

People with tuberculosis, infections of the teeth, the tonsils or the sinuses, with high blood pressure, kidney disease, or diabetes may have symptoms affecting their eyes directly related to the other diseases that have been mentioned, and the diseases of the eye will not be improved until the other conditions are brought under control.

Inflammation of retina. The tissues of the eye behind the lens are also subject to infections and inflammations. There are the delicate membranes of blood vessels and pigments, the rigid outer coating, and the retina or membrane of light perception. The large cavity is filled with *vitreous,* the fluid of the eye. Normally, rays of light pass through the vitreous without any hindrance, but occasionally there are small pieces of tissue in the vitreous which cast a shadow on the retina, such shadows being seen constantly as specks. Inflammations which affect the retina and the delicate membrane associated with it may be associated with the changes that take place in the blood vessels or tissues in old age, with infections elsewhere in the body, and with specific damage to the tissue itself.

The physician uses the ophthalmoscope to look into the eye and to observe any changes that have occurred in these tissues. Sometimes he sees changes in the retina which indicate a systemic disorder, such as *diabetes, tuberculosis,* and *high blood pressure.* Obviously that condition must be taken care of before any attempts are made in relationship to the eye itself.

Detachment of retina. Sometimes the retina itself is loosened, so that the condition called *detachment of the retina* occurs. As soon as any part of the retina becomes detached from its bed, the vision controlled by that part is disturbed, and unless it is reattached in a short time the vision is lost permanently. The person who has had detachment of the retina should go to bed immediately. Sometimes competent control of fluid intake helps the situation. In other instances operations have been developed which appear to be useful in aiding reattachment of the retina. Several competent authorities say that reattachment with recovery of vision occurs in about 15 per cent of the cases. A device called a *laser* has been invented which throws a beam of light to the retina and causes reattachment by coagulation.

Cataract. The lens does not have blood vessels or nerves but receives its nourishment from the fluid material in the eye. The lens is entirely surrounded by a capsule which acts as a filter, keeping out undesirable material. Should this capsule be broken, the lens is infiltrated with material from the fluid of the eye; then it becomes cloudy, and the person has what is called *traumatic cataract.* As people get very old, the capsule gradually becomes less efficient, and the nutrition of the lens is interfered with. As the lens becomes clouded, it gradually becomes cloudy from the outside toward the center. When finally the center becomes clouded, it is exceedingly difficult for the person to see. This condition is called *senile cataract.*

It must be remembered that the human eye is like a camera. It has a lens; it has a shutter, which is the iris. The pupil is the hole in the shutter through which the light enters. At the back of the eye is the retina or sensitized plate on which the image is cast.

Most cases of cloudiness or cataract of the lens, such as have been described, occur in people between fifty and seventy years of age. The only treatment for senile cataract is surgical. There are no drugs, no drops of any kind, no exercise or treatments which are successful in stopping the slow development of a cataract. Nevertheless, such methods of treatment have been used by vast numbers of quacks to get money from people who fear approaching blindness because of cataract.

There are numerous operations now developed which are relatively simple and which are quite safe in the majority of instances. Moreover, good vision follows in 97 per cent of the operations for cataract. After the cataract is removed, the person wears what are known as *cataract glasses.* These are made so that they help in focusing the image properly on the retina. By use of a hormone called *chymotrypsin* the tissues surrounding the lens may be softened and this has greatly facilitated the operation for cataract.

Tear ducts. Tears keep the eyes moist so that the delicate tissues, of which they are made, are preserved. If the eyes are not constantly kept moist, the tissues dry and are much more easily attacked by bacteria.

In a little bony notch on the inner side of the eye there is a gland called the *lacrimal gland.* From this, six or more little tubes carry the tears to the eyes. There is another tube, which is known as the *nasal duct,* which carries fluid from the eyes to the nose. Hence, whenever a person cries or his eyes water, his nose runs simultaneously. When the amount of moisture is so great as to overflow, the excess comes down through the nasal duct until there is so much that it falls on the cheeks. Most of the time there is just enough moisture to keep the eye in the proper state of softness and luster.

Occasionally a tear duct becomes blocked because of the presence in it of a cinder or a hair. Under such circumstances, it is necessary to open it up. This requires special instruments and the care of a physician who knows how to do the unblocking correctly.

In other instances the gland and the duct become infected. Then there is a reddened swelling in the inner corner of the eye and the discharge of a small amount of pus. Pressure over the swelling will force out most of the pus. It is sometimes possible to get relief by treatment, but in other instances it may be necessary to cut into the gland, and there are instances in which it has to be removed surgically.

In 1581 a Latin writer described a girl sixteen years old whose tears resembled blood. Other cases have been described in many countries. Apparently in such cases there has been a leaking of red blood cells out of the blood vessels into the lacrimal gland. In some instances in which bloody tears appeared, the women concerned had not experienced the normal changes that occur to girls. In other cases there were tumors of the eyelids.

Transplanting the cornea. One of the most sensational medical procedures has been transplantation of the transparent membrane which covers the surface of the eye and which is known as the *cornea.* Sometimes a scar appears in this tissue as a result of an infection or an injury or a burn, and as a result the vision is prevented as if a curtain were drawn over the pupil of the eye.

Not every case of scarring is suitable to such an operation. Failure of the operation may lead to severe emotional disturbances. Hence the surgeon and the specialist must choose the cases according to a wide variety of considerations which vary with every case. There are many diseases of the eye in which the scarring over the pupil is simply incidental. If there are severe scars, such as result from powder burns or burns by lime, involving all of the layers of the cornea, the transplant is seldom successful. Certain eyes are exceedingly sensitive to surgical procedures, and secondary inflammation may result in complete loss of sight.

Eye banks have been established from which the ophthalmic surgeon obtains the necessary material for use in the transplant. Frequently the material to be transplanted is obtained from the eyes of stillborn infants. Of special importance is the great amount of care necessary to be given to such eyes following an operation, because obviously secondary infection might not only damage the results of the operation but leave the patient with an eye worse off than the eye he had before the operation. The eye bank in New York City now supplies about twenty-five eyes each year, but its facilities have been increased so that tissue for transplantation is now available for as many as two hundred eyes each year. The operation of an eye bank is an exceedingly costly and difficult matter, requiring technical services that are not generally available.

Black eye. One of the most common disturbances of the eye is injury caused by a blow of some type. Indeed, these injuries are so common that they have become common material for the cartoonist. The immediate effect of a blow on the eye with a blunt instrument may not be serious, but the later effects may be extremely serious. It is, therefore, best to treat every severe blow of the eye as a serious condition until sufficient time has passed to indicate the extent of the damage. Sometimes there is merely bleeding of the small vessels in the white of the eye. An x-ray picture may show that the bones of the skull which surround the eye have been broken.

It is safe, whenever one has had a blow on the eye, to go to bed immediately and to put an ice-bag on the eye and to have competent medical attention as soon as possible.

Penetrating injury. Much more serious than a blow with a blunt instrument is the penetrating injury, such as may be brought about by a sharp probe, or by flying particles of glass, steel, or similar material. If any of the fluid material of the eye has escaped through the injury, the condition is especially serious. Fortunately, the x-ray is now of great aid in indicating whether or not a substance has actually penetrated the eyeball.

The removal of the foreign substance from the eyeball is a most difficult process, and one of which only trained physicians are capable. The use of a magnet is sometimes helpful. There are many substances which are not attracted by a magnet and which may cause great harm if they remain in the eye. Sooner or later destruction of the tissue occurs around the foreign substance. Sometimes there is infection, and not infrequently complete loss of vision.

Flying particles of hot steel are usually free from infection. However, even when germs are not carried into the eye with the foreign substance, they may be brought to the eye by the blood and localize in the spot which has been damaged by the irritation.

Sympathetic ophthalmia. Most serious in connection with any penetrating injury of the eye is the serious inflammation of the other eye, known as *sympathetic ophthalmia*. This occurs some fourteen days after the injury to the first eye, most frequently in from four to six weeks, but may occur many months or even years later. The appearance of the eye first injured helps the physician to determine the possible onset of such an inflammation in the other eye. In the majority of cases, proper preventive measures are taken immediately. If the first eye is severely damaged and inflammation is serious, it is customary to remove the injured eye promptly before any signs of inflammation have appeared in the second eye. In some instances *cortisone* has been helpful.

No one knows yet just why sympathetic ophthalmia occurs. It is such a serious condition, however, as it means loss of both eyes rather than of one, that the physician must give the benefit of the doubt to the patient. If the vision of the eye first injured is destroyed, if the eye is soft, if it is painful, and if the condition seems to be progressive, the physician may feel that to remove the eye immediately is safest for the patient.

Guarding eyesight. Here are a few simple rules helpful in guarding eyesight:

1. Do not face bright windows or bright light when at work.

2. Never cleanse the eyes with a towel used by others.

3. Do not place hooks, doorstops, or other projections at the level of children's eyes. If such objects are placed near the floor or above children's eye level, there are less likely to be serious accidents involving a child's eyes.

Prevention of eye injuries in industry. Blindness or impairment of vision is one of the most serious and costly of all nonfatal accidents which workers may suffer.

Some eye disorders are known to be definitely associated with processes involving intense light and heat. For instance, a cataract occurs in the eyes of glass workers, who are exposed to the heat and glare of a furnace for many hours each week. All sorts of devices have been developed to prevent exposure of eyes of glass workers to this and other hazards. Fortunately the introduction of machinery for making glass bottles and other machinery to take the place of hand operations has minimized the dangers of furnace glare. Workers in other industries, like steel making, who are regularly exposed to glare from furnaces should wear appropriate glasses to shut out the light.

Workers in electric arc welding sometimes have inflammation of the eyes, with pain and headache. Similar symptoms affect workers in studios where photography, such as motion picture and television photography, is the chief occupation. Here again, careful attention to prevention of overlong exposure to powerful lights is imperative to overcome the hazard.

Certain industrial poisons are dangerous to the eyes, including ammonia, phosphorus, derivatives of lead, benzene, and methyl alcohol. At least fifty known poisons that can affect the eyes are used in industrial processes. Inhalation of poisonous dust or vapor and direct action of the poison on workers who have not throughly cleansed their hands is possible.

Adequate provision for frequent washing of hands by workers, and the use of exhaust fans for getting rid of dusts and gases are the best means of eliminating industrial eye hazards. The prevention of accidents to the eyes involves protection against flying fragments of metal, stone, and grit, and against burns from acids or strong caustics.

Properly made goggles, helmets, and shields are part of the safety program of well-managed plants.

Safety rules in eye injuries.

1. Under no circumstances should an untrained or inexperienced person attempt to remove any foreign body from the eye.

2. Immediately after an accident, the eye may be bathed with suitable mild aseptic or sterilized solutions, preferably a weak solution of boric acid made with sterilized water.

3. The eye should be covered with a sterile bandage moistened with this solution.

4. The person whose eye is involved should be sent immediately to a physician in charge of such cases.

Removing foreign bodies. Hundreds of superstitions suggest how best to remove foreign bodies from the surface of the eye. They concern sneezing or rubbing the other eye or similar notions. It is actually much safer to rub the other eye than the one in which the foreign body has lodged. Usually rubbing pushes the foreign substance farther into the eye.

Those persons who understand how to remove foreign bodies make certain that their own hands are clean and that every instrument or other material used is clean or sterilized. The eye itself must be handled with the utmost delicacy. The person examining the eye carefully studies the eye, while the affected person first looks upward so that the lower lid may be pulled down; then downward, while the upper lid is turned back. The upper lid cannot be turned back safely while the person is looking up or moving the eyeball constantly. With practice, skill can be developed in turning back the upper lid.

If the foreign substance is not seen, the examiner then looks at the surface of the eyeball, changing the light so as to catch the reflection of any foreign substance which may be imbedded in the cornea. Great care must be taken to prevent infection, as secondary infections may incite ulcers which may destroy the sight of the eye.

Viewing television.

1. Make sure that you are getting clear reception.

2. Adjust tone setting before tuning the picture to desired brilliance. An unsteady image or too much light will produce visual discomfort.

3. Avoid intense darkness or bright light in the room in which television is viewed. Mild, indirect light is preferable.

4. Sunglasses should not be worn for viewing because they adapt vision to unnatural conditions.

5. Avoid excessively long periods of concentration on television.

6. Find the most comfortable distance for your own eyes.

7. In case of discomfort, have your vision examined. Many older persons who wear bifocal glasses may find neither segment suited to television viewing.

See also ASTIGMATISM; BIFOCAL; CATARACT; CONTACT LENSES; CORNEA; CORNEAL TRANSPLANTATION; EYEGLASSES; MYOPIA; OCCUPATIONAL HAZARDS IN INDUSTRY; PRESBYOPIA; GLAUCOMA; TRACHOMA; SQUINT. *See* MEDIGRAPHS pages 325, 433, 687, 1331.

EYE BANK, a repository in which an ophthalmic surgeon may secure a cornea, to be used in an eye-grafting operation. The eye bank, in turn, secures its materials from a variety of sources, such as the eyes of a stillborn infant or on the death of an older person. Many persons now will their eyes for such transplantations. To operate such a bank is not only expensive but demands that the members of the staff possess extraordinary technical skill. However, the results are frequently so good as to justify all costs. *See also* CORNEA; CORNEAL TRANSPLANTATION; EYE.

EYEGLASSES, lenses used to correct and aid inadequate vision. They may supplement the diminishing capacity of the eye to adapt itself to distance, adjust the difficulty caused by the pull of various eye muscles, or aid in correcting poor vision caused by faulty anatomy of the eye.

Anomalies in anatomy are responsible for *astigmatism,* in which the image fails to focus properly on the retina, the part of the eye which receives the image. A person is *farsighted* when the rays of light focus behind the retina, a condition usually corrected by a convex lens. If the person is *nearsighted,* so that the focus occurs in front of the retina, the adjustment can be made with a concave lens. *See also* ASTIGMATISM; BIFOCAL; CONTACT LENSES; EYE; MYOPIA; PRESBYOPIA.

F

FACE, the front part of the head, including the eyes, cheeks, chin, forehead, nose, and mouth. The facial skin, although not thick, contains numerous blood vessels and glands for the passage of oil, sweat, and other secretions. The tissue underneath the skin is thickened only in the vicinity of the chin; elsewhere it tends to be rather loose. Because of this looseness, space is available for swelling.

Many facial muscles, some near the surface, others far beneath, are used in facial expressions. These muscles coordinate with muscles in the forehead. In the act of eating, a muscle in the cheek poises the food between the teeth while it is being chewed and prevents food from gathering between the teeth and on the inside surface of the cheek. One of the principal nerves, the seventh or *facial nerve,* controls these muscles.

The main *artery* of the face moves upward and then forward. One of its branches is directed toward the tonsil and two other branches to the upper and lower lips respectively. Since these branch arteries to the lips are joined by two parallel arteries from the other side of the face, bleeding of the lip is difficult to control except by compressing the mouth at both ends.

The *facial vein,* which sometimes runs parallel with the facial artery, is connected with the cavernous sinus located inside the skull. Because of this connection, any serious infection of the face can transmit its poison to the veins in the skull. A facial infection should always be taken care of by a physician.

Complexion denotes the color and texture of the facial skin. Many ailments and conditions can affect the complexion. In *chloasma,* commonly known as *liver spots,* discolored patches appear on the skin. It is often, though not necessarily, associated with pregnancy. Similar patches may occur which are not chloasma. Facial ruddiness has a variety of sources. If permanent it may be a birthmark. It may be associated with fever or with the hot flashes which sometimes accompany menopause. Redness in the vicinity of the nose often accompanies a type of acne, *acne rosacea*, which is produced by digestive ailments. In alcoholics, the nose may be red and the network of blood vessels chronically swollen. Prolonged exposure to weather can cause the skin to take on a red appearance. A bluish tinge to the facial skin may result from persistent *bronchitis* or *asthma* or prolonged heart disease. *Anemia* may cause the complexion to be pallid. Any of these color tones to the complexion may be perfectly normal. In a healthy person, the gums and inside of the lower eyelid are a rosy color and, as with the skin, a deviation from this may indicate the presence of some undesirable condition. The appearance of the complexion may also be affected by such afflictions as *acne, eczema, or impetigo.*

A large amount of fat is packed under the facial skin. When this tends to diminish, as in old age or sickness, the skin becomes less elastic and begins to show wrinkles. *See also* ACNE; ACNE ROSACEA; CHLOASMA; COSMETICS; SKIN.

FACIAL NEURALGIA. *Trigeminal* or *facial neuralgia* is characterized by a sharp shooting pain passing across the face. This pain usually occurs when the patient is washing, shaving or otherwise touching his skin. The condition is sometimes associated with severe malocclusion of the jaws. Trigeminal neuralgia is more common among women than men, among persons over 40 years, and among persons who are minus a number of teeth. Pain is felt because an irritating stimulus passes along the facial nerve. In attempts to treat this condition the use of vitamin B_{12} injections and also of cortisone seems to have been effective in some cases. *See also* NEURALGIA; TIC DOULOUREUX.

FAINTING, may be defined as a temporary suspension of consciousness. Originally a depression occurs in the action of the heart. This can be caused by something environmental, such as cold, heat, or hunger, or by mental shock, perhaps from pain or fright. As a consequence, the flow of blood to the brain is interrupted. Dizziness, difficulty in vision, a ringing in the ears, pallor, and an unsteady appearance may follow. The climax is a falling or sinking to the ground, possibly with a long sigh. Momentarily the victim may hardly seem alive. The breathing and pulse beat, for example, are sometimes almost imperceptible.

Treatment must encourage the flow of blood to the brain. This means that the patient's head should go down between his knees, or his entire body placed in the prone position. It is equally important that the victim should have plenty of air; the coolest place, especially in a hot and crowded room, is undoubtedly near the floor. Clothes should also be loosened, particularly those which are wound around the neck or across the chest. Brandy, whiskey, ether, ammonia, or smelling salts are often administered. Under intelligent treatment the patient will soon begin to breathe again in a normal fashion. At the same time color will come back into his face and his eyes will open. *See also* DIZZINESS; FIRST AID.

FALLEN ARCHES. *See* ARCHES, FALLEN.

FALLOPIAN TUBES, the two tubes lying close to each of the two *ovaries* and leading into the *uterus.* Their function is to transport the egg cell or *ovum,* liberated each month by one of the ovaries, into the uterus. They are also called the *oviducts.*

The potency of the Fallopian tubes is essential to pregnancy. They may, however, like other tissues, become affected by various disorders which interfere with their normal function. Painful twisting and blocking, for instance, may occur and be followed by secondary infection.

Sometimes a fertilized egg cell will begin to develop abnormally in one of the Fallopian tubes rather than in the womb. The condition, *tubal* or *ectopic pregnancy*, demands prompt surgery since unchecked growth of the developing embryo within the tube will rupture it, and serious hemorrhage within the abdominal cavity may follow, which may be fatal.

Gonorrhea is the most frequent infection of the Fallopian tubes, accounting, it is estimated, for 70 per cent of Fallopian infections. The symptoms of the acute stage resemble those of acute appendicitis. The temperature rises, the white blood cells increase, and the abdomen is tender to the touch. The infection may become chronic without acute manifestations, causing long-lasting ill health and eventually sterility.

Antibiotic and sulfa drugs are effectively used to treat gonococcal infection of the Fallopian tubes whereas formerly surgery was required. In the most serious cases, however, surgery may still be found necessary.

Tuberculosis or other infectious diseases may also attack the Fallopian tubes. Infection associated with inflammation of the tubes is known as *salpingitis. See also* ECTOPIC PREGNANCY; OVARIES; REPRODUCTION SYSTEM. *See* MEDIGRAPH page 995.

FALLOUT PROTECTION. Fallout consists of tiny particles of dust and debris that are made radioactive by nuclear explosions. When an atomic or hydrogen bomb is exploded close to the ground thousands of tons of these particles are sucked up into the air and help form the mushroom cloud seen when the nuclear explosion occurs. As the cloud disintegrates, many of the radioactive particles accumulate in the atmosphere and are carried by the wind for thousands of miles. This is the widely publicized nuclear fallout which later returns to earth, perhaps over a period of years, contaminat-

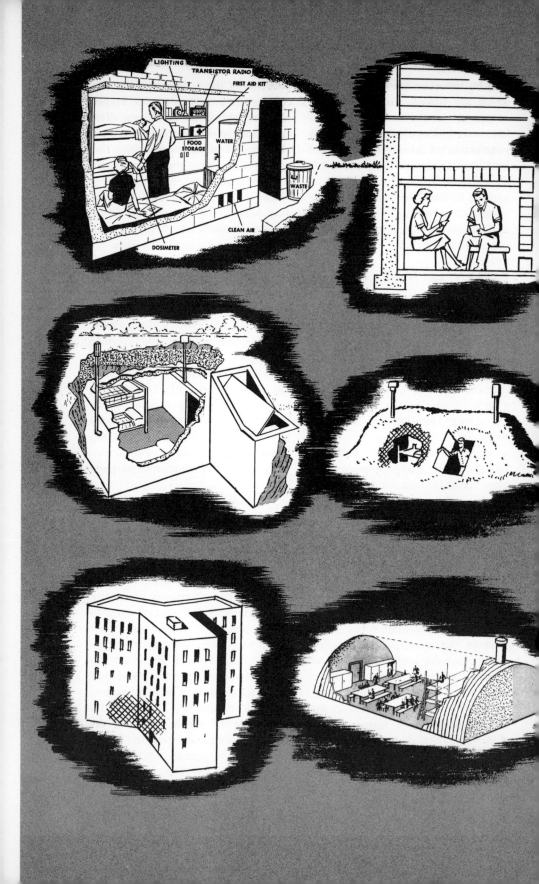

ing by its cumulative effect water, milk and other foods. However, the remainder of the radioactive fallout presents a danger directly after the explosion. This fallout descends within an area that can extend for hundreds of miles, and can bring widespread death and injury over a period of days or weeks. It is this fallout, dangerous immediately after the detonation, that is urgently serious.

In the actual vicinity of a nuclear explosion, almost all life not protected in strong blast-proof shelters would be destroyed by blast, heat, or massive radiation. Survivors outside this area of destruction would be subjected to dangerous radioactive fallout, usually without knowing it. This fallout may sometimes be seen in the form of fine ash or dust, but the rays emitted by the radioactive particles can neither be seen nor felt. Only weight or mass of material can give protection against these radioactive rays.

The best protection against radioactive fallout is an underground shelter with at least three feet of earth or sand above it. Two feet of solid concrete will provide the same amount of protection. Solidity is essential; hollow concrete blocks should be filled solidly with cement mortar. An underground shelter of such mass provided with an adequate door and air filter will give almost complete protection. Fallout

after a nuclear explosion will usually give a little time for one to reach his fallout shelter. It will not arrive at a location where there are likely to be a number of survivors until after about an hour. In more distant locations the time may be as much as 8 or 10 hours after detonation, depending on terrain, wind and weather conditions. Defense authorities agree that in planning a protection program it can generally be presumed that survivors of the immediate blast will have about one hour to go to their homes or other place of protection from fallout. Since transportation may not be available, the time of one hour allows for the distance one can travel on foot.

A program of protection against fallout is based on three characteristics of fallout radiation. The first is that radiation dissipates with passage of time. Although early radioactivity is extremely high, the intensity level declines after seven hours to about ten per cent and after two days to about one per cent. The second characteristic is that radiation diminishes with distance. Radiation is only one-quarter as harmful at a distance of 200 feet as it is at 100 feet. Thus, by getting away from the fallout material— by going to the intermediate floors of a tall building, or by clearing the fallout out of an area—the damaging effects of radiation can be

Fallout Protection—Protection against radioactive fallout is feasible if fallout shelters are available. Designs vary but all well-built shelters use shielding materials. Among the types of fallout shelters are the basement shelter

(top left, right); underground shelter (center left); earth-covered, pre-shaped metal shelter (center right); central ground floor area and basement in apartment house (bottom left); group shelter (bottom right).

greatly reduced. Thirdly, radiation is reduced by shielding.

Shielding is the key to a protection program against radioactive fallout. Radiation easily penetrates ordinary materials such as clothing, glass or the walls of the average frame house. The more dense the material interposed between the individual and the fallout, the greater the protection. In an emergency, stopping up doors and windows helps, and stacks of books, magazines, newspapers or filing cabinets provide some protection. Earth and concrete, however, are the safest. If no underground or two-foot concrete shelter is available, staying in a house basement will cut down exposure to about one-tenth the outside exposure. In such an eventuality, sandbagging the windows provides a further reduction. In a house that has no basement, staying on the first floor near the center of the house would cut down the radiation to about one half. A good rule to remember is that if caught in a building that has no specially provided fallout shelter—in office building or apartment house—basements, inside rooms, or corridors are safest.

A person who suspects he may have been in a fallout area should wash himself and his clothes thoroughly. If the clothes and the water cannot be disposed of, the clothes should be left outside. Some experts advise that outer garments be removed and left outside the shelter and the water used for washing be thrown outside. If unpackaged food has been exposed to fallout, it should be decontaminated by peel-

ing and washing. It should not be discarded. In emergency it is preferable to eat it, though contaminated, rather than starve.

In planning for maximum safety against fallout, Civil Defense experts advise that important survival requirements for individuals and families are: shelter from radioactive fallout, a two-week supply of food and water, cooking and eating utensils and equipment, fuel, clothing, bedding, first aid supplies, special medicines (if required by chronic illness), sanitation supplies and equipment, and a battery-powered radio. Two types of simple, inexpensive radiation instruments are also recommended: a dose rate meter to show the intensities of radiation at different locations in and around the shelter, and a dosimeter for each individual to indicate the cumulative dosage of radiation received during the emergency. If the survival items are not stored in the home shelter, they should be in a convenient place where they can be quickly moved to the shelter, or to the car in case of evacuation.

The fallout shelter itself has no fixed design but may be compact or roomy, according to the needs and desires of the individual family. Some shelters can be built as a do-it-yourself project, others require contractors. It is estimated that for family shelters 10 square feet per person is adequate. Concrete or bricks, earth or sand are some of the materials suggested; there is about the same amout of shielding in 8 inches of concrete as in 12 inches of earth, 16 inches of books or 30 inches of wood. If built in a completely exposed location, the shielding should be the equivalent of concrete 18 inches thick. Information on fallout shelters and fallout protection may be obtained from local Civil Defense offices, or by writing to the Office of Civil and Defense Mobilization, Washington 25, D.C. *See also* RADIATION SICKNESS; ATOMIC BOMB.

FARSIGHTEDNESS. *See* EYE; PRESBYOPIA.

FASTING, abstinence from food, or limiting food, for religious, political, or medical purposes. For medical reasons, resting the stomach may aid in the relief of indigestion. Water, taken abundantly during a fast, may serve to rid the body of accumulated waste. A period of fasting is often required of diabetics, as a preparation for undertaking a diet.

Green vegetables are sometimes permitted during a partial fast. They provide necessary vitamins, help to move the bowels, and also allay the discomforts of hunger. Hunger, incidentally, does not constitute a serious problem in fasting. It is a minor inconvenience after the first day; and usually, after the second, it is hardly noticeable. The individual lives on his own reserves of fat, until these are exhausted. Vitamin injections should be given in conjunction.

If a fast is planned for a period of more than two days, it is well to consult a physician in advance. He may suggest that the person fasting should remain in bed as much as possible, to conserve his energy and to keep warm. When the fast is broken, the consumption of food should at first be light and slow.

FAT. To be well-nourished, the body should have enough fat in storage or reserve for nutritional purposes and for padding and insulating material—no more and no less. Excess fat is simple dead weight. The skeleto-muscular system, like all the other systems of the human body, is capable of withstanding stresses over and above expected maximum loads. But the long-continued strain of bearing an excessively heavy burden of fat is often partly responsible for the joint changes characteristic. of *osteoarthritis,* the form of arthritis most common in middle and old age. Indeed the joints most frequently affected in this crippling disease are those which have the hard usage of weight bearing—for example, the knees and the spine.

Ordinary experience teaches us that the carrying of heavy burdens may not only be "back-breaking," but also put a strain upon vital functions of the body. We are all familiar with the signs of physical strain. For example, we puff and pant and sweat, our hearts beat faster, our faces get red with exertion. Occasional temporary periods of strain ordinarily do no harm. Indeed we might say that they are expected, since the body is so lavishly supplied with factors of safety in structure and function. The healthy heart, for example, has a superabundance of volume and force, and cunning and varied are the devices for obtaining extra supplies of oxygen and fuel food and for stepping up the elimination of metabolic wastes. But the very functional adaptations required to move excess fat with every step and motion during long periods of overloading may bring about changes in structure—organic defects—that seriously impair health and even threaten life. The sequence of events leading to such changes is frequently obscure, but overweight is too often associated with it to admit of any doubt that excessively fat individuals are taking a chance of speeding up the deterioration of their hearts and their arteries and their kidneys and their pancreases or other vital body organs—and often of shortening their lives.

Experience has shown that moderate overweight among young people in their teens and among young adults is not particularly harmful. It may sometimes help to increase resistance to certain diseases (particularly tuberculosis) which are most commonly encountered in youth. But overweight, even at these ages, is becoming less desirable now that measures taken to control such diseases are meeting with increasing success.

It will always be foolish, however, for young people in their desire to be fashionably slender to allow their weights to reach a dangerously low level. Extreme underweight—20 per cent or more below average—undermines efficiency, saps physical endurance, is often as socially embarrassing as overweight, and constitutes a definite health hazard. Rapid excessive loss of weight is always to be looked upon with suspicion, since it nearly always characterizes the development of certain diseases such as tuberculosis, diabetes, and malignant tumors.

True leanness, which persists throughout life as an hereditary type of body build, is not ordinarily detrimental to health. Indeed the moderate underweights have the best longevity records in middle life and beyond—that is, better even than have those of average weight. The tall, willowy (asthenic) type of constitutional leanness, however, may be characterized by lack of endurance and chronic fatigue because of a lack of tissue reserves. A person of this type will find that he feels better and looks better when he increases his weight to within the average range for his height and body build. This can sometimes be accomplished under medical guidance.

There are actually no "best" or "ideal" or "normal" weights for health. All that we have to go on at present are the average weights of individuals of three different body types who have good longevity records. These weights, according to insurance studies, are those which are within the range of average weights for height of various body types at age twenty-five.

We have plenty of negative evidence of the adverse effect on health of excessive overweight in figures that show its close association with the development of various degenerative diseases and conditions which are most common in middle age and beyond. We know also that extreme underweight interferes with health, efficiency, and good looks.

Finally, if we dismiss disease, the ultimate end of which is death, whatever its causative factors may be, and concentrate on health, the ultimate meaning of which is life in the fullest and most complete sense of the word, we may find that our looks and our feelings give us practically as good an idea of desirable weight for health as scales and tables do. It is not stylish to be stout or fashionable to be emaciated. Bulges and angles annoy us—worry us— make us uncomfortable in mind and body.

When we set about getting rid of excess fat or of gaining needed pounds under medical supervision and week by week see ourselves and feel ourselves getting thinner or fatter as the case may be, we like what we see and feel. It delights us. And the measure of our delight as we reach the point of weighing what the doctor wants us to weigh is certainly the most agreeable measure of desirable weight for health. *See also* FOOD FATS; WEIGHT, NORMAL FOR HEALTH; WEIGHT, FACTORS WHICH INFLUENCE; WEIGHT-REGULATING MACHINERY OF THE BODY; UNDERWEIGHT, HAZARDS OF; CARBOHYDRATES; PROTEIN; NUTRITION; FASTING; FATS, UNSATURATED; OBESITY.

FATIGUE. The cells and tissues of the body have a remarkable power to recover from ordinary fatigue, but excessive, prolonged, and accumulated fatigue is dangerous. Fatigue is a warning that the person is attempting to do too much and if this warning is ignored the fatigue may develop into *exhaustion,* a condition in which the body is severely depleted.

A proper diet is a good preventive against fatigue. Muscles use sugar in performing their functions; numerous vitamins are essential for satisfactory functioning of the nerves; iron is required for the blood. A deficiency of these as well as other substances the body needs brings on fatigue more rapidly than when the body is receiving an adequate diet.

Fatigue can result from too little rest and sleep, from infection and disease, poor nutrition and physical and mental overwork. Some of the numerous symptoms of fatigue are a tendency to yawn, drowsiness, sweating without previous exertion, easy irritability, depression, general slowness of action or forgetfulness. Chronic fatigue induces loss of appetite and weight and increased irritability. When fatigue has progressed to this point, a doctor should determine the degree and cause of the fatigue. Rest, a change of diet, or perhaps a change of occupation may relieve the fatigue.

Four common-sense rules follow:

(1) The best treatment of fatigue is rest.

(2) Stop physical activity before exhaustion is manifest.

(3) Don't take stimulants like coffee, "pep" pills or other pick-me-ups. The feeling of relief is only temporary and induces further fa-

tigue. Taking stimulants is like whipping a tired horse.

(4) If exhaustion is evident, medical care, including a special study of the glands, is desirable. *See also* EXHAUSTION.

FATS. *See* FOOD FATS.

FATS, UNSATURATED. Medical statistics have been accumulated which seem to suggest that the countries of the world with the highest standards of living have the highest incidence of *arteriosclerosis* (hardening of the arteries) and consequently a proportionately high mortality from coronary occlusions and other types of heart disease. Conversely, in many of the countries where the standard of living is comparatively low, the rate of deaths attributable to arteriosclerosis is far less. The United States and the Scandinavian countries—with two of the highest living standards in the world—are the places where diseases brought on by arteriosclerosis are highest. However, in China and southern Italy where the great mass of the people are poor, the statistics show that these diseases are a relatively minor cause of death.

Cholesterol has long been known to be associated with arteriosclerosis. It is manufactured by the body and stored in the body where it participates in certain necessary physico-chemical functions. The body's supply of cholesterol may be increased by heavy consumption of certain animal fats which are high in cholesterol content. When the cholesterol level in the blood rises above normal, the excess is deposited on the inner linings of the arteries narrowing the passageways and thereby making it necessary for the heart to work harder to maintain circulation. Narrowed arteries also increase the danger of clotting, especially in the network which supplies the heart itself.

Since cholesterol is found primarily in fats, and especially in animal fats, eggs and dairy products, the first controlled experiments on the subject tended to suggest that the danger of recurrent heart attacks to people who had had previous attacks could be at least partially avoided by sharply reducing the amount of fats in the diet. Since the body needs fats in order to maintain its balance, it was recommended that wherever practicable, vegetable fats be substituted for animal fats.

However, further experiments in the field, particularly those made in subsequent years in Great Britain and the United States, indicated that there is still another important factor to consider. Fats have been broken down chemically into two basic divisions, *saturated* and *unsaturated*. The research indicated that, in these experiments, unsaturated fats did not as a general rule increase the cholesterol content of the blood, while the saturated fats did. Another interesting discovery was that unsaturated fats, added to the normal diet containing saturated and animal fats, actually tended to *lower* the blood cholesterol.

Since there are several types of vegetable fats in each category, further breakdowns had to be made. It was found that certain saturated vegetable fats, such as coconut oil and to a lesser extent certain oleomargarines, when added to the diet raised the blood cholesterol level. Butter had the same effect. Unsaturated vegetables fats such as cottonseed oil, safflower oil, corn oil, and in some cases, olive oil, when added to the diet, either did not increase the cholesterol level or actually decreased it.

However, it is still premature to draw sweeping conclusions as to the preferability of unsaturated to saturated fats in the diet from the results of these early experiments. The simple fact that the Eskimoes subsist on a diet tremendously high in saturated fats, yet suffer little from arteriosclerotic diseases, should tend to cast suspicion on such overgeneralized theories. Subsequent investigations have tended to indicate that excessive consumption of highly refined carbohydrates—sugar and foods high in sugar content, such as cakes, pies, candy, soft drinks, etc. —and of alcoholic beverages, especially whiskey and other hard liquors, may be more closely connected with excessive blood cholesterol levels than is the consumption of saturated fats. Consumption of such refined carbohydrates and alcohol is also very high in the United States and Scandinavia and low in China and southern Italy! Much more research needs to be conducted in this field before any definitive conclusions can be drawn. *See also* ARTERIOSCLEROSIS.

FEAR, a feeling of agitation caused by the presence of danger or pain. It is common to distinguish fear from *anxiety,* a reaction that is out of proportion to any actual danger involved and the causes of which may be subconscious. However, many psychiatrists use the two terms interchangeably.

Fear invariably expresses itself in certain bodily changes. For example, the adrenal glands become more active, the gastrointestinal tract may cease functioning, the heartbeat usually increases in rate, and breathing becomes more rapid. Modern proponents of the "emergency theory" of fear see in these changes an attempt of the entire organism to prepare itself in such a way as to enhance survival.

Normally, fear is present from birth, with the general purpose of protecting the infant from various stimuli of the outside world. There is, for instance, fear of loud sounds, fear of bright lights, of food that is too hot or cold, and so forth. Reactions of fear to such stimuli are essential in the very young infant because his undeveloped nervous system cannot tolerate extreme stimulation for any prolonged period. Many psychiatrists believe the reaction to such stimuli in the newborn is the basis for fearful reactions expressed throughout the early years of life and extending into adulthood.

Parental attitudes play a decisive role in the childhood expressions of fear. As soon as the child leaves the crib and begins to explore his surroundings, he is trailed by his parents and warned of the dangers in objects he may encounter. If a needle or a pin in the child's path on the floor is picked up by the parents, the child will come to share the anxiety of such an object with the parents. The same may occur with respect to articles of furniture that may fall on the child, dirt that may make him sick, drafts, heat, etc. The average infant experiences all these natural defenses against harmful objects. Whether he will "outgrow" or retain the fears associated with them depends upon how much emotion is invested in the warning. Normally, fear is also related to conditions outside the home. For example, inclement weather often becomes associated in the infant's mind with harm. Later, vehicular traffic, other children, and adults other than the parents may arouse fear in the child. Parents should remember that the things which they themselves fear most are the unknown. If a child is given an adequate explanation of the meaning of the dark, if he is told about such animals that might arouse fear, if he sees his parents view small cuts, bruises and pains with equanimity, he is likely to have the same attitude toward them.

There are some children who display unusual sensitivity to fears, even though the parents train the child within the normal range of concern. The child often clings violently to the parents and is only at ease in their presence. Such children may go through the early grades of school being handed over directly by the parent to the teacher and back to the parent. While in class the child may experience nervousness before the simplest tasks. He often finds that with recognition of his condition he can gain certain advantages over other children in compensation for his apparent weakness. In later life he may still employ the same methods, fear being aroused by a vast array of things in the environment unless some sort of parental figure accompanies him.

A *phobia* is characterized by an overwhelming fear of special situations, such as closed or open spaces, animals, the dark, etc. Most people have relatively unimportant fears of this type, but in some individuals these fears become so intense as to inhibit normal functioning of the person. The fears are attached to objects that are often harmless in themselves but which may represent unconscious feelings which are the true basis of the fear. The person, to keep his unconscious fear from coming into consciousness, displaces or projects the fear onto the outside world in the form of the phobia. Thus, being alone or in any high place may come to represent abandonment. In this way the connection between the unconscious feelings and the phobia are often hidden. In effect, the phobic individual blames the external situation instead of his unconscious fear which maintains the phobia.

Fear is often closely associated with feelings of guilt. Many of these guilt feelings can be likened to the feelings of a phobia in that they are unconscious. Sexual impotence and frigidity frequently may have their origin in unconscious guilt which may be expressed in their fear of the sexual act. Here an early attitude of disapproval of and guilt toward sexuality in general, as well as parental fear of sex which has been transferred to the child, play a significant role. Since these generalized fears are actually symptoms involving the whole evaluation of oneself and others, treatment of these conditions is difficult and involved. Psychotherapy has proved successful when the treatment involves the whole personality and not just the symptom of fear alone. *See also* ANXIETY; EMOTIONAL HEALTH; STRESS.

FEBRILE, a descriptive term meaning feverish.

FECES, the excretion from the bowels. It consists of undigested residue from food, bacteria and substances secreted from the intestinal walls and from the organs connected with the digestive tract. *See also* URINE.

FEEBLE-MINDEDNESS, mental deficiency or mental defect, a condition in which average intelligence either is not present or fails to develop. It must be clearly distinguished from *mental disease,* such as *neurosis* and *psychosis,* in which functions of a mind of normal capacity become disordered.

Different degrees of mental defect or feeble-mindedness are recognized. A person with an I.Q. below 20, who doesn't advance past a mental age of three, is considered an *idiot.* Custodial care of idiots is necessary. They usually present no

special problem, since only a few live to adulthood and those who do cannot procreate as they are infantile. *Imbeciles* have I.Q.'s below 50. Often they can be taught to do certain tasks, but they may require protective supervision. *Morons,* who have I.Q.'s below 70, generally can be trained to take care of themselves, and may even be able to support themselves. As well as doing domestic tasks, morons have held jobs in factories. Training of the feeble-minded involves sensory stimulation and development of muscular coordination. Good physical condition is important to help compensate for the mental limitation.

Symptoms of feeble-mindedness tend to manifest at an early age, although it is essential to have expert opinion regarding each individual case. A baby's failure to be as responsive to sounds and sights as normal, delay in teething and other phases of development may indicate a tendency to feeble-mindedness. However, variations in development are so great that such symptoms are certainly not inevitable indications of mental defect. The condition becomes more apparent as the child grows older and cannot adjust to other children or compete with them in studies or at play. The mentally defective person tends to remain infantile even though he grows physically.

Much can be done to prevent mental defectives from being hopeless and helpless burdens on others. Such capacity as they do have should be developed to the fullest rather than deprecated and neglected. They should be taught physical coordination to the greatest possible extent. They should be schooled as far as their capacity permits, but removed from situations in which repeated unsuccessful competition with children may give them acute feelings of inferiority and defeat. Special institutions for training the feeble-minded are available.

Individual attention is essential in caring for the mentally defective. Attempts to apply the same routine to a large group of feeble-minded persons are ineffective, because each one responds quite differently, depending on the extent of his ability.

Feeble-mindedness has a hereditary tendency. Normal people, in no sense mentally defective themselves, may be carriers of mental defect; that is, they are genetically capable of transmitting the defect to offspring. Feeble-minded persons should not marry, and those who have had a feeble-minded ancestor should recognize the potentiality of having a defective child.

Recent research has demonstrated that factors other than heredity may be responsible for feeble-mindedness. Sickness of the mother during pregnancy and injury during delivery of the infant have been suggested as possible causes, and still others may be found. Parents should not feel themselves to blame when a mentally defective child appears in the family.

The term *mental retardation* is currently socially preferable to *feeble-mindedness* when discussing this disorder.

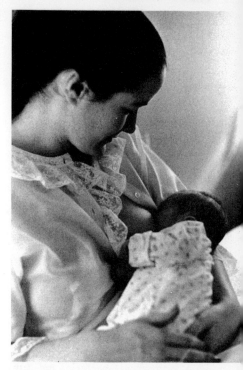

Breast-Feeding — Breast-feeding offers the mother freedom from the formula preparation associated with bottle-feeding. She need not worry if the breasts take a few days to give milk, after the birth of the baby. Good care of the breasts and attention to her diet and health are essential.

FEEDING, BREAST. Conflicting ideas about breast-feeding a baby— that is, feeding directly from the breast—as opposed to bottle feeding have produced some confusion in the minds of mothers, especially those who are having their first child. The weight of opinion favors feeding at the breast. A formula in the bottle, if the doctor's prescription and the mother's preparation are correct, will provide adequate nourishment, but human milk contains valuable qualities which are not present in other forms of milk. Also, the latest investigations indicate that the breast-fed baby probably has a psychological advantage over the bottle-fed baby. Even though the mother who feeds her baby by bottle holds him tenderly and affectionately, the bottle does in some way impede the direct communication between mother and child. However, breast-feeding when it is done with a hurried and indifferent attitude can be emotionally unsatisfactory to the child, just as bottle feeding can give the child the feeling of security and love he needs. Above all, the attitude of the mother is important.

During the months of pregnancy much can be done to prepare the prospective mother for the task of breast-feeding her baby. The doctor can recommend special care of the breasts, diet, massage, techniques for adjusting the shape of the nipples. A hospital can be selected which offers special facilities for the nursing mother.

The first days of nursing are a time in which the mother and child come to know each other. The child may at first refuse to take the breast, but if the mother is relaxed the child will probably begin to suck as soon as the nipple is introduced into his mouth. The first substance which is received is not milk but a yellowish thick liquid called *colostrum*. Under the stimulus of the infant's mouth the breasts quickly begin to release a thin blue milk. The nursing mother should keep in touch with her doctor during the first few weeks. The milk may not agree with the child; the child may get too much or too little milk at a feeding; he may

eruct part of the intake, get colic pains, or other situations may arise which should be brought to the attention of the doctor. In general, the doctor will want to be sure that the mother is in good health and receiving the proper rest and food, exercise and recreation, and that the infant is progressing normally.

Occasionally breast and bottle feeding may be effectively combined. This may be necessary if the mother is sometimes absent from home during feeding time or if she cannot keep up the necessary supply of milk. Such a combination should be arranged with the help of the doctor. The combination of breast and bottle feeding usually will facilitate weaning.

The mother must decide which method will be used to feed the child. As stated, breast-feeding is usually better for the baby, both physically and psychologically. It also eliminates the daily chore of cleaning bottle equipment and preparing the formula. Whatever method the mother decides to follow, the feeding should be administered with love and affection. *See also* CHILD CARE.

FEET, Feet are subject to a great variety of ailments. These include sprains, strains, dislocations, fractures, excessive sweating, warts, chilblains, ringworm, hammertoes, painful heels, ingrown toenails cracked toes, blisters, bruises, circulation disturbances, fallen arches, corns, bunions and calluses, and many others. Some of these are incurred during athletic activities, some are

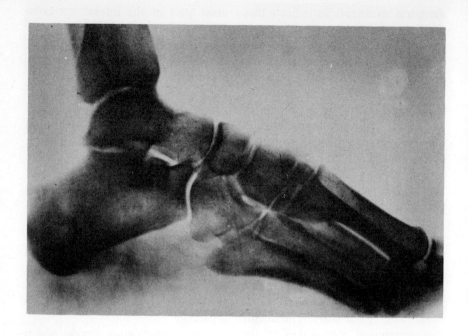

Feet—(*Top*) X-ray of a normal foot. (*Below*) X-ray of a normal foot in high-heeled shoes.

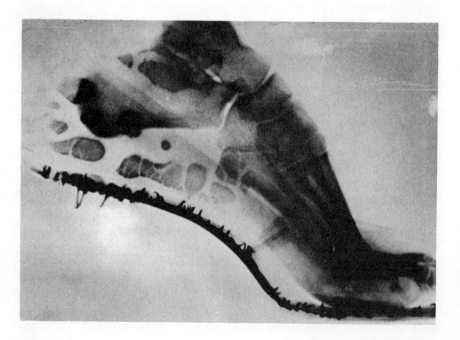

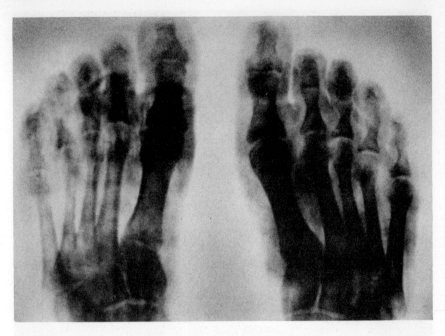

Feet—(*Top*) X-ray showing the natural position of the bones in normal feet. (*Below*) X-ray of the abnormal position of foot bones due to ill-fitting shoes. The bones are cramped because the shoes are too narrow, too short and pointed at the toes.

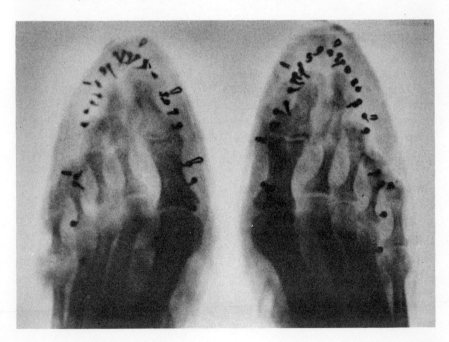

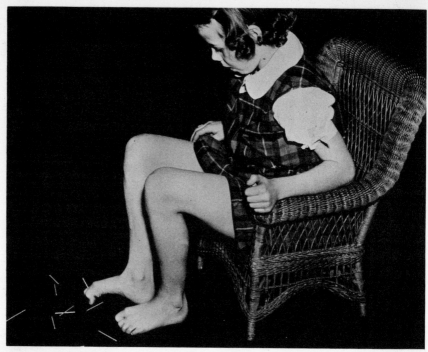

Feet—A young girl demonstrates a good exercise for keeping the foot flexible and strengthening the muscles. Exercises of this type are highly recommended by chiropodists.

due to faulty footwear, and others are present at birth.

Fallen arches refers to a painful condition affecting the main bone of the foot, the *astragalus*. This affliction is especially common among people whose work requires many hours of standing or walking. The pain is due to the spasmodic efforts of certain muscles to overcome the strain which is placed on the tissues. Often the person can terminate the pain simply by getting off his feet.

Ordinarily, however, fallen arches require special treatment. Hot applications and massages taken at the end of the day are beneficial. Even more important is the appropriate choice of shoes. Generally shoes

should be specially fitted with a medium-width rigid shank which supports the arch.

Among the most common of all foot complaints are *calluses, corns,* and *bunions.* When the skin is persistently rubbed, it tends to thicken. Such thickening, *callus,* develops most frequently on the bottom of the foot. usually at a point where constant pressure is exerted. For example, the golfer may develop a callus at the place on his foot where he pivots when driving the ball. A callus can be removed by the doctor. The real problem is how to prevent its return. Sometimes this can be done by padding the shoes in such a way as to shift the point of pressure on the foot.

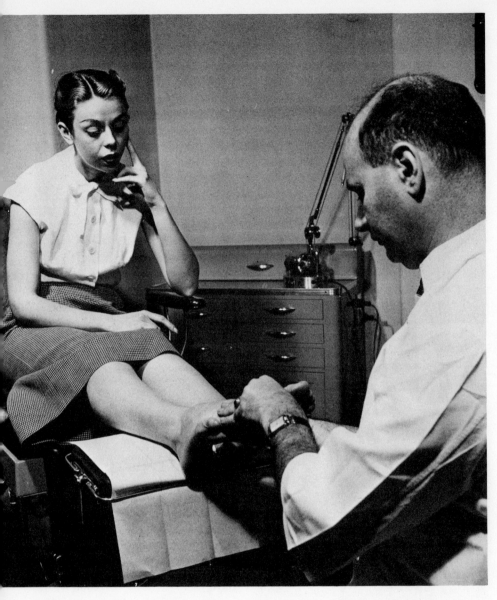

Proper care of the feet is much more important than many people realize. The feet are subject to a wide variety of disorders, all of which are seriously aggravated by neglect or improper treatment. A chiropodist (podiatrist) should be consulted at any sign of disturbance in the feet. Disturbances of the feet include sprains, dislocations, *hyperhydrosis* (excessive perspiration), fallen arches, ingrown toenails, corns, bunions, calluses, warts, chilblains, and ringworm. The feet may be subject to circulatory disturbances, such as phlebitis, peripheral arteriosclerosis, or Buerger's disease. It is important to wear proper shoes. Shoe soles should be of sturdy flexible leather to permit the proper evaporation of perspiration. It is advisable for men with hyperhydrosis to wear wool socks. Women with this problem can use *Fuller's Earth®* powder.

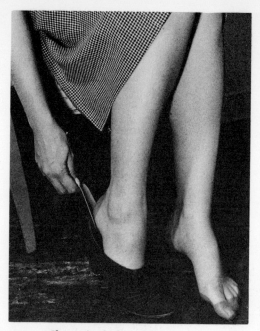 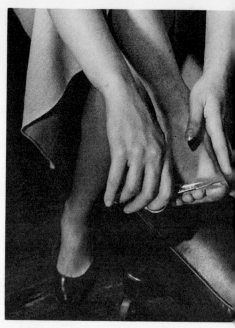

Shoes should be soft and supple to allow for normal foot expansion. Putting on shoes with a shoe horn *(above, left)* helps the foot to adjust more easily to the shoe, for a comfortable fit. Toenails should be cut straight across *(above, right)*. Ingrown toenails may result from improper cutting. Arch supports and other corrective devices should be fitted by a chiropodist *(below)*. The feet should be cared for properly.

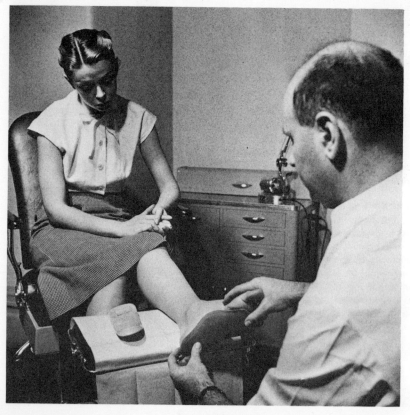

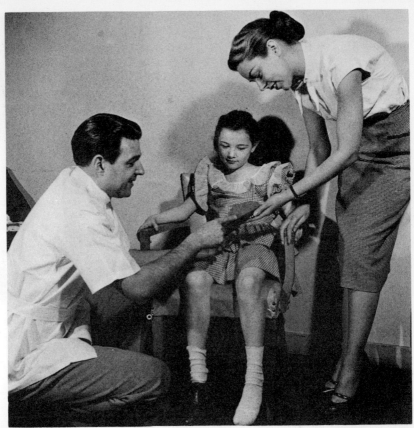

Wool socks and shoes with porous leather soles can mitigate hyperhydrosis (excessive perspiration). Children's shoes should never be purchased without preliminary fitting, since the foot size changes rapidly. The feet should be examined at regular intervals as a precautionary measure.

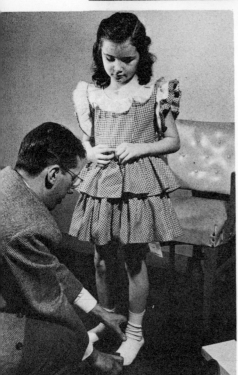

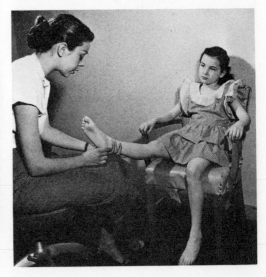

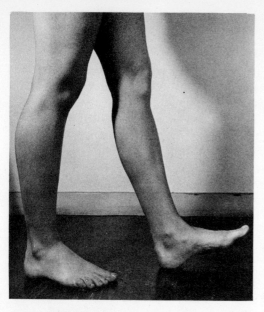

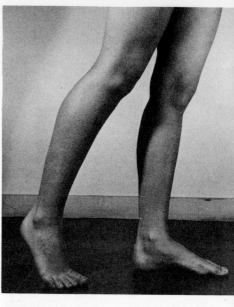

Many people walk improperly. In particular, women who wear high-heeled shoes (and that includes most women) may encounter difficulties due to excessive pressure on the soles and toes. Barefoot exercises can serve a useful remedial purpose. Posture is important in proper ambulation. Feet pointed straight out *(below, left)* are preferable to the position at right, which may result in awkward gait.

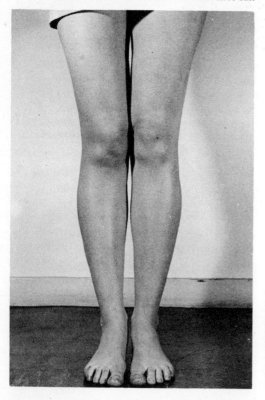

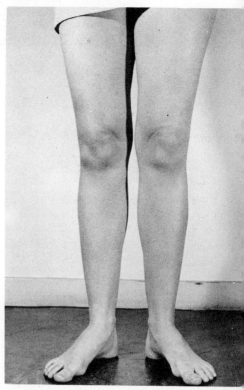

A callus on the toes, between the toes, or—especially—on the outer part of the little toes, is a *corn.* The soft corn, produced by a rubbing together of the little toe and the fourth toe, is a frequent point of infection, especially of *ringworm.* A majority of the numerous commercial cures for corns make use of *salicylic acid,* a drug which if given sufficient time will cause the corn to fall away. The only cure is an operation, seldom done, which removes not only the corn but also a part of the bone beneath the corn.

A *bunion* is a swelling produced by the inflammation of a *bursa,* a fluid-containing sac located between the tendon and a bone which serves to facilitate action. Bunions are found most often on the outer part of the big toe. They may also appear, however, in the middle of the top of the foot, where the person may have laced his shoes too tightly. This type of bunion can be relieved by inserting pads under the laces or by avoiding shoes which lace. Bunions resemble corns in that permanent relief may be found only in surgery. However, surgery for bunions is frequently and successfully done.

Care of the feet. The feet should be bathed once a day, then carefully dried and perhaps dusted with talcum or a germicidal powder so that moist areas will not rub together and produce infection. The general health of the feet may be improved by use of the so-called *contrast bath.* The person places his two feet first in one pail filled with hot water, and then in another filled with cold water. The feet should remain in each pail for about one minute, and the entire operation should continue for ten minutes. The purpose is to open and close the veins in such a manner as to encourage blood circulation. Massage of the feet is also beneficial and should be done with a circular movement of the fingers. If the skin is unusually sensitive, cold cream may be used in the massage.

For the general health of the feet, nothing is more significant than careful selection of shoes, properly fitted to the individual foot. The most crucial measurement is that from the back of the heel to the middle of the big toe. Many persons, including shoe salesmen, speak of breaking in a pair of tight shoes. This is an incorrect notion; it is the feet which are broken in. This is especially dangerous if the tightness of the shoe is longitudinal, where the tendency is to force certain toes into a right angle position, causing the *hammertoe.* A hammertoe may become so serious that it can only be relieved by an operation. Healthful shoes will always have round toes and shanks of only medium width. Extremes in the height and location of heels ought to be avoided. Specialists usually recommend a daily change of shoes. Shoes which are not being worn should be kept in shoe trees to retain their shape. Rubber heels possess therapeutic value because they decrease the shock effect on both feet and body. *See also* ARCHES, FALLEN; ATHLETE'S FOOT; BUNION; CALLUS; FLATFOOT.

FELLATION, oral stimulation of the penis. *See* HOMOSEXUALITY; IRRUMATION.

FELON, an infection at the bottom of a fingernail which may be caused by staphylococcus or another pus-forming germ.

Home remedies like painting with iodine and other antiseptics or the application of hot wet packs soaked in boric acid solution are not always effective and the condition may get worse. If the infection penetrates muscular tissue, the bone covering, or the bone, the condition is serious and should be treated promptly by a doctor.

The doctor prevents pus and infection from penetrating deeper by soaking the finger in hot water to soften the tissue. Then by surgical procedure he releases the pus from the infected area. Hot packs soaked in boric acid are then applied and followed by painting with iodine.

If a felon is not controlled, the infection may spread along the lymphatic ducts and tissues into other parts of the body and produce a generalized infection. Indication of such diffusion is the appearance of red inflammatory lines running upward through the hand and wrist.

FEMININE HYGIENE. Hygiene in women differs from hygiene in general only as it concerns itself with certain qualities which are special to the female. Specifically these include the well-being of those parts of the body associated with reproduction throughout the entire life of a woman and particularly during pregnancy. The emotional or social well-being of women is discussed here only when these aspects are closely interwoven with the physical.

Infancy. Good hygiene is closely associated with ordinary common-sense cleanliness. This starts at birth with the diapering of the baby girl. Leaving soiled diapers on too long may lead to uncomfortable irritation, the usual reaction of sensitive skin to acid secretions. A baby with a sore itchy "bottom" is not a happy baby. We use the term "bottom" frequently to refer to the entire anal-vaginal region, including the excretory opening and the genitals. Actually there is no one medical word which covers this entire area.

Diaper rash can generally be avoided by cleansing a baby girl's skin with mineral oil and changing the diaper's frequently. If a rash does develop, the diapers will need special attention such as boiling and rinsing in a solution that inhibits bacterial growth. A commercial diaper service is better than home washing because it provides sterilized diapers that are less likely to cause irritation.

Irritated skin needs protection. Bathing the affected area with cool water containing a little starch and powdering with borated talc usually prove soothing. Soap should be avoided at this time since it can irritate an already inflamed skin. If these simple measures do not lead to prompt relief, consult the doctor.

Childhood. As a baby girl grows older, other causes of irritation may appear in the genital area. Even a very young child can acquire worms; this in turn can lead to intense itching around the anus.

Itching is a violent sensation which demands relief. This is usually achieved by rubbing or scratching and such rubbing may be falsely interpreted as *masturbation*. By directing attention to the sensitive genital area, however, the irritation may lead to masturbation.

Babies explore all parts of their bodies and in doing so explore their genitals too. This casual handling of the genitals as well as actual masturbation often causes great concern among parents. For some reason our society associates sin and uncleanliness with this practice. Parents should realize that masturbation generally does no harm and is widely practiced by almost all children at one time or another. Physically it causes nothing more serious than an occasional local irritation. Genuine emotional suffering, however, can come to a child who has been told by an adult that masturbation will bring horrible results such as insanity or blindness or sterility. If parents can look upon childhood masturbation as a normal part of sexual growing up, they will be able to be more casual about it. But excessive masturbation, when a girl seems to be withdrawing too much within herself for satisfaction, presents a real problem. This will rarely occur in an otherwise emotionally sound and happy child. In this case the problem of masturbation is only a symptom of a more complicated emotional disturbance

which will probably need the help of a professionally trained consultant.

Of course, sensible physical measures should be taken to relieve any irritation and itching around the genitals. Soaking the "bottom" in tepid water to which a small amount of baking soda has been added usually affords gentle relief. If the vulvar area—the tissue surrounding the vaginal opening—is acutely inflamed, however, expert advice will be needed. In dressing the little girl, always remember that tight clothing, particularly panties, can start or aggravate an irritation in the genital area.

Sometimes a little girl is brought to a doctor because of a discharge that soils her underwear. The mother is afraid that her daughter has acquired a venereal disease. Venereal disease does occasionally occur in children of both sexes, either spread accidentally from a diseased person or by actual sexual contact. But it is exceedingly rare among children if there is proper supervision of their activities. Other infections are more common in little girls. The mother may have some type of vaginal infection accompanied by discharge. If she is careless about her towels, the germs may be carried from mother to daughter and the infection spread in this way. Although not serious, the discharge is odorous and the irritation unpleasant. Generally this type of inflammation can be quickly corrected by suitable treatment.

Probably the most common cause of a yellow malodorous discharge in a little girl is a foreign body in the vagina. Girls frequently insert small objects into the vagina, the most frequently found objects being buttons, hairpins, small pencils, and pieces of paper. This object generally becomes "lost" and sets up a rather violent reaction with odor and discharge which persists until the foreign body is removed.

The presence of any excessive discharge, particularly a malodorous discharge, is not normal during childhood and should be brought to the attention of a physician for treatment.

Adolescence. As the little girl matures and approaches puberty, certain changes become obvious. The breasts develop, hair begins to grow in the armpits (*axilla*) and over the genital area (*pubis*), and skin pimples may appear for the first time. In addition, an increase in vaginal secretion may occur for a few days each month and a more distinct body odor develops for the first time. All these changes are perfectly natural; the little girl is being transformed into an adult. Before long she will have her first menstrual period, the herald of sexual maturity. With *menstruation,* the child becomes a biological adult; she is now physically capable of being a mother. The growth of breasts and hair, and the development of odors are all a normal part of her growing up. But the girl should be prepared ahead of time for what is coming, particularly for the onset of menstruation.

Many people have an erroneous idea that menstruation is a process by which the body rids itself of "bad" blood. That is absolutely false. Menstruation has been graphically described as "weeping of the disappointed womb." Each month, from puberty until the *menopause,* an egg matures in the ovary and is available for fertilization. At the same time, the uterus (womb) prepares a suitable bed to receive that egg if it is fertilized. If the egg is not fertilized, the bed or lining of the uterus is cast off—the menstrual flow. The process is repeated month after month throughout the mature life of a woman in hopeful preparation for the times when fertilized eggs will appear.

When she is approaching sexual maturity, the explanation of why she will bleed for a few days every month should be given to the girl. She should also be instructed in advance in the use of a sanitary belt and pad to avoid needless soiling and embarrassment.

You will probably find that your daughter has been briefed by her schoolmates for what is to come. You will want to check on this and be sure that she has not picked up false information and also to allay her fears and answer her many questions. If you do not feel up to doing this, turn to someone who can, but do not ignore the situation. Evasion only brings unnecessary anxieties. And your daughter may turn to others, usually youngsters whose information is deficient and distorted. A good book or pamphlet is helpful, especially in showing how the reproductive organs work. But nothing can take the place of a friendly and frank discussion between mother and daughter.

Here are some common questions that arise in connection with puberty and menstruation:

What can be done about perspiration and body odors? Odor goes with perspiration. After puberty, the sweat glands and sebaceous glands, particularly in the armpit and groin, secrete substances which have a characteristic odor because these areas are not exposed to the free circulation of air and secretions are easily decomposed by bacterial action which sometimes leads to offensive odors. This is all normal but nevertheless undesirable. Odor from the body in general can be minimized by frequent bathing and frequent changing of underclothes. Odor from the armpit is at times difficult to control. Shaving the underarm is esthetically desirable and makes it easier to apply antiperspirants and deodorants. The many antiperspirants now on the market vary from powder to salves and pastes and also liquids in spray bottles. Most of today's commercial preparations are time-tested, effective, and relatively nonirritating. In their advertising, most emphasize the deodorant qualities and minimize the antiperspirant because actual suppression of perspiration is much more difficult to maintain. In stubborn cases, it may be advisable to use a combined treatment: shaving and bathing the area, then applying either a liquid or salve and finally a deodorant powder.

Perspiration and sebaceous secretions in the vulva and vagina may create the same problem as armpit perspiration. Sometimes, during warm weather, clipping or even shaving the hair in the pubic region may be advisable. A deodorant powder effectively controls odor from this source.

Occasionally a woman suffers from malodorous feet. Here the problem is usually more than one of lack of cleanliness. Malodorous and excessive perspiration of the feet is not a condition easy to eradicate. It usually requires the attention of a skin specialist.

What can be done for undesirable hair? An excessive or dark growth of facial and body hair may result from many causes, some normal, some abnormal. Many normal women are subject to the growth of facial and body hair that they find unattractive. Hair on the arms and legs can easily be removed by depilatories, by wax, or by shaving. Superfluous facial hair, however, requires expert treatment and generally is best removed by electrolysis. But electrolysis creates some practical problems. The hair is removed very slowly, the treatment is costly, and often there is a tendency for the hair to regrow. The high cost alone may call for another method of hair removal. One can turn to chemical *depilatories* but there is always the danger of skin irritation which is particularly noticeable on the face. There are also specially prepared waxes for use on the face. But perhaps the simplest and best solution is shaving. Shaving does not make the hair grow more rapidly or cause it to become coarser.

What sort of sanitary pads should be used? The external, Kotex-type of pad is the most commonly used nowadays. The wick, internal, or Tampax-type of protection is less widely used because it cannot be used under all circumstances. In virgins, the vaginal orifice may not be large enough to admit its insertion. Normally a thin membrane, the *hymen,* covers this orifice. Normally also there is an opening in this membrane which permits the escape of menstrual blood. But in some girls this opening may not be large enough for the insertion of the wick. Whether there is adequate room can best be determined by a physician. After marriage, the opening usually becomes large enough for insertion of the wick. During the first two days of a menstrual period, however, the amount of flow often is more than the wick can absorb. Many women, therefore, use the ordinary pad during the days of heavy flow and the wick as the flow tapers off. Properly used, internal protection is safe, comfortable, and convenient.

May one bathe or go swimming during menstruation? The answer is yes, providing the water is not too cold. A chilling bath is apt to bring about a sudden cessation of menstruation; but there isn't the slightest objection to showers or tub baths in warm water. Swimming presents different problems. What about the bulkiness and wetness of the pad, or the possibility of blood escaping?

Both problems are readily solved by using the internal wick, if it is anatomically possible and the flow is not too heavy. Otherwise, it is best to forego swimming for this period.

What about going to dances and parties during menstruation? It can do no harm at all.

Marriage. With marriage, a new series of problems and questions concerning feminine hygiene present themselves. In books and advertisements, a great deal of space has been devoted to the subject of douching. It is *sometimes* recommended as a hygienic measure following sexual union. But actually there are very few circumstances when a douche is needed and as a general practice douching is physiologically unsound and illogical because the vagina is a muscular pouch that must remain moist in order to serve its function. This moisture comes from the mucous secretions of the *cervix* (the opening of the womb) and from the cast-off lining cells of the vagina. The amount of secretion, particularly of the cervical mucus, varies normally during the menstrual cycle, being most abundant during the midcycle when the egg is passed. In addition, sexual stimulation increases the secretion from accessory glands before and during the sexual act. In other words, the female secretions during and after intercourse are quite normal and necessary. Following the climax, male semen is deposited in the vagina. But since the vagina is a muscular organ and drains by gravity, this secretion will run out naturally upon completion of the act, leaving no need for a douche.

Perhaps douching has been recommended to you as a contraceptive agent. If so, it is an extremely poor choice. Even when used purely as a cleansing agent following coitus, a douche is ineffective since nothing remains to be cleansed. If you feel like it, a bath or shower after intercourse is a much better idea. Unfortunately many women have been raised to consider douching an essential part of their daily toilet and must be re-educated to accept the fact that douching does not serve a useful function.

Two other occasions for which douching has been thought useful are the completion of the menstrual period and when a diaphragm has been used in intercourse. Here again douching is not the answer. If the period is truly finished, the last vestige of blood disappears rapidly without douching. If a diaphragm is used, there is no reason to douche; simply wash the diaphragm after it is removed and bathe if you wish.

What about douching if one suffers from *leucorrhea* or excessive vaginal discharge? The answer again is no. There is a cause for these conditions and to treat the condition properly the cause must be determined. Excessive discharge may be the earliest sign of cancer of the female organs; it may be due to excessive sexual stimulation or to one of several microscopic organisms which are not too serious but extremely annoying. Leucorrhea may be due to venereal infection, to foreign bodies, to erosion of the cervix, or, as already mentioned, the flow may be a perfectly normal phenomenon. Only a physician can advise proper treatment. Certainly washing out the secretion by douching does not do permanent good.

But doesn't douching get rid of vaginal odors? The answer again is no! In health, there are no offensive vaginal odors. Offensive odors arise from disease or from failure to keep the vulvar and anal areas clean. Dribbling urine leads to a urine odor; improper cleansing after a bowel movement leads to a fecal odor; the presence of a cancer or a foreign body causes a fetid odor; infections due to yeast or to an organism known as *trichomonas* cause characteristic unpleasant odors. None of these conditions is relieved by douching, except perhaps temporarily. And none of them can be cured by douching, only by removing the cause.

All too frequently a physician encounters patients who lack the basic knowledge of how to cleanse the anal area. Proper cleansing is best attained by using water, tissue, or by actual bathing, using a non-irritating soap. Dry cleaning is second best.

Many people wonder about the danger of having sexual relations during the menstrual period. There is nothing harmful about having intercourse during menstruation, but the practice is messy and may thereby hurt the relationship.

Pregnancy. Many questions arise about pregnancy. May I take tub baths? May I wash my hair? Is intercourse proper? What about excessive vaginal discharge and odors?

Bathing is not only proper but desirable. There was a time when tub baths were considered dangerous during the latter weeks of pregnancy, but nowadays the water supply in most modern communities is pure and the fear of contamination is unwarranted. The only danger from a tub bath is the risk of a fall while getting in or out of the tub; a little caution will prevent this.

Washing the hair is quite harmless and so is having a permanent. During pregnancy, however, the permanent does not hold well and the results may not justify the time and money expended.

Intercourse is proper during pregnancy but precaution should be taken during the early and late periods to refrain from roughness. Early in pregnancy, the stimulation may cause miscarriage; late, it may lead to premature labor. Generally, however, with gentleness harm will not ensue.

The problem of the vaginal discharge in the pregnant woman is the same as in the nonpregnant. While the congestion of late pregnancy leads to increased secretion, this is a nonirritating and odorless flow. An irritating odorous secretion is abnormal and calls for medical investigation.

After the baby arrives. Before childbirth, the breasts do not require any special care. The watery secretion which may be expressed from the nipple from the earliest months of pregnancy can be removed by or-

dinary bathing. After the milk flow is established, the problem is not different. The breasts should be washed with mild soap and tepid water daily and the nipples should be cleansed with plain water before each feeding.

"Hardening" or conditioning the nipples prior to actual nursing has been attempted through many different procedures for years. But there does not seem to be any benefit from this. The secret of good nursing and preventing the nipple from cracking is to nurse frequently and not to permit the baby to bite the nipple. This is accomplished by carrying the nipple forward so that it rests on the baby's tongue.

Bathing either with tub baths or showers can be resumed shortly after childbirth. The warm water imparts a sense of well-being, relieves the achiness in the region of the stitches, and does much to wash away the odorous secretions which always follow childbirth. The vaginal discharge or *lochia* persists up to four to six weeks and the odor may be disturbing. In addition to bathing, a deodorant salve may be applied to an external pad. Internal wicks should not be used until the doctor has given his permission. *See also* BODY ODOR; BREAST; DIAPER RASH; FEEDING, BREAST; LEUCORRHEA; MASTURBATION; MENORRHAGIA; MENSTRUATION; CHILDBIRTH AND PRENATAL CARE; POST-NATAL CARE OF THE MOTHER; VAGINA; VULVA.

FERMENTATION. When a *ferment,* or *enzyme,* induces an alteration in any substance involving decomposition or effervescence, the process is known as *fermentation.*

Alcohol is produced by a ferment known as *yeast.* When yeast is added to a solution of water and grape sugar, a froth consisting of carbon dioxide is formed. In the midst of this process, the sugar content is converted into alcohol. Wine is the result. Beer is produced by the action of yeast on grain. If any of these alcoholic beverages later acquire a sour or vinegary taste, it is due to another enzyme, known as *mycoderma aceti,* which has changed part of the alcohol into acetic acid (vinegar). To further illustrate the process of fermentation: if the lactic acid bacillus is added to milk sugar instead of grape sugar, *lactic acid* results. This occurs in the process of souring milk and also in the production of artificial buttermilk. If this enzyme produces fermentation in the stomach, the resultant carbon dioxide may lead to the formation of gas. The process of fermentation is also important in the production of bread and many other foods and industrial materials. *See also* ENZYME.

FERTILITY, the power of reproduction, has been noted in females as young as eight years and as old as sixty. Among males, fertility has occurred as young as thirteen and has been reported in men of advanced age.

Fertility varies greatly from one person to another. In many instances, the male may be infertile with one woman but not with another. Similarly the woman may or may not be fertile, depending on the male. Accordingly fertility should be viewed as depending on the reproductive ability of both man and woman and not on one of them alone.

The likelihood of giving birth to more than one child at a time has been estimated as: twins, once in 90 births; triplets, once in 10,000; quadruplets, once in 750,000; quintuplets, once in many million, and the recorded delivery of sextuplets includes at least a few instances which are authentic.

By the use of x-rays, a multiple birth may be anticipated early enough so that proper preparations can be made for the arrival of the infants. Fecundity is apparently a hereditary characteristic. *See also* BIRTH, MULTIPLE; STERILITY.

FETUS, a term designating the unborn child in the mother's womb and applied usually from the end of the third month of pregnancy until birth. *See also* CHILDBIRTH AND PRENATAL CARE.

FEVER, the abnormal rise in temperature of the human body. Normal body temperature is 98.6° F. or 37° C. To determine whether or not a person has fever and its degree, a thermometer is used. Thermometers are generally graded from 92° to 108° F. Normal temperature is indicated by a tiny red arrow on the thermometer. To measure temperature, the mercury in the thermometer should always be well shaken down before the thermometer is used, and the thermometer left in the mouth at least three minutes. A thermometer placed under the arm records about one degree lower, and a thermometer placed in the rectum about one degree higher than one placed in the mouth. Human beings seldom survive if the temperature by mouth exceeds 110° F. or falls below 90° F.

In certain diseases the form of the fever is distinctive. In many infections such as pneumonia and typhoid fever, the temperature becomes high and stays high. In other conditions, as for instance tuberculosis, the fever may be low in the morning and high in the afternoon. In some forms of malaria a fever occurs which lasts about eight hours and develops every other day. In other forms of malaria the fever lasts about eight hours but occurs only every third day. Physicians who have studied the various forms of disease can learn a great deal from a case record of the temperature made every four hours.

Fever may result not only from a disturbance of the heat-regulating mechanism of the body but also through disturbances of the blood or the rate of breathing. Indeed, there are records of a rise of the temperature of the body in which the fever is the sole manifestation of some mental or emotional disturbance, which in turn causes tissue changes that bring about an increased temperature.

When the body is invaded by germs, an infectious fever results.

This is due to the fact that the mechanisms which in health prevent a fall in temperature when the body is exposed to cold are affected by the poisons produced by the infecting germs. The loss of heat from the body is prevented by constriction of the blood vessels, as seen in the fact that the skin is cold, pale, and slightly blue. There is also a feeling of chilling and shivering, which in turn is due to the fact that the tissues in the skin which provide a feeling of warmth are not stimulated by the warm blood which ordinarily would be coming to them. The chills of fever are due to the spasm of the vessels in the skin and the exclusion from these blood vessels of the warm blood that comes from deeper in the body. In fever, the blood volume being reduced, there are also changes in the concentration of the blood and in its content of salts and other materials. Drugs which produce a fall in temperature are those that increase elimination of heat from the body through drawing water from the tissues into the blood vessels, increasing the blood sugar, and dilating the blood vessels.

A fever is, therefore, not necessarily detrimental to the human body. It may be an important aid in combating disease. In fact there are some germs which cannot live in the presence of a temperature above that of the normal temperature of the human body.

Fever causes a definite increase in the speed of the chemical changes that go on within the human body. For every rise of 1 degree Fahrenheit in the temperature of the body, there will be an increase of about 7 per cent in the speed of the chemical changes. The excretion of nitrogen in the urine is greatly increased in most fevers. The nitrogen comes from the protein of the human body, so that from 300 to 400 grams or almost a pound of protein may be destroyed daily by a fever. Therefore it has now become customary to feed a fever by increasing the total amount of calories taken into the body and also by increasing particularly the amount of protein that is given. In order to reduce the waste of the body tissue in fevers, a liberal diet is given containing foods that are not contra-indicated by any special feature of the disease. The sugar and fat are also drawn on during starvation as well as in fever. The amount of calories taken by a patient with a fever may be twice the amount normally required to maintain the person at his normal weight. Because people sometimes find themselves unable to take food during a fever, sick people usually lose weight.

There is a section in the brain that is known as the heat-regulating center. A hemorrhage or a tumor in the brain at this point may be accompanied with an exceedingly high fever. Such cases are, however, extremely unusual.

The extent to which a fever is to be prevented or controlled, therefore, depends on the physician's judgment as to just how much control he wishes to exercise. He is likely to provide plenty of water to the patient because the body will evaporate more water from its surface. Frequently the best technique for lowering an ordinary fever is a simple sponge bath with warm water, 85 or 90 degrees or even slightly warmer. The sponge bath should never be given in a cold room. Any of the drugs used to control fever, including aspirin, sodium salicylate, phenacetin, as well as the more dangerous acetanilid, are to be used only when the doctor prescribes them and only in the amount prescribed. *See also* CONVULSION; THERMOMETER.

FEVER BLISTERS. *See* HERPES SIMPLEX.

FIBRILLATION, the name of the condition in which a muscle develops a slight shivering or tremor. In certain degenerative diseases, such as *amyotrophic lateral sclerosis*, muscles fibrillate, but the term is applied particularly to *auricular fibrillation* in the heart. Instead of having a smooth powerful beat, the heart action and pulse become irregular in relationship to each other. This weakens the force of the pulsation. The condition is treated either with *digitalis* or with *quinidine*. If the fibrillation is associated with thyroid disease, surgery of the thyroid may be indicated.

Ventricular fibrillation, an extreme form, occurs in the ventricles of the heart in coronary thrombosis. Since little blood, if any, can be poured into the aorta from the heart, the condition is usually fatal. *See also* HEART.

FIBRINOGEN DEFICIENCY. Fibrinogen is one of the essential blood proteins manufactured by the liver. In severe liver disturbance this function may be disordered and restrict the clotting ability of the blood. *See also* COAGULATION.

FIBROMA, a tumor of fibrous tissue. Most fibromas are *benign,* as opposed to cancerous tumors which are *malignant.* However, some tumors have both fibrous and cancerous tissue and are known as *mixed tumors. See* MEDIGRAPH page 1315.

FIBROSITIS, inflammation of fibrous or connective tissue of the muscles anywhere in the body outside of the joints. *Muscular rheumatism* is a form of fibrositis. While rheumatic toxins may be responsible for fibrositis, other toxins, such as those from septic teeth or throat or from some other form of infection may be the underlying cause.

The condition is frequently related to exposure to damp or cold weather, and, in the case of middle-aged or older persons, to overexertion or fatigue. Many people suffer from fibrositis after a slight draft or after an electric fan has played on a part of their body even for a short time.

Fibrositis in the lumbar region of the back may be a form of *lumbago.* Frequently it is involved in cases of stiff neck and sometime affects the scalp, the buttocks, and less often the muscles between the ribs. Occasionally the tendons are inflamed; and the bursas, or fluid-bearing sacs, in certain joints may also be affected.

The most common symptom is pain, increasing in intensity and lasting from a few days to a few weeks. The condition tends to become chronic, and is worse after periods of inactivity.

Temporary relief may be obtained by moderate exercise or massage. Aspirin and other salicylates may be beneficial. A combination of heat and massage as well as the application of liniment is also helpful.

If fibrositis is accompanied by fatigue or exhaustion, an attempt should be made to find the specific cause, such as infection, error in diet, or undue exposure. People with fibrositis should be protected against catching cold, chilling, dampness, or sudden changes in temperature. Wool or a wool mixture should be worn next to the skin, and drafts avoided.

Fibrositis affecting the bursa may sometimes be effectively treated by x-ray. In other instances anesthetic substances injected directly into the affected area have been successful. *See also* ARTHRITIS; RHEUMATISM.

FILARIASIS, an infection caused by a threadlike worm *filaria* which invades the human body. The female filaria gives birth in the human body to embryos which migrate through the body to the blood vessels and skin. From the skin, they are taken by blood-sucking flies and mosquitoes. In the insect's body they mature and migrate to the salivary glands. When the insect bites a person, the larvae get into or near the tiny wound inflicted by the insect's bite, and eventually penetrate to the interior of the person's body and travel through blood or lymph vessels until they find a permanent living site.

Perhaps the best-known form of filariasis is the tropical disease *elephantiasis* (*Bancroft's filariasis*), in which the legs and other parts of the body become grossly swollen. The worm lives in the lymph vessels and associated tissue in the groin and in tissues associated with the external genitalia. Inflammation is followed by acute pain in these areas, then by apparent but temporary recovery. The symptoms reappear, alternating with the seeming recovery until a chronic stage is reached when lymph glands and ducts become obstructed by the worms, and the more pronounced forms of elephantiasis are observed. The larvae or *microfilariae* circulate in the person's blood at night when he is quiet, typically between midnight and two o'clock, and blood samples are taken by the doctor at this time. The larvae leave the blood during the active, daytime hours. The legs, groin glands, and male genitalia swell and the process sometimes extends to the interior of the body. On the surface of the skin, blood circulation is seriously impeded, cracking occurs, and finally secondary infection by bacteria and fungi sets in.

Satisfactory treatment for this infection was unknown in the past. Recent reports, however, describe favorable results with *naphuride sodium* and *hetrazan*. Sulfonamides are used against secondary infection

and surgery for deformities of overgrown tissue. Prevention against filariasis consists mainly of eliminating the mosquito-breeding areas, the use of screens, and of DDT to protect persons from the infected mosquitoes.

Another filarial disease is caused by the burrowing migrations below the skin of a threadlike worm, the *eye worm,* which is found mostly in Africa. This, too, is transmitted by insect bite, that of the *mango fly*. The worm leaves an irritated, raised serpentine track as it passes on its slow way, perhaps an inch a day. It typically takes a route almost straight across both eyeballs and the bridge of the nose, down the temple and neck to the other side. Treatment consists of removing the worm with a hooked needle. The victim usually recovers.

An acute condition, *onchocercosis,* caused by filaria produces tumorous growths of coiled worms under the skin, sometimes as large as an orange. It is found in some parts of Central and South America as well as Africa. The microfilariae of this infection can create serious disturbances in the eye and sometimes blindness. Surgical removal of the growths and administration of the drugs used against *Bancroft's filariasis* are employed against this condition.

FINGER. The human hand terminates in four fingers and a thumb. The fingers are known as the fore or index, the middle, the ring, and the little finger, the first being the most mobile and sensitive. The movements of the fingers are performed by small muscles in the hand, controlled by the ulnar nerve. If this becomes paralyzed, a loss of function and inability to spread the fingers results. The other movements of the hand are controlled by the muscles in the forearm which connect with the fingers. Sometimes an infection of the little finger will result in an abscess in the forearm, traveling along the connecting sheaths covering the tendons in the finger, palm, and wrist.

Various congenital deformities affect the fingers: too many fingers, too few fingers; adjoining fingers united by a thin or even fleshy web; contracted or bent fingers.

Various distortions of the fingers resulting from burns or accidents may be successfully treated by plastic surgery. Certain diseases, such as endocarditis or tuberculosis may induce clubbed fingers which are swollen at the ends. Arthritis may cause hard nodules to form, and deposits at the joints may result from gout.

FINGERNAILS. *See* NAILS.

FIRST AID, emergency treatment given in case of accident or sudden illness. It is necessary on innumerable occasions. Certain principles of first aid should be known to everyone, since immediate treatment before a doctor arrives may prevent more serious developments or even save lives.

Here are a few suggestions on what to do in an emergency situation:

1. Give a stricken person space—people have a tendency to crowd around the victim. Be sure he has air so that he can breathe freely.

2. Don't try to make someone who has fallen sit or stand. The effort to stand or sit may cause grave injury. Do not move the person; a bone may be broken. If the person must be moved, splints should be improvised and applied beforehand.

3. In case of bleeding, try to find the source. Merely placing a thumb on a bleeding cut and keeping it there has saved lives. Never give alcohol to a person who is bleeding externally or internally; it will only increase the bleeding.

4. When a person has fainted, keep his head below the level of the rest of the body so that the blood will flow more easily to the head. Loosen clothing about the neck and chest.

5. Since most accidents involve shock, the victim should be kept warm with extra clothing or blankets. A light massage of the limbs may be helpful.

A doctor should of course be summoned unless you are absolutely sure that the injury is slight.

Every home should have a really adequate first-aid outfit. It should include the following items kept in their original containers in a tightly shut tin box: 1 yard of 2″ gauze: ½ yard oiled silk; absorbent cotton; 2 triangular bandages; finger bandages; and clean scissors.

Also essential in the home is a properly supplied medicine chest which should include: 1 ounce bottle tincture of iodine; 1 ounce boric acid powder; aromatic spirits of ammonia; 1 ounce epsom salts; enema syringe; and clean scissors. *See also* ACCIDENTS; MEDICINE CHEST; POISONING; RESUSCITATION; SHOCK.

FISH. Many persons in the United States believe that a diet of fish is not as nutritious as one of meat. This is wholly untrue. Entire nations subsist largely on fish and thrive on it. Some investigators tend, in fact, to support the view that a diet high in fish is more healthful than one high in meat. At any rate, arteriosclerotic and coronary diseases are far less common in countries like Japan, where fish is the main protein staple, than in the United States, where meat is the main protein staple. It is entirely possible that the protein of fish is more readily assimilable by the human body than that of meat. Further research remains to be conducted in this field.

The protein content of most of the fish most commonly eaten, such as halibut, cod, whitefish, salmon, trout, pickerel, and perch, averages from 15 to 18 per cent as contrasted with approximately 21 per cent for mutton, beefsteak, and pork.

The flesh of fish generally contains, in addition to protein, water, fat, mineral salt—particularly iodine and phosphorus—and vitamins. It is especially valuable as a source of vitamin A and vitamin D which is significant in relation to the use of calcium and phosphorus by the body. Cod liver oil and other fish liver oils, notably halibut and salmon, are also rich in vitamins A and D. Fish roe contains vitamins B and E as well. Most of the fat in the leading fish is stored in the liver, except for salmon, mackerel, tuna, bonito, sardines, and herring which have about 10 to 15 per cent in the flesh. Studies of the vitamin content of various edible parts of fish indicate that oysters give the most complete vitamin value, followed closely by salmon and herring. Fish, while rich in all these things, lack calcium. Lobster has a high manganese content.

FISSURE, a division or groove between adjoining parts of similar substance. The brain contains many fissures. The term is also properly applied to certain narrow abnormal pathways, such as those which occur in the nipple or anus.

A fissure of the nipple is seen most frequently when the mother is nursing and is commonly due to lack of care, though a certain stiffness of the skin over the nipple may accentuate the breaking of the skin. To avoid this type of fissure, the mother should wash and dry the nipple with care after every feeding. Any rigidity of the skin in this area can be prevented or reduced if an appropriate ointment is applied.

The presence of an anal fissure is usually accompanied by severe pain when defecating and often reaches down into the thighs. Blood or pus or both may also be seen in the feces. An anal fissure ordinarily occurs at the lower end of the bowel and probably near the rear. A hemorrhoid is often seen where it reaches the anal opening.

The pain of an anal fissure may be somewhat relieved if the person will take laxatives as needed to soften his bowel movement. The surface should then be cleansed with soft paper or cloth, and the anus and adjoining parts should be washed after every movement. After the area is dried, a soothing ointment is beneficial. Most physicians are convinced that surgery is the only successful treatment for anal fissure. *See also* ANUS; HEMORRHOIDS. *See* MEDIGRAPH page 743.

FISTULA, an abnormal narrow passage which leads from some cavity of the body to the outside skin and which may connect one cavity with another. Such an opening if not a narrow passage is not, strictly speaking, a fistula. Nevertheless, it may properly be described as fistulous.

A fistula present at birth indicates that some passageway, normal while the infant was in the womb, failed to close after birth as it should have done. Sometimes a child is born with an aperture at the navel through which urine escapes. Similarly this opening, normal in the fetus, ordinarily closes after birth.

A fistula may also stem from a wound or abscess which cannot heal because it persistently receives the contents of some body cavity. An *anal* fistula often originates in this manner. Two types of anal fistulae are the *complete,* which opens from the rectum and travels outside the bowel to the skin, usually terminating close to the anus; and the *incomplete,* so-called because it lacks

either the surface or the rectal opening.

The incomplete anal fistula may also lead from the surface to some abscess which is created and occupied by germs which have seeped through the wall of the bowel. Early treatment of such an abscess may avoid the development of a fistula. However, if the fistula already exists it will drain persistently to the surface. The patient will not suffer pain unless the passage becomes clogged. However, at the point where the fistula reaches the skin he may experience discomfort and itching.

Another common type of fistula travels from the wall of the stomach to an abscess near the appendix, and still another is the *vaginal* fistula. If the lining of the vagina has been damaged in childbirth, this type of fistula may arise between the vagina and bladder or between the vagina and rectum. A fistula may also arise from either one of the *parotid glands,* which are under the ears, and move to a point where it enters the cheek. This is known as a *salivary* fistula.

If a fistula persists beyond the early stages, surgery is the only cure.

FITS. The word *fit* without a modifier simply means a sudden attack or seizure of any kind. The term is commonly used, however, to designate an attack of *convulsions*. Fits are associated not only with epilepsy but may also occur in connection with asphyxia, poisoning, lockjaw, rabies, apoplexy, meningitis and in slow-pulse diseases such as anemia of the brain. They may also appear, together with subsequent coma, as a disturbance of late pregnancy. The type of fit known as *infantile convulsions* may sometimes be a reflex action associated with teething, worms, rickets, fever or diarrhea.

Hysterical fits are of special interest because they do not involve such symptoms as loss of consciousness or incapacity to control the bladder or bowels. Usually they occur to a person in the company of others, which seems to indicate that the victim is subconsciously trying to gain attention. Though hysterical fits are seldom physically dangerous, they do indicate a tense emotional conflict which may require the attention of a psychiatrist.

Regardless of the cause, the first step in giving relief to a convulsive patient, while awaiting the doctor, is to place him on his back. It is necessary to prevent him from doing harm to himself but use of force should be kept to a minimum. A piece of wood should be wrapped in a handkerchief and placed between the teeth so that he will not bite his tongue. His clothes should be loosened, especially around the neck and across the chest. If he vomits, he should be placed on his side. Gradually as the person recovers, every effort should be made to communicate with him and to reassure him. The patient is only half conscious at this stage, however, and must be treated with caution since he might suddenly become physically dangerous. *See also* EPILEPSY; ECLAMPSIA; CONVULSIONS.

FLATFOOT, a common foot disorder which may be the result of an occupation that requires long periods of standing or walking, overweight, disease, injury, or paralysis. The condition may be based on weakness of the foot arch that is inborn, or it may be acquired through overstrain and poor position. Poorly fitting shoes may also promote the sagging of the arch. These faults which do not seem great nevertheless cause the ligaments to stretch, relax, and become incapable of returning to their original flexibility. The bones are then affected and the arch flattens, and soreness, pain, and fatigue result.

If some flexibility is retained, much may be done by proper shoes, arch supports, pads, manipulation, training, and by exercise to strengthen the muscles and other parts of the foot. All of these exercises and the course of treatment should be under the supervision of a foot specialist since slight variations of adjustment are sometimes notably effective. Even surgery may be necessary to break up the fibrous adhesions which form in rigidly flat feet. *See also* ARCHES, FALLEN; FEET.

FLATULENCE, an excess of air or gas in the stomach or intestines or in both. Often painful, this accumulation of air may adversely affect breathing, as well as the normal action of the heart.

Flatulence can be caused occasionally by fermentation in the stomach, or more often by eating of certain types of food such as beans. Most frequently it results from swal-

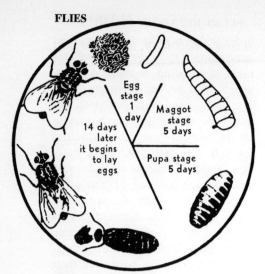

Flies—The life cycle of a fly. During the cold weather, the fly usually stays in the pupa stage. In warm weather it can become an adult fly within five days.

lowing air while eating or drinking.

Drugs taken for relief of flatulence are *carminatives*. Ordinarily their active component is peppermint, ginger, dill, or anise. Any of these serve not only to expel the accumulated air but also to soothe the stomachache associated with flatulence.

To avoid swallowing air, chew food with the mouth closed. This is most effective when peace and harmony are encouraged during eating. *See also* INDIGESTION.

FLIES. Flies are one of the commonest and most dangerous pests known to man. Such species as the common housefly, stable flies, greenbottle flies, bluebottle flies, blowflies, fruit flies, and others feed on contaminated garbage and may spread viruses and germs. Such filth-feeding flies have been incriminated in the spread of epidemics of typhoid, dysentery, diarrhea, cholera, infectious hepatitis, and other diseases.

A female housefly can lay as many as 2000 eggs during its lifetime. In warm weather these eggs hatch in from eight to ten hours and the new flies go right on breeding. Here are some simple recommendations for getting rid of filth-feeding flies:

Clean up yards, vacant lots, and all surroundings.

Flies—The fly is one of the most dangerous animals known because it feeds and breeds on filth and spreads disease-producing organisms.

FLIES CARRY FILTH

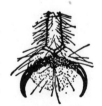

BECAUSE
BRED IN
FILTH

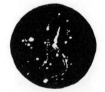

Hairy foot of a fly

Bacteria colony in fly's footprint

A FLY OFTEN CARRIES 6,600,000 BACTERIA ON ITS HAIRY BODY

FROM
Manure pile
Garbage can
Privy vault
Spittoon
Sickroom

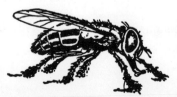

TO
Milk
Baby's lips
Baby's bottle
Food
You

Get rid of accumulations of decaying material.

Keep all garbage cans covered and wash them frequently.

Don't spill garbage around the can or permit it on the sides of the can.

Fill in all low spots where water is accumulated after rain.

Screen all doors and windows in the home and keep the screens in repair.

Cover the baby carriage with mosquito netting when the baby is sleeping outdoors.

Keep flies out of any sick room.

Be sure that all food is kept covered and do not buy food where it is constantly exposed to flies.

Swat the fly and be sure the fly swatter is scrubbed once in a while.

Always wash your hands with soap and water after handling a fly.

Outdoor privies should be soundly constructed and screened. Application of quick lime or crude oil or a 5–10 per cent solution of DDT in oil should be made frequently to the contents of the pit. Of course, running water toilets are vastly preferable and should be installed whenever possible.

Remember, if there is no exposed debris or filth there will probably be fewer flies.

FLU. *See* INFLUENZA.

FLUID RETAINED IN THE BODY. Ordinarily the body contains a certain amount of water which is distributed in the cells of the different structures that make up the body. Extra water is a problem.

It may collect in or around the cells in small amounts, or it may collect in large amounts in the different body cavities. The word *edema* is used to describe extra fluid in the tissues beneath the skin. Its presence is determined simply by pressing with the finger, in which case the indentation or pit remains. Fluid in the abdomen is called *ascites* and fluid in the chest is known as *hydrothorax*. When there is excess fluid everywhere in the body the term *anasarca* is used. One sign of excess fluid accumulation may be rapid gain in weight.

A variety of conditions may be responsible for these disturbances of handling of water by the body. The trouble may be with the blood, or the blood vessels, or the blood pressure. The difficulty may be in the composition of the tissues themselves. There may be blocking of the flow of lymph. Finally, the kidneys play an important part in the elimination of fluid.

Actually the taking of an excess of water as fluids or in food is not the chief or important factor in water accumulation. Ordinarily the excess of fluid is simply eliminated by the kidneys which can get rid of twenty times as much fluid as they usually eliminate. An excess of sodium or salt is more likely to cause accumulation of water in the body since the ability of the kidneys and sweat to get rid of excess salt is much less than for water. Since the adrenal glands are important in controlling the salt-water balance, disturbances of these glands may be responsible for excess fluid.

651

Swelling of one leg or arm is likely due to an obstruction of circulation affecting that organ. When both swell the difficulty is probably a general one. Swelling of eyelids and face in the morning is associated with insufficient protein intake. *See also* NEPHROSIS.

FLUORIDATION, the addition of chemical salts—*fluorides*—to the water supply. It has been carried out in many communities in an effort to reduce dental decay. Fluorine is a chemical element found in the enamel of teeth, bones, and in minute quantities in other body tissues. Experiments with schoolchildren, each one receiving a regular intake of one part per million of flourides in drinking water, have established that there is a definite reduction in dental decay in children when water is fluorinated. No such results have been established for adults. Fluorine occurs naturally in the water supply of some parts of the world in the form of *calcium fluoride*. Its artificial addition to the water supply in other communities has usually been in the form of *sodium fluoride,* which has precipitated widespread controversy. However, no definitive proof has yet been adduced to show that the use of sodium fluoride is actually harmful.

FLUOROSCOPY, the act of using a fluoroscope; of observing, on a specially coated screen, the shadows of objects which are being x-rayed. This diagnostic technique has the advantage of offering a moving picture rather than a static photograph. The intestines may be examined in action, or the setting of a fractured bone can actually be followed with the eyes. The disadvantage of the fluoroscope is the fact that the image is less precise than that of a photograph. *See also* X-RAYS.

FOOD ALLERGY, a disturbance affecting people who are sensitive to one or more particular foods. When eaten, such foods cause symptoms of irritation of the stomach and bowels, and often a skin rash such as hives, erythema, eczema, or perhaps asthmatic symptoms.

White of egg is a frequent cause of such allergy, as are fish, cheese, tomatoes, pork, shellfish, and other foods. The protein contained in them is most often responsible.

Food allergies in infants generally result in eczema or diarrhea and may be caused by egg white, milk, or cereals. The symptoms usually appear the first time the infant is fed these foods, and ordinarily disappear by the end of the second year. In children, sensitivity to eggs, wheat, and milk occurs less frequently as the child grows older and should disappear between the ages of four and twelve. The symptoms are dry and itchy skin eruptions. Scratching causes thickening and intensified itching, and broken skin. Because of the danger of infection, childhood eczema should be carefully watched. *See also* ALLERGY; ECZEMA.

FOOD, BASIC REQUIREMENTS. The human body grows from approximately seven pounds at birth to many times that weight in maturity. Then, after full growth is attained, the body must maintain itself by a process of constant replacement for the duration of life. The body constantly replaces itself with new cells and destroys the old ones.

The body requires certain conditions to carry on this process of growth and replacement.

Quantity of food. Food energy is measured in calories. One calorie is the amount of heat needed to raise the temperature of a liter of water from 15° to 16° C. By knowing the number of calories in a particular food, the amount of energy contained in any quantity of that food can be calculated. This tells how much energy the body will be able to get from that food. (Calories are measured by actually placing the food to be tested in a miniature furnace and accurately measuring the energy released as heat. In the human body foods are burned by a process of chemical digestion; but the amount of energy released by any food when used by the body is almost exactly the same as the amount of energy released when the same food is burned in the testing furnace.)

Different foods contain different amounts of calories (energy). Fat foods are fattening because a piece of fat contains more than twice as many calories as a piece of protein or carbohydrate of the same weight. An ounce of pure fat provides 288 calories, while an equal amount of protein or carbohydrate would give only 128 calories.

The number of calories which the human body needs depends upon the person's weight, his age (growth rate), the climate in which he lives, his individual chemical makeup, and the amount of physical activity he is engaged in. An adult requires 13 calories for each pound of body weight just to keep the body alive for twenty-four hours—the wear and tear of destroying and rebuilding body tissue. An infant requires three to four times that number of calories, and a growing child about twice—or 26 calories—per pound of body weight to build the new muscle, bone, and skin which make the body grow larger. The person who performs hard physical labor needs more calories than someone whose work keeps him sitting at a desk all day. Heavier people frequently require more food than lighter people. Hot weather decreases and cold weather increases the calories required. An additional 10 per cent of the total calories needed are used for digestion of food. In the last three months of pregnancy an extra 450 calories per day should be added to the diet, and during lactation a woman who is nursing her baby needs an extra 1000 calories daily. *See also* NUTRITION.

FOOD FATS. Fat is a white or yellow substance, greasy to the touch, found in both animals and plants. When pure, fat has no odor, taste, or color. It exists both as a liquid and as a solid and may be dissolved in chloroform, ether, or benzene, but not in water or cold alcohol.

As a food, fat is valuable primarily as fuel, a source of energy. The most concentrated food we have, it possesses more than twice the caloric value of carbohydrates. Every ounce of fat has the same value as every other, whether it be an ounce of butter or an ounce of cottonseed oil. One type of fat, however, may be more accessible or assimilable than another. In the United States, fats are consumed most frequently in the form of eggs, butter, margarine, cream, meat, olive oil, vegetable oil, and nuts. *See also* NUTRITION; FATS, UNSATURATED.

FOOD POISONING, an illness due to disease-causing organisms or harmful foreign substances, such as chemicals, in food. Misconceptions and confusion are common regarding food poisoning. For example, there is actually no such illness as "ptomaine poisoning." Ptomaines are products of putrefactive organisms which, because they were toxic to experimental animals when given by injection, were long considered responsible for the effects of food poisoning. Later studies established that ptomaines are destroyed in the human digestive process and almost certainly do not have any connection with the symptoms of food poisoning.

Disease-causing bacteria are the commonest source of food poisoning, the most frequent probably being the *staphylococcus*. The same type of bacteria is responsible for many local infections of the skin involving abscesses and formation of pus. Perhaps the most severe type of food poisoning from bacteria is

botulism, which occurs much less frequently than staphylococcal poisoning. As with botulism, poisoning by staphylococci is actually the effect of a toxin produced by the organisms. Probably everyone is affected by it at some time or other. Possibly what was once called ptomaine poisoning was actually caused by staphylococci. Putrefaction by itself, the process carried on by the organisms which produce ptomaines, is not harmful. Limburger cheese and other putrefied foods are safely consumed. Such foods will, of course, become poisonous just as other foods, if when poisonous substances or organisms enter them.

Although not all staphylococci produce a substance toxic to human beings when ingested, those that are involved in boils and abcesses do, and such an infection on the hands or arms of a person preparing food can be a source of poisoning to many people. Cream and similar foods like custard and ice cream, Chedder cheese, potato salad, many kinds of sauces and prepared meats are especially susceptible media for these organisms. The poison itself is heat-resistant, but whereas botulinus toxin is ineffective if boiled for a few minutes, staphylococcus toxin retains its potency even after half an hour's boiling.

Staphylococci are found in the human nose and throat under ordinary conditions, although they are normally kept in check by natural balances. Another organism responsible for food poisoning is a type of bacteria called *salmonella*. Its effects may be more severe than those of

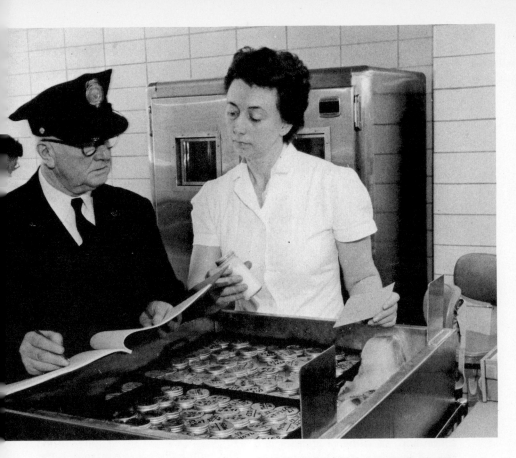

Government inspectors maintain a constant vigil against the possibility of food contamination. Above, milk is inspected to ensure its purity from microorganisms. Below, left, strawberries are inspected to determine the residue, if any, of injurious insecticides or fertilizers. Below, right, an inspector of the Federal Food and Drug Administration checks shipment of fish against possible decomposition.

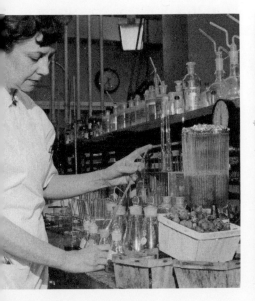

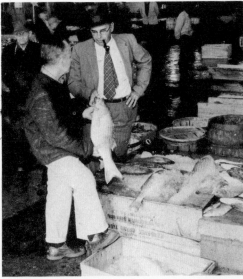

the staphylococci, and salmonella outbreaks have occurred in which 10 per cent of those stricken died. This, however, is extreme and the usual fatality rate is about 1 per cent.

A few varieties of mushrooms may prove fatal if eaten. *Mussel poisoning* has been traced to a protozoan, a one-celled microscopic organism, toxic to human beings, which is sometimes eaten by the mussel. *Cadmium poisoning* may occur when acid food is consumed which has been left in cadmium-plated containers, such as ice trays.

Food poisoning manifests its symptoms within six hours after consumption of the poison-containing food. Symptoms are similar to those often present in intestinal disturbances, nausea, cramps, diarrhea, vomiting, and frequently headaches and sweating. Fatalities are rare. The acute symptoms tend to abate after five or six hours. Prostration may occur, generally due to loss of body fluids. The physician usually prescribes remedies directed more toward ridding the body of the poison rather than merely relieving the symptoms. Removal of the infectious or poisonous matter from the stomach is probably necessary unless it has already been evacuated by natural processes. Water and salt in the appropriate form is administered to overcome the depletion of both, and general exhaustion treated with drugs which aid circulation and heart function. *See also* BOTULISM; MUSHROOM POISONING; POISONING.

FOOT-AND-MOUTH DISEASE, an acute febrile (fever) disease, characterized by an eruption of blisters about either or both the feet and mouth. It affects chiefly cattle and other animals with cloven hoofs. The disease is contagious, involving a virus which may be spread by the infected animal, or, indirectly, through contact with the animal's straw or milk.

This affliction seldom attacks man. When it does, symptoms do not appear before three to five days after exposure. Fever and headache are followed by the appearance of characteristic blisters. In man, these appear on the hands, as well as on the feet and mouth. Treatment of human beings is primarily concerned with reducing the fever and applying antiseptics to the blisters and to the open sores which appear when the blisters break. Since foot-and-mouth disease is contagious, the patient—man or animal—should be isolated until a physician can be consulted.

FOREIGN BODIES. Any strange substance that does not belong in the human body but gets in and stays there for a length of time is known as a foreign body. All sorts of substances can get into the body accidentally or purposely. Children are always swallowing substances that should not be swallowed, and poking them into the nose or ear. Sometimes adults push foreign substances into the openings of the body, such as the genitals or the rectum.

Needles, nails, toothpicks, bullets, shell fragments, and pieces of glass have been found in the heart. Out of 109 cases which one doctor collected, needles were present in 18 and bullets and shrapnel in 85. A nine-months-old girl swallowed a piece of wire with some food because her mother used an old wire strainer for sieving vegetables. She had noticed that several small pieces broke off but she continued to use it. Eventually it was found by the use of the x-ray that the child had a piece of the wire in the heart. Still later this passed out of the body. Two years after the x-ray showed the wire to be in the heart, the child suddenly coughed up an old blood clot in which was a piece of corroded wire. The x-ray was used again and showed that the wire had passed out of the heart.

Surgeons group foreign bodies found in the gastrointestinal tract or elsewhere in the body as hardware, jewelry, pins, seeds, bones, buttons, dental and surgical objects, ammunition, toys, or coins. All sorts of means have been developed for retrieving such bodies. Magnets are used to retrieve steel or iron foreign bodies. Tubes have been invented that can be passed down the throat or into other openings and are thus available for reaching into the farthest corners of the esophagus, the windpipe, the bronchial tubes, and even into the lungs.

When foreign substances get into the nose, more harm is usually done by attempting to dislodge them with improper instruments than by letting them alone until a doctor can be called. If blowing the nose will not remove a foreign substance, sneezing will usually accomplish this. The doctor usually washes out foreign substances or removes them with special forceps.

The toothpick is almost wholly a North American institution. There are many cases on record, however, in which people chew toothpicks and swallow portions, subsequently requiring a surgical operation for their removal.

Most important in detecting a foreign body in any portion of the body is the x-ray. By the use of the x-ray all kinds of materials have been found in the stomach and in the intestines, including hair balls, collections of seeds, or pieces of glass.

A foreign body in the ear is best removed by turning the head to one side and filling the ear with warm oil by means of a spoon. This will help to float the body out of the ear. If an insect is in the ear, the warm oil will suffocate the insect and permit it to float out. After the use of the warm oil, the ear can be syringed with warm water. The water is sprayed against the side of the entrance to the ear rather than against the eardrum. No one should ever attempt to remove a foreign body from the eye or the ear or the nose or any portion of the body without being certain what he is doing.

FRACTURES. Breaking of a bone or cartilage is a fracture. Fractures may be classified by the type of bone or the type of break. If a

the injury and its causes An injury is described as a fracture when there is any break in the continuous line of the bone. It may be a complete fracture, which means right through the bone, or an incomplete one in which the break is partial. When the ligament tears a small piece of bone at the point where it is attached, it is called a chip or sprain fracture. A compound fracture is one in which the broken bone protrudes through the skin. Other fractures are identified by the direction of the break and the position of the fragments.

A fracture is usually the result of violence to the part involved and occurs most often to the young age group exposed to accidents, and older people subject to falls. However, it also can be caused by weakness of the bone structure, local bone disease, rickets, and old age.

A dislocation of a bone always occurs at a joint. This, too, may be complete or partial. The patient cannot move the part involved, and there is deformity which disappears when the dislocation is corrected.

symptoms Most often the patient is involved in some kind of accident and feels a sharp pain at the point of the fracture as it happens. He may even hear the snap of the bone. There is swelling, pain, and tenderness along with bruise marks. The bone moves at some point where it should not, in a direction different from its normal one. There can be deformity of the part, and the patient will not be able to use it freely. Sometimes a grating sound is heard at the site of the fracture. In severe cases there is shock.

The symptoms of a dislocation are similar, except that there is no grating sound, and the deformity is usually much more obvious.

complications "Fracture fever" may develop, a condition which begins a day after the injury and can last several days. Infection is not an unusual development in cases of compound fracture. Other complications depend on how well the fracture heals. It is not unusual to have destruction of the local blood vessels and nerves when there is poor healing, and this may result in serious vascular and nerve disorders.

Dislocations can result in neuritis or palsy of the affected part. Or else the joint can become so loose that it dislocates at the slightest provocation.

prevention (or lessening of impact) Obviously, there is no way to prevent development of a traumatic fracture. Patients with bone disorders can only exert extreme care so they are not placed in a position where they are more susceptible to injury. Once the fracture has occurred, adequate and careful medical management is necessary to prevent poor healing and future problems. The diagnosis and the course of healing are followed by X-Ray.

These same factors also apply to the prevention or lessening of impact of dislocations.

Fractures and Dislocations

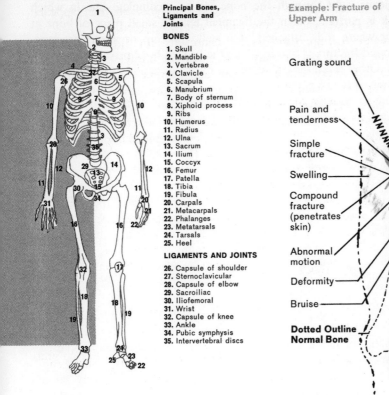

Principal Bones, Ligaments and Joints

BONES

1. Skull
2. Mandible
3. Vertebrae
4. Clavicle
5. Scapula
6. Manubrium
7. Body of sternum
8. Xiphoid process
9. Ribs
10. Humerus
11. Radius
12. Ulna
13. Sacrum
14. Ilium
15. Coccyx
16. Femur
17. Patella
18. Tibia
19. Fibula
20. Carpals
21. Metacarpals
22. Phalanges
23. Metatarsals
24. Tarsals
25. Heel

LIGAMENTS AND JOINTS

26. Capsule of shoulder
27. Sternoclavicular
28. Capsule of elbow
29. Sacroiliac
30. Iliofemoral
31. Wrist
32. Capsule of knee
33. Ankle
34. Pubic symphysis
35. Intervertebral discs

Example: Fracture of Upper Arm

Grating sound

Pain and tenderness

Simple fracture

Swelling

Compound fracture (penetrates skin)

Abnormal motion

Deformity

Bruise

Dotted Outline Normal Bone

Example: Dislocated elbow

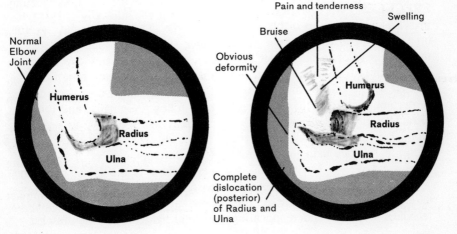

Normal Elbow Joint

Humerus

Radius

Ulna

Pain and tenderness

Swelling

Bruise

Obvious deformity

Humerus

Radius

Ulna

Complete dislocation (posterior) of Radius and Ulna

659

broken bone penetrates the skin, the condition is a compound or open fracture. If it does not penetrate the skin, it is a simple fracture. Careless handling of an injured person may change a simple fracture to a compound one. For this reason, the patient should never be moved until a physician has advised it, unless absolutely essential.

Some fractures have descriptive names, such as a *march fracture,* which involves the breaking of a small bone in the foot, a type of fracture which a soldier on a long march could sustain. A *greenstick* or *hickory stick fracture* occurs when one side of the bone is broken and the other side only bent.

A broken bone will not always be evident to an untrained person. A fracture may exist even though the victim is capable of moving the injured part. Anyone who has suffered a fall or injury with ensuing discomfort should seek medical advice promptly. *See also* BONES; RIBS; SKULL; SPINAL FRACTURE. *See* MEDIGRAPH page 659.

FRECKLES, are harmless small brown pigmented spots or blemishes on the skin, caused by exposure to the sun's rays or to ultraviolet light from artificial sources. They are formed by the cells of the skin as a protection against further action of ultraviolet rays. People with red or blond hair and light skin are more prone to freckles than those whose skins are dark.

Freckles appear about the seventh or eighth year and remain for life, receding in winter and reappearing in spring and summer. If the skin is shaded from the sun their appearance will be retarded.

Ointments for the skin which screen off the ultraviolet rays of the sun and prevent freckles from appearing are available, as are cosmetics which conceal freckles. Freckles may be removed with ointments containing skin-peeling properties. However, these ointments include substances that are poisonous and may cause dangerous irritation to the skin. Such preparations should not be used, especially on children. Freckles may be removed with these preparations, but they cannot be prevented from recurring. *See also* PIGMENTATION.

FRIEDREICH'S ATAXIA, a rare hereditary nervous disorder which may affect several members of a family. The difficulty usually appears in childhood or early youth with a lack of muscular coordination beginning in the legs and gradually involving the whole body.

The gait becomes shambling, almost drunken, the feet deformed as in claw foot. The child will walk with the heel raised, and on the outer side of the foot. The speech is also impaired and curvature of the spine to one side is noticeable. Paralysis of the whole leg muscle may follow eventually, and the victim may never be able to walk.

The disease is caused by imperfect development of bundles of nerve fibers in the spinal cord, and so far a cure is not known. However, attempts should be made to prevent tightening of the muscles.

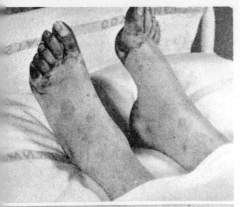

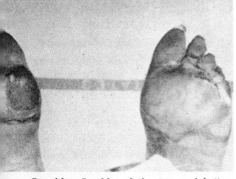

Frostbite—Frostbite of the toes and bottom of the feet. Picture was taken about seven days after freezing took place. Some of the areas are gangrenous. Patient was not aware he had a frostbite injury until the toes started to become black and hard.

Although there may be a gradual hunching position, disturbance of sensation or wastage of the muscles does not occur apart from that due to the action of the disease. Death comes not from the disease itself but from pneumonia or other secondary infections.

FROEHLICH'S SYNDROME, named after the scientist who first described it, is a disturbance of the glandular system in which sexual organs remain infantile. The disease is rare.

If the disease occurs in early childhood, it causes *dwarfism,* but if it appears in children before puberty, the boy or girl will be fat. The victim will be lazy mentally and have a voracious appetite for food. The sexual organs will be undeveloped. Most fat children do not suffer from this condition, and are more likely to be obese because of bad dietary habits.

The adult male becomes effeminate, his skin is soft, and the distribution of flesh around the thighs and breasts has a woman's appearance. Female patients become exceedingly fat, sometimes weighing as much as 300 pounds.

Modern hormone therapy can relieve many of the symptoms if the disease has not progressed beyond control. Treatment includes medical care and administration of hormones, such as pituitary extract. Proper therapy will reduce excessive weight, correct deformity, and restore sexual development.

FROSTBITE, a condition caused by exposure to extreme cold or cold and wind. The toes, fingers, ears, and tip of the nose are usually the first parts of the body to be affected. The frostbitten areas turn pale, the blood and moisture in the tissues freeze, and the circulation is cut off. Frostbite is dangerously deceptive since there is no feeling of pain and the victim is usually unaware of what is happening.

The old theory that a frostbitten area should be rubbed with snow or ice is completely false; such a procedure can actually cause harm. The best rules to follow in cases of frost-bite are simple: warm the affected area slowly by immersing it in tepid water or bundling it up in woolen cloth. Warming too fast produces severe pain. Do not under any circumstances rub the frostbitten area as the friction can break down the cell structure of the tissue. If the skin is warmed immediately the color will usually return. However, if the frostbite is severe, the area will remain white, indicating that the cold has contracted the blood vessels to such an extent that normal blood circulation cannot immediately be resumed. A doctor should be called immediately. In time the blood will seep back into the tissues, and the affected area will appear purplish or black. In a day or two, these areas may become acutely inflamed and painful from the pressure of fluids in the skin coming through the lower layers, and *blisters,* characteristic of frostbite, will appear. The blisters may leave ulcers on rupturing, and the affected tissues may die. Blisters should be treated with ointments after being opened, and then covered with dry sterile dressings. In severe cases of frostbite, the tissues may be irreparably damaged and *gangrene* result. Amputation of a toe, finger, or entire limb has been known to be necessary in such cases.

To prevent frostbite, outdoor activity should be postponed or limited when the temperature is below 8° F., particularly when there is a strong wind. If the temperature is between 8° F. and 15° F., some danger of frostbite exists. Clothing should be warm, wind-resistant, and properly fitted. Tight shoes, socks, and gloves restrict circulation and encourage frostbite. People who must work outdoors during extremely cold weather should not stay out longer than two hours at a time without intervening rest periods of half an hour. People with diabetes or any form of heart or circulatory disease are especially susceptible to serious damage from frostbite. *See also* CHILBLAINS; GANGRENE; SKIN; HAZARDS OF COLD.

FUMIGATION. Fumigation is done with disinfectants which employ smoke or fumes. The method is used, for example, against domestic insects or as a means of cleansing the sickroom of a patient who has suffered from an infectious disease.

When a room is to be fumigated, any metallic articles present must be washed with a disinfectant and removed. Likewise cupboard doors must be opened and all drawers pulled out. The window sashes should be sealed with gummed paper, and if the room contains a fireplace, the chimney should be stuffed with newspapers. Finally, after igniting the disinfectant, the doors ought to be sealed with gummed paper from the outside.

For general purposes, the best fumigant is *sulphur*. This is not effective, however, unless moisture is present. Therefore, before fumigating is begun, the walls, ceiling, and floor and also the furniture should be sprinkled with water. The next step is to fill a large basin partly with water and place it on a table in the center of the room. The sulphur, in a small bowl, is then set in this larger basin. The sulphur may be either in the form of candles or roll sulphur. Roll sulphur to be inflammable must be moistened with wood alcohol.

A more recent type of fumigant, and in some ways a more effective one, is the *freon bomb* which was first used by the armed forces in World War II. This contains an insecticide, such as *pyrethrum* or *DDT*. Immediately upon being opened, this fumigant penetrates to every corner of the room.

Approximately twenty-four hours after fumigation, the doors and windows can be opened wide and the room aired for a day or more. The wallpaper, if any, may be removed at this time and burned, and it is also advisable to limewash the ceiling and to scrub the floor, the woodwork, and the furniture with soap and water. *See also* BEDBUG; DISINFECTION; VENTILATION.

FUNGUS, a form of plant life. Fungi, a widespread group of simple plants commonly known as *mushrooms, molds,* and *yeasts,* do not have any chlorophyll of their own and depend upon green plants or other organisms for their food sources. Fungi which invade another living organism and obtain their food at the expense of this organism are *parasites.* Fungi which live on dead or decaying organisms are *saprophytes.* They flourish in the soil and in all sorts of warm damp places where they hatch and develop prolifically.

Some fungi are many-celled and reproduce by spore formation, each spore being capable of forming a new plantlike growth similar to the parent plant. Others, like the yeasts, are unicellular and reproduce by budding. The buds break off and form new cells.

Thousands of varieties of molds have been isolated and identified. Most of them are quite harmless to man and in some cases are highly beneficial. Some varieties are used as the source of the *antibiotics* which have saved countless thousands of lives since the development of penicillin. Many fungi, however, constitute a serious threat to mankind.

Disease-bearing molds are most prevalent in the soil, although they have also been found in such diverse sites as unpasteurized milk, cellars, animal excrement, cattle, and even in some community water supplies. Dangerous or undesirable fungi sometimes infest plant crops raised for food, causing potato blight and wheat rust. Some initiate and intensify certain types of asthma or hay fever; others cause the fungus or mycotic diseases which are quite common in human beings as well as in many domestic animals. These infections may be superficial, affecting only the skin, hair, and teeth, as in ringworm of the scalp, feet, and nails. More invasive fungi penetrate the tissues of internal structure and produce serious diseases of the mucous membranes, heart, lungs, and other organs. Among the more prevalent of these infections are *actinomycosis, blastomycosis, histo-*

the disease and its causes Fungi are responsible for many types of common skin disorders. These include athlete's foot, ringworm, and so-called jock itch or rash. They are contagious, although the individual reaction varies greatly. Perspiration, irritation from clothing, generalized illness, and skin sensitivity or allergy all play a role.

symptoms ATHLETE'S FOOT This type of fungus infection begins with the formation of small, watery blisters on the hands or feet. Itching is usually quite intense. The blisters dry and go through the peeling stage, but new areas of fresh lesions usually appear at nearby sites. Scratching or rubbing causes a spread of the infection, local irritation, and occasionally secondary infections. The areas between the toes are most frequently involved, and deep cracks or fissures frequently develop. It is not unusual to have athlete's foot spread to the soles and top of the feet. Allergic reactions to medications used in treatment are not unusual and may make the diagnosis and treatment more difficult.

RINGWORM OF THE BODY This is characterized by the development of a lesion which is usually round or ringlike in nature, has a scaly surface, and spreads from its red outer margin. The inside portion frequently appears clear. Again perspiration, with the increase of skin moisture and heat, appears to be an important factor.

Ringworm may involve any part of the body, and it differs somewhat in appearance depending upon the area affected. In men the beard area is a common site, and the lesion, while still round in appearance, frequently includes watery and pussy blisters. On the head it is associated with hair loss in the area involved, and the patches are usually grayish in color. The early stage of infection may be overlooked until a bald spot appears. The hair is found to be broken off near the skin, and the latter gives the impression of being coated with cigar ashes. The lesions are usually bean sized, but may involve larger or smaller areas. It is frequently difficult to see areas involved with the naked eye, but they are apparent under examination with a specific fluorescent light.

JOCK ITCH This eruption appears on the upper, inner surface of the thighs, extending almost to the buttocks. It also occurs in the armpits and beneath the breasts in women. The skin is inflamed, usually brownish red in color, with a deeper red toward the edge. Excessive perspiration can give it a very raw appearance. It is common during the hot weather.

complications The only complications are secondary infections. But the unsightly effect, when the head or face is included, can also be distressing.

prevention (or lessening of impact) Fungus infections are contagious and spread from human to human and animal to human. Contact with infected people or animals should be avoided and good hygiene practiced. Unsterilized barber tools should be avoided, and clothing should not be exchanged. Patients with athlete's foot should avoid group showers, wear protective slippers, and bathe their feet frequently.

Fungus Infections of the Skin (Athlete's Foot, Ringworm, Jock Itch)

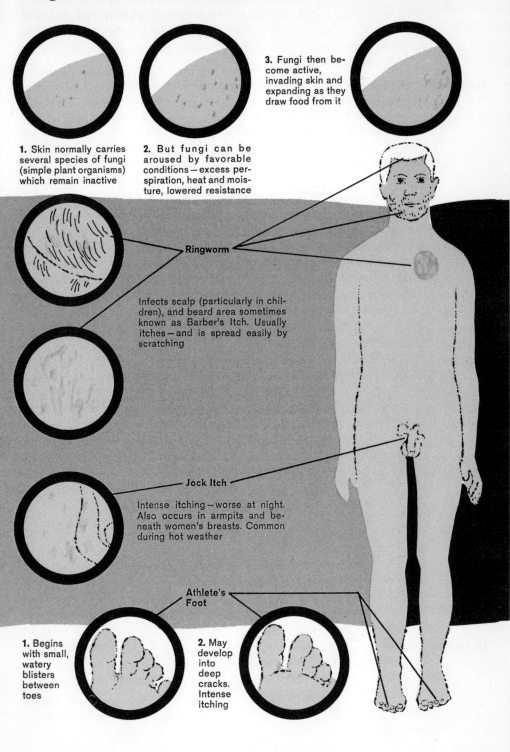

1. Skin normally carries several species of fungi (simple plant organisms) which remain inactive

2. But fungi can be aroused by favorable conditions—excess perspiration, heat and moisture, lowered resistance

3. Fungi then become active, invading skin and expanding as they draw food from it

Ringworm

Infects scalp (particularly in children), and beard area sometimes known as Barber's Itch. Usually itches—and is spread easily by scratching

Jock Itch

Intense itching—worse at night. Also occurs in armpits and beneath women's breasts. Common during hot weather

Athlete's Foot

1. Begins with small, watery blisters between toes

2. May develop into deep cracks. Intense itching

plasmosis, coccidioidomycosis, moniliasis, and *sporotrichosis,* all found throughout the southern and southeastern United States and in scattered areas throughout the world. *Maduromycosis,* a disease affecting the feet, occurs chiefly in tropical countries. *See also* ANTIBIOTICS; and names of specific fungus diseases. *See* MEDIGRAPH page 665.

FURUNCLES. A furuncle, or *boil,* is a painful, pus-producing inflammation of the skin, with a central core, caused ordinarily by certain types of bacteria which enter the skin through hair follicles or sweat glands. Usually such an infection does not occur unless resistance has been weakened by *diabetes, Bright's disease,* or a *fever.* Likewise, anyone suffering from undernourishment, fatigue, or constipation is vulnerable.

The skin may also be weakened by local irritation, such as the persistent rubbing of a starched collar on the neck.

Boils in the vicinity of the nose or in the ear should be examined promptly by a doctor. Others, unless they get large, may be permitted to follow their own course. Larger boils may be painful and often require surgery. An appropriate antiseptic may be applied to the general area to prevent the infection from spreading and creating another set of boils.

When the entire body is afflicted with boils, a physician will sometimes administer sulfonamides, penicillin, or other antibiotics. X-rays and ultraviolet rays, as well as vaccines and similar preparations, have also been used with success against persistent boils. *See also* CARBUNCLES. *See* MEDIGRAPH page 315.

G

GAIT, a characteristic manner of walking. Certain diseases are associated with a characteristic gait. Coordination between the two feet may be distorted—for example, by a degenerative disease of the spinal cord known as *locomotor ataxia.* The victim of this disease will lift each foot abruptly and higher than necessary, after which he pushes it forward and lowers it with a sudden thump. At the same time, he seems compelled to lean out and observe these movements, in order to finish them.

Another disease of the spinal cord, involving the lateral columns of the cord, produces a wooden gait in which the feet are pulled across the ground. This often involves a kind of crisscrossing of the feet, as they are dragged forward.

Several other types of paralysis have special effects on the manner of walking. When certain muscles of the leg are paralyzed, for example, a kind of drooping of the foot results. To prevent his toes from dragging on the ground, the person lifts his foot high in the air before every forward movement. Again, paralysis on one side may necessitate twisting the entire body so that the leg on the opposite side can be swung around before it advances. In *paralysis agitans,* the person seems to hustle and shuffle as if being shoved from behind. At the same time the body careens forward in advance of the feet, as if the person were attempting to avoid falling on his face. In *muscular* or *pseudohypertrophic paralysis,* growth occurs in the calf of the leg. Although the muscles become enlarged, they are weak. The result is a waddling gait, resembling that of a pregnant woman.

The best known of all abnormal gaits, the *limp,* is often caused by stiff muscles, localized pain, or a difference between the length of the two legs. *See also* ATAXIA; PARALYSIS.

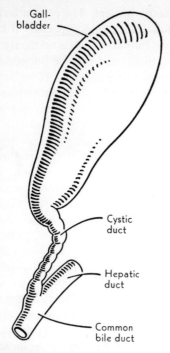

Gallbladder—The gallbladder lies under the liver in the right upper abdomen. With disease it may enlarge sufficiently so that it can be touched quite easily during physical examination. Occasionally the sac is so large it may extend to the right lower abdomen. The gallbladder stores the bile it receives from the *liver*. A tube, the *hepatic duct*, transports the bile to the gallbladder and the common *bile duct* conveys the bile from the gallbladder to the intestines. *Bile*, a necessary fluid for proper digestion in the intestines, varies in color from brown to greenish-yellow.

GALLBLADDER, a baglike, pear-shaped sac lying usually on the underside of the liver. It stores bile and neutralizes the acid semidigested food coming from the stomach.

The gallbladder is susceptible to infection and to obstructions in the tubes carrying bile, particularly by the formation of stones. The probable cause of gallstones is interruption of the bile flow by infections and digestive changes. Gallstones may range in size from that of a poppy seed to that of an egg. The stones will float in water and are soaplike to the touch. They consist largely of cholesterol, a fatlike substance found in the blood and other parts of the body, and of bile pigments. These are derived from the bile itself, but the nucleus around which they coalesce seems to be a foreign substance, such as a small cluster of bacteria or of infected discharge. Approximately 5 to 10 per cent of all adults have gallstones, and they occur in women five times oftener than in men.

Gallstones are not always troublesome, but they may block a *gall duct* and induce an attack of *biliary colic* without warning. The pit of the stomach is seized with pain which may be agonizing and so severe that the patient collapses. Such attacks are likely to be accompanied by vomiting and fever, and usually end when the stone slips back into the gallbladder or proceeds into the intestine whence it is excreted with the solid wastes. Another attack may not occur for months or years. When the colic symptoms are repeated, the stomach feels full, pains are felt after eating fatty foods, and gas is present.

Removal of the gallbladder is advisable if the person suffers from frequent attacks of gallbladder colic. Not only is ordinary comfort restored, but certain definite risks are thus avoided. Infection, with dangerous formation of pus, or cancer may develop if stones persist. Some persons, however, cannot undergo the surgical operation and must have continuous medical treatment and care.

Cholecystitis is the serious condition incurred by infection and inflammation when interruption of the flow of bile occurs. Acute pain in the upper right abdomen, abdomen distended by gas, and sometimes jaundice and fever accompany cholecystitis. When such attacks become a major problem, the solution is surgical removal of the gallbladder, preferably not during an acute episode. Nevertheless, if continued vomiting, rapid pulse, and indications of poisoning ensue, it may be necessary to operate immediately.

Chronic infection and inflammation of the gallbladder induce a tendency to formation of stones, and symptoms of chronic indigestion are constantly present. The patient feels too full after eating, especially if he has had fatty foods. Pain on the right side is likely, and may be intensified by stooping or bending. Heartburn often accompanies this condition and medical examination reveals hyperacidity in the stomach.

A special technique for detection of gallstones is one of the outstanding achievements of medical science. A substance, *iodophthalein,* when ingested or injected into the blood stream, renders the gallbladder visible on an x-ray photograph, so that the functions of the liver and gallbladder may be evaluated. The substance is carried by the blood to the liver, then in the bile to the gallbladder. If the x-ray plates do not reveal the gallbladder, further studies are made to determine whether or not

Gallbladder—Gallbladder and surrounding areas are visualized by x-ray after the administration of a radiopaque substance into the body. The substance goes into the liver and then into the gallbladder. The gallbladder is clearly defined and appears to be normal. Tube-like structures leading into and away from the gallbladder are definitely outlined. This technique aids in detecting a defect or disease in the gallbladder and tubes.

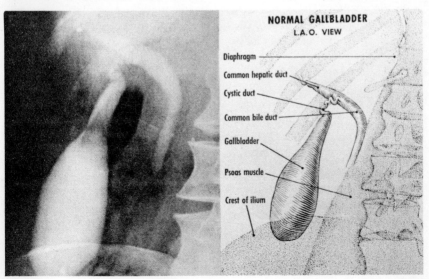

NORMAL GALLBLADDER
L.A.O. VIEW

Diaphragm
Common hepatic duct
Cystic duct
Common bile duct
Gallbladder
Psoas muscle
Crest of ilium

the disease and its causes   It is not yet known what causes stones to form in the gallbladder. Chemically, gallstones are made up of a combination of bile pigment (bilirubin), cholesterol and calcium, although occasionally pure stones of a single chemical are found.

Gallstones are very common, occurring in up to 25% of the older age group. Stones, varying widely in size and number, are seen more in women than in men, particularly among those who are overweight.

symptoms   Many people with gallstones have no symptoms whatsoever. But there can be a variety of symptoms, including belching, bloating, and attacks of abdominal pain. The abdominal pain is severe and knife-like, radiating from the right upper abdomen to the back. It is caused by the movement of a stone into the duct carrying bile to the intestine. A gallstone attack may follow a fatty meal, or it may have nothing to do with what the patient has eaten that day. At its peak there is severe nausea and vomiting, and the patient may find it difficult to breathe. The upper abdominal wall is tender and tense. Medication may help stop the attack, or it may stop of its own accord. Between attacks the patient may be in excellent health. Some patients may have some difficulty in digesting fatty or fried foods. When a gallstone attack does not subside or respond to medication, surgery may be necessary.

complications   Inflammation and gangrene of the gallbladder are the most common complications. Others are related to the blocking of the drainage duct of the gallbladder and liver by gallstones. This can cause liver infection, abscess, a form of cirrhosis, or yellow jaundice. Cancer of the gallbladder is another complication.

prevention (or lessening of impact)   There is no way known to prevent the development of gallstones, and no medications are available that will dissolve them. The effects of low-cholesterol diets and weight control are hard to evaluate, but it would be worthwhile to follow these practices where there is a strong family history of gallstones. A patient who knows he cannot tolerate fatty or other foods should stick to a diet that excludes them.

When a routine examination reveals the presence of gallstones, although the patient has had no discomfort, the doctor will consider the advisability of preventive surgery in the light of many factors, including the patient's age and general health.

Gallstones

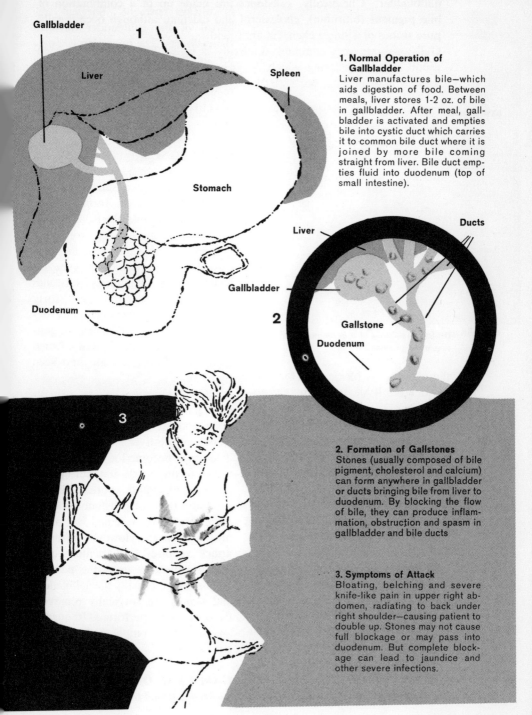

Gallbladder

Liver

1

Spleen

Stomach

Duodenum

Gallbladder

2

Liver

Ducts

Gallstone

Duodenum

3

1. Normal Operation of Gallbladder
Liver manufactures bile—which aids digestion of food. Between meals, liver stores 1-2 oz. of bile in gallbladder. After meal, gallbladder is activated and empties bile into cystic duct which carries it to common bile duct where it is joined by more bile coming straight from liver. Bile duct empties fluid into duodenum (top of small intestine).

2. Formation of Gallstones
Stones (usually composed of bile pigment, cholesterol and calcium) can form anywhere in gallbladder or ducts bringing bile from liver to duodenum. By blocking the flow of bile, they can produce inflammation, obstruction and spasm in gallbladder and bile ducts

3. Symptoms of Attack
Bloating, belching and severe knife-like pain in upper right abdomen, radiating to back under right shoulder—causing patient to double up. Stones may not cause full blockage or may pass into duodenum. But complete blockage can lead to jaundice and other severe infections.

671

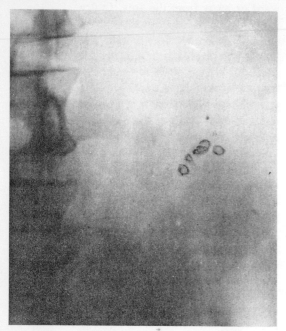

Gallstones—X-ray of a gallbladder containing several large stones.

is always present. Surgical removal of the gallbladder obviates these threats. The operation is a major one, usually successful. Symptoms promptly disappear, but diet regulation is desirable. *See also* GALLSTONES. *See* MEDIGRAPH page 671.

GALLSTONES, small masses of a substance composed most frequently of cholesterol, bile salts, and pigments. They often form in the gallbladder or bile ducts, and may cause symptoms varying from mild colicky pain to rupture of the gallbladder and peritonitis or even infection of the pancreas. Gallstones usually occur after the age of forty although younger women may develop them after pregnancy. In general, women are more often affected than men. Gallstones are best seen by x-ray.

Gallstones cause colicky pain as they pass into and along the bile ducts and are often followed by infection in the liver and by jaundice. They may become lodged at the entrance to the duodenum, causing intense jaundice and severe itching.

Mild attacks of gallstone colic are often treated by rest and hot packs on the stomach. However, a severe attack requires the attention of a doctor who may prescribe pain-relieving drugs. Usually the gallbladder and stones are surgically removed; the operation is performed frequently and is rarely complicated. *See also* GALLBLADDER.

GAMMA GLOBULIN, a chemical substance found in the protein globu-

the bile duct is blocked. If the gallbladder is visible in the roentgenograms, most of the stones will also be seen. Some stones are visible by x-ray without the aid of iodophthalein.

Jaundice in severe cases may be active but does not always accompany chronic gallbladder infection. Infection of the gallbladder produces a great range of internal symptoms which incriminate almost any organ but the one actually responsible. A tightness of the chest, palpitating heart, or shortness of breath may be quite confusing in these circumstances. Medical examination is indispensable to determine the exact cause and condition. Many persons live for years with a chronically inflamed gallbladder and without serious consequences. The risk, however, lins of the blood plasma. The blood has the power to develop antibodies to combat disease. The antibodies in gamma globulin have been found useful in developing immunity to measles in children as well as in hepatitis and other infections. Commercially available serum containing globulin has been used to advantage both in developing temporary immunity to measles and also to lighten an attack of measles in a child who has been exposed and develops the disease. *See also* BLOOD.

GANGLIONS, nodes or lumps which usually form in the sheaths encasing tendons. They are frequently seen on the wrist but may occur elsewhere. It has been found that a suspension of *hydrocortisone acetate* may be injected directly into the cavity of such a cyst; in many instances the injection promotes absorption of the fluid and disappearance of the ganglion. *See also* CYST.

GANGRENE, the death of tissue, caused by interruption of circulation. It can result from accidental damage to the tissue, as in burns, wounds, crushing or poisoning of the flesh. Interruption of circulation with the ensuing death of the flesh can be caused by other conditions—for example, a hernia—or by a section of lung failing to receive its supply of blood. Diseases such as diabetes, hardening of the arteries, or Bright's disease may affect circulation in a similar way.

Gangrene is generally classified as *dry* or *moist,* depending on whether or not certain fluids flow to-

ward or away from the area. In dry gangrene the tissue gradually shrinks and the color becomes brown and finally black. In moist gangrene the tissue is swollen, often blistered, and has the colors characteristic of a bruise. Moist gangrene is more dangerous than dry because it offers greater opportunity for infection. Since the infection can be fatal the doctor takes special precautions against bacterial invasion. The skin is thoroughly and regularly cleaned, particularly the skin around fingernails and toenails where germs might find a breeding place, and the nails themselves are usually clipped as short as possible. Antiseptic dressings are frequently applied.

Eventually a red line, the line of demarcation, will appear on the skin. This line separates the dead tissue from that which can heal. The doctor will try to save the tissue capable of healing, and stop the progress of the deteriorating tissue. Sometimes amputation is the only means of stopping rapidly deteriorating tissue. However, it may be advisable to operate without waiting for the appearance of the line of demarcation, even at the sacrifice of potentially healthy tissue.

Injury of tissue, as in wounds, encourages certain types of bacteria which cause *gas gangrene*. These germs behave as ferments and break up the sugars in the tissues so as to produce a gas which soon spreads through the muscles. The area becomes severely inflamed, and in later stages the color changes to yellow and then black. The progress of gas gangrene varies among patients; in some it is rapid, in others slow. As yet there is no full explanation for this difference, although the severity of the wound seems to be a primary consideration.

During World War I when gas gangrene became a serious problem, the only medical solution was to remove all damaged tissue from the body as soon as possible. However, during World War II a serum was developed which could be injected into a person threatened with gas gangrene; and, if the infection had already started, sulfa drugs were ordinarily sufficient to bring it under control. *See also* FROSTBITE.

GARGLE, a liquid solution used to rinse the throat, pharynx, and nasopharynx, and held in this area by a stream of air from the lungs. Since some of the liquid may be accidentally swallowed, anything which might be internally harmful should never be used as a gargle. If an inflammation is so severe that gargling causes pain, the liquid may be held in the throat for a few minutes, or merely swished around, or sprayed in with an atomizer. For a slightly irritated throat, a pinch of salt or bicarbonate of soda diluted in warm water is often helpful.

GASTRIC, a term derived from the Greek word *gastro*—stomach. In medicine many words beginning with *gastro* are used which relate to medical conditions affecting the stomach. Accordingly *gastritis* is an inflammation of the stomach, *gastroenteritis* an inflammation of the stomach and intestines, *gastrectomy* the removal of all or a part of the stomach, *gastroscope* a device for looking inside the stomach.

GASTRIC ULCER. *See* PEPTIC ULCER.

GASTRITIS, a common form of stomach upset, is inflammation of the stomach wall. When the lining of the stomach is irritated or infected, it becomes red and swollen and in a severe inflammation may even bleed.

Gastritis may be *acute* or *chronic*. Acute inflammation is often caused by food poisoning, eating spoiled food, or simply overeating. The lining of the stomach may also become seriously inflamed following the swallowing of irritating substances like lye, acid, or poison, and quick action by a physician to remove the substance is imperative. This must be followed by neutralization of the poison or the stomach wall will be perforated and acute peritonitis will set in. Surgical treatment may also be necessary.

Symptoms of *acute gastritis* include loss of appetite, a sense of pressure and fullness in the pit of the stomach which is unrelieved by belching, nausea, headache, and a slight rise in temperature. Vomiting then follows, producing a sense of relief. However, the person will feel extremely fatigued afterward. Examination of the material from the stomach enables the doctor to determine the nature and severity of the inflammation. Relief of acute gastritis is usually brought about in a few days by eliminating the irritating substance.

Diagnosis and treatment of constant or *chronic gastritis* are difficult. Many different conditions may produce these repeated irritations of the stomach lining, and treatment requires observation and control by the physician over a long period of time. Certain vitamin deficiencies in the diet produce a tendency to irritation and inflammation. Disorders of the secretion of gastric juice may also be the cause. Gastritis is generally part of the development of an ulcer in the stomach, and a chronic ulcer is likely to produce chronic gastritis. Alcohol taken in excess produces irritation, followed by inflammation.

In treatment of chronic gastritis, small meals of easily digested foods at frequent intervals are prescribed. Irritating foods must be avoided, and drugs to reduce excess stomach acidity will be administered. The physician treating chronic gastritis must carefully examine the entire system and general health of the patient. If the condition is severe, it may be desirable to begin treatment with a few days of rest in bed and a milk or light bland diet. Medication to promote regularity of the bowels may be prescribed, and later substances to promote appetite and digestion. *See also* DIET IN DIGESTIVE DISORDERS; DIGESTION; DIGESTIVE SYSTEM; STOMACH.

GASTROENTERITIS, a general term that applies to a variety of gastrointestinal disturbances. In this inflammatory condition of the stomach and intestines, nausea, vomiting, and diarrhea occur, generally accompanied by cramps.

Acute gastroenteritis of a nonspecific nature occurs in alcoholism, malaria, acute hepatitis, and as a sensitivity reaction to certain foods. Food poisoning by staphylococci is a form of gastroenteritis.

Treatment of gastroenteritis may vary from temporary change of diet in mild disorders to surgery in extreme cases. See appropriate heading for discussion of specific symptoms and treatment. *See also* AMEBIC DYSENTERY; BACILLARY DYSENTERY; DIARRHEA; FOOD POISONING; GASTRITIS.

GASTRO-INTESTINAL SYSTEM. *See* STOMACH; INTESTINES.

GASTROPTOSIS, dropping of the stomach, a condition caused by downward displacement of the stomach which may be seen by x-ray.

GATOPHOBIA, a morbid fear of cats.

GELATIN, a transparent substance, colorless, odorless, and almost tasteless, produced by boiling the skin, bones, and ligaments of animals and treating with acid. It is firm when dry and jellylike when moist. Gelatin is considered a protein, but it does not possess all of the amino acids which are necessary for growth. Gelatin is the basis for such products as glues and jellies. When used in desserts it is usually flavored and sweetened. It is medicinally used in accelerating coagulation of blood by intravenous injection, and experimental work is being done with gelatin as a blood substitute. Gelatin also stimulates growth of nails.

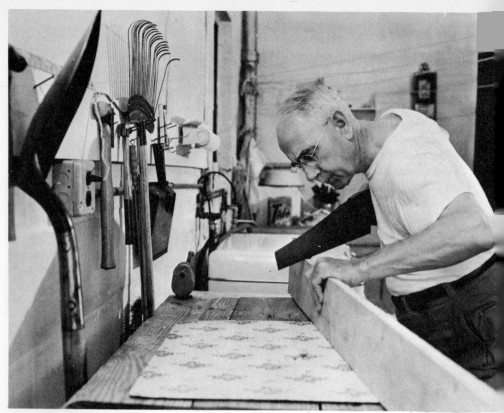

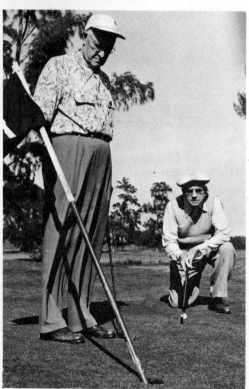

The conquest in this century of infectious diseases by antibiotics, vaccines, and other drugs, and the remarkable improvement and refinement of surgical techniques, have allowed many more people to live to an advanced age than ever did so in previous times. This unprecedented host of elderly people in our society has given rise to the serious study of *geriatrics*—the professional care of the aged and their problems. Properly speaking, geriatrics concerns the medical aspects of old age, but insurance companies, real estate enterprises, educational and recreational facilities, and the government are all directly involved with the life and welfare of the aged.

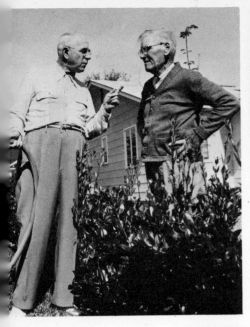

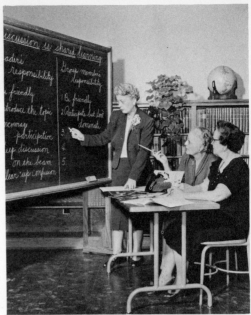

Physical activity is important for the continued well-being of older people. An interest in personal appearance, world events, gardening, and recreation promotes a continued enjoyment of life, prevents discouragement, and obviates loneliness. Most people retire by the age of 65 or 70. It is advisable to initiate preparations for retirement many years in advance. Wise savings and investment during their working years can protect those envisaging retirement from the ravages of inflation, rising costs, and reduced income, and afford a salutary sense of independence.

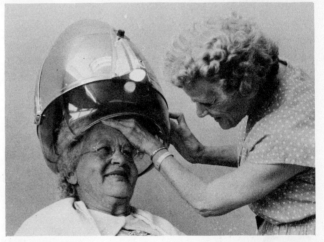

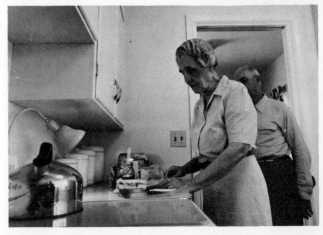

GENETICS. *See* REPRODUCTION SYSTEM.

GENITALS. *See* PENIS; TESTICLES; SCROTUM; VAGINA; VULVA; CLITORIS.

GENITO-URINARY SYSTEM. *See* REPRODUCTION SYSTEM.

GENIUS. Persons who achieve distinction in life usually reveal in childhood some evidence that they are of unusually high intelligence.

Psychologists at a leading university who studied the records of three hundred eminent men and women of history to evaluate the factors that make for success concluded that those who achieve eminence are not only endowed with high intellectual gifts but also motivated by persistence of effort, self-confidence, and great strength or force of character. A genius usually appears in a well-endowed family in which he has superior opportunities for education and other inspirational factors in his environment. Great ability thrives in a cultured atmosphere. While hardship and resistance may stimulate intensive effort, the capacity must be present or genius will never be manifested. *See also* INTELLIGENCE.

GERIATRICS, the science of medical and hygienic care of aged people. It has broadened and expanded in recent years because of the increased number of older people. In 1890, the number of persons in the United States over sixty-five was about 3 per cent. Today, more than 20 per cent of the population is over sixty-five. Geriatrics must therefore be-

come more and more significant in the future. *See also* SENESCENCE; SENILITY.

GERMAN MEASLES, also known as *three-day measles* or *rubella,* a mild but highly infectious virus disease. German measles occurs in epidemics at three- to four-year intervals, often in early spring, together with an outbreak of *measles*. It affects persons of all ages, though it is uncommon in infants and children under four, and generally occurs most frequently in older children and young adults. German measles during pregnancy may be harmful to the fetus.

German measles, like measles, is transmitted most commonly by droplet infection and direct contact. The incubation period is from fourteen to seventeen days, occasionally ranging from ten to twenty-one days. The infectious period is generally a day or two before before the rash appears.

The first symptoms in younger people are slight: a scant rise in temperature, perhaps a running nose and some soreness of the throat. In older persons, German measles may be accompanied by headache, weakness, slight fever, sore throat, and swelling of the glands at the back of the head and neck, with some tenderness. Usually the rash is the first symptom noted by the patient. It appears after twenty-four to forty-eight hours, first on the face, forehead, scalp, and behind the ears, then spreading over the body. The rash resembles scarlet fever rash more than measles rash. Itching may aggravate the rounded rose-red spots, which are separate at first, then tend to run together. The rash lasts about three days and fades with a fine scaling. Koplik's spots do not appear in German measles.

The general treatment is similar to that for measles. The person should remain in bed until his temperature is normal and the rash has disappeared. As in measles, he should be isolated, since he is infectious for about ten days after the appearance of the rash. German measles is not dangerous, but all efforts should be made to avoid secondary infections, since encephalitis is a rare but possible complication. *Gamma globulin* is sometimes given to help resistance. One attack of German measles confers lasting immunity. The patient's bedding and linens and bedclothing should be disinfected and the sickroom thoroughly aired. Children who have been in contact with German measles should be kept out of school for at least three weeks from the date of the last contact.

In 1968, the National Institute of Allergy and Infectious Diseases in Washington, D.C. announced the development of an experimental vaccine against German measles. Originally developed in the Institute's laboratories in 1966, it underwent its first major test in the spring of 1968 in Taiwan, where 9,000 schoolchildren were inoculated. By chance, an epidemic of the disease broke out in that country shortly after the administration of the vaccine to these children, giving scientists an excellent opportunity to evaluate its effectiveness. The results were reported as being highly encouraging. The Institute subsequently announced plans to administer the vaccine to schoolchildren in several leading American cities. It is expected that the vaccination of the children will prevent the disease from being transmitted to their mothers.

If German measles occurs during the first third of pregnancy, the possibility is great that the child may have congenital defects, such as cataracts, heart malformations, deafness, or mental retardation. These serious complications have been known to occur in more than 50 per cent of such cases. Therefore, it is essential that an obstetrician be notified immediately. *See also* MEASLES. *See* MEDIGRAPH page 681.

GERMICIDE, any substance that kills germs. There is a significant distinction between germicides and antiseptics; antiseptics destroy poisonous material as well as germs and also inhibit and prevent multiplication of germs.

GERMS. *See* BACTERIA; VIRUSES; RICKETTSIAL DISEASES.

GIANTISM. *See* ACROMEGALY.

GILCHRIST'S DISEASE. *See* BLASTOMYCOSIS.

GINGIVITIS, an inflammation of the gums. *Pyorrhea* is a form of gingivitis with pus, and the condition called *Vincent's disease* or *trench mouth* is also gingivitis. *See also* PYORRHEA; VINCENT'S ANGINA.

679

the disease and its causes German measles is a mild but highly contagious disease caused by a virus present in secretions such as nasal discharge and saliva. It is spread by direct contact and almost never through objects or a third person. One attack usually give lifelong immunity. It occurs most often in winter and early spring, and follows a pattern of epidemics every three to four years. The incubation period is 2 to 3 weeks. The disease is most contagious from a day or two before the rash appears until the rash leaves. It is rare to find it in anyone over 40. Infants under six months are probably immune if their mothers are immune.

symptoms The symptoms are mild, and the whole disease is usually over in 2 to 4 days. There may be a low fever, mild aches and pains, a running or stuffed nose, red running eyes, and swelling of the glands, as shown in the accompanying Medi-Graph. The throat may be sore. But often the symptoms are so mild that the patient doesn't know he has German measles until the rash breaks out. The rash starts with individual rose-red spots on the face or neck, then spreads onto the head, arms, trunk and, in small amounts, onto the legs. It disappears in the same order in which it began. The glands remain swollen 5 to 7 days after the rash clears.

complications These are very rare, although during severe epidemics, cases of ear and kidney infections, arthritis, and encephalitis are occasionally reported. However, a serious complication of German measles can occur when a woman contracts it during the first three months of her pregnancy. The virus may attack many parts of the unborn child, such as the eyes, heart, ears, or brain; and serious defects occur in as many as 50% of such births. When a pregnant woman learns she has been exposed to this disease, she should notify her doctor immediately.

prevention (or lessening of impact) As a rule, very little treatment is required. There is generally no itching and the patient is comfortable with bed care for a day or two. While there is a difference of opinion as to the advisability of deliberately exposing a child, and girls in particular, to this disease, it is hardly necessary to go to great lengths to prevent a child from getting it.

German Measles

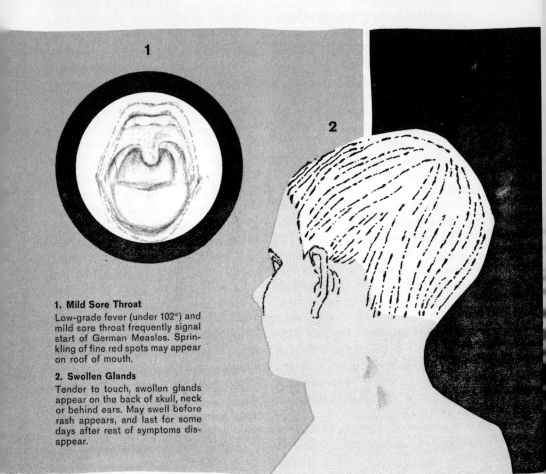

1. Mild Sore Throat

Low-grade fever (under 102°) and mild sore throat frequently signal start of German Measles. Sprinkling of fine red spots may appear on roof of mouth.

2. Swollen Glands

Tender to touch, swollen glands appear on the back of skull, neck or behind ears. May swell before rash appears, and last for some days after rest of symptoms disappear.

3. Rash

Faint, blotchy rash appears—first on face or neck, then spreading to rest of body. Usually fades within 2 days in children, takes a day or two longer in adults.

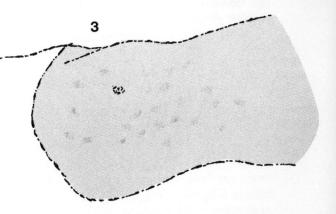

GLANDERS, a contagious disease of animals, involving swellings under the jaws and an abundant discharge of mucus from the nostrils. This disease, although found ordinarily among horses, mules, and donkeys, is occasionally communicated to human beings, primarily to persons who work with horses. This happened more frequently in the past when horses were more commonly used.

When the germ gains entrance into human tissue, it may be weeks before the first signs of the illness appear. A test exists, similar to the Wassermann test, by which the presence of the germ can be recognized. High fever, vomiting, and diarrhea accompany this disease. Where the germs localize, a swelling occurs and large ulcers and abcesses of the lymph glands appear rapidly. The latter are first seen as small knots under the skin, known as "farcy buds."

If this disease becomes chronic in a person, severe damage to the cartilage and bones is likely. In the chronic form, there is constant fever and abnormal thinness. So-called chronic glanders, as contrasted to the acute form, is sometimes curable. Antibiotics, antitoxins, and surgery are all usually necessary.

When this disease is contracted by a human being, he should be isolated at once, and all discharges from his body should be removed on materials which can be easily burned. These precautionary measures are necessary because the disease is highly contagious as well as dangerous. For the same reasons, animals infected with glanders are always destroyed.

GLANDS, organs of the body which develop a secretion, a substance which performs a specific function, as in digestion. Many of the body's most important processes are effected through the glands and their secretions.

The glands are of *external* and of *internal* secretion. The glands of external secretion include the *digestive* glands and the *sweat* glands of the skin. Those of internal secretion, also known as the *endocrine* glands, secrete their products, called *hormones,* into the blood. These are carried to other parts of the body where they exert specific effects on other glands or organs. Some glands of external secretion also produce substances which penetrate the blood as internal secretions or hormones.

Glands of external secretion include the *liver,* which produces bile; the *stomach,* which gives hydrochloric acid and pepsin for digestion; the female *breasts,* which secrete milk; the *salivary glands,* which produce the saliva that moistens the mouth and contains digestive substances; the *pancreas,* which produces trypsin used in digestion and also insulin, an internal substance which regulates the use of sugar; and the *sex glands.*

The glands of internal secretion are more complex in operation and more far-reaching in effect than the glands of external secretion. For example, whereas hydrochloric acid found in the stomach acts directly on food, the products of the endo-

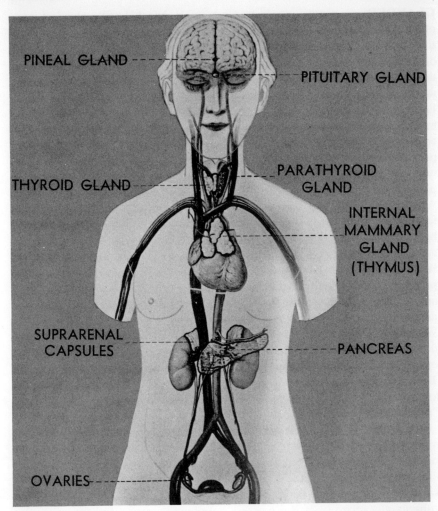

PINEAL GLAND

PITUITARY GLAND

THYROID GLAND

PARATHYROID GLAND

INTERNAL MAMMARY GLAND (THYMUS)

SUPRARENAL CAPSULES

PANCREAS

OVARIES

Glands—The endocrine glands of the body. These glands secrete their hormones directly into the blood stream. In the male the sex hormone is produced by the testicles (*not shown*). Some of these glands produce more than one hormone and feature prominently in other body functions in addition to their endocrine activity. These glands regulate many functions of the body. The growth of the body, mental development, personality, masculinity or femininity are some aspects influenced by the endocrine system.

crine glands function indirectly. Together they form a system which regulates many of the body's most vital processes.

The glands control growth, the body's response to stress of all kinds, and initiate its defenses, and govern the development of sexual maturity. They induce the secondary physical characteristics which distinguish men from women, such as hair on the face and the deeper voice. They regulate the delicately balanced expenditure of energy that persists continuously in the tissues, and are intimately involved in metabolism.

The endocrine glands include the *pituitary,* sometimes called the "master gland" because it performs a multiplicity of functions and helps regulate other endocrine glands such as the *thyroid gland* involved in the consumption of oxygen; the *adrenal gland*—divided into two parts, the *medulla* and the *cortex,* which among other functions assist the body in emergencies; the *testes* and *ovaries,* male and female sex glands which affect both sexual processes and, even more, general body conditions; the *parathyroids* which control the calcium and phosphorus content of the blood; and the *pineal* and *thymus* glands which are less well understood than others.

Endocrine disorders may have profound effects. A pituitary gland which is not functioning properly may cause *giantism* or *dwarfism* or permanent enlargement of the chin, hands, and feet. A thyroid gland deficient at birth retards the growth of the body and mind, and causes *feeble-mindedness.* Later thyroid disorder may greatly accelerate or abnormally retard various processes, reacting unfavorably on the heart or other organs. Lack of the hormones of the cortex, which is the outer layer of the adrenal glands, produces death in a few days if they are not replaced. Disturbances of the sex glands and their hormones may cause a woman to assume male attributes or a man to develop feminine characteristics. If a duct of a gland is blocked the secretion continues. The accumulation of fluid causes the gland to dilate and form a *retention cyst.* An *adenoma* is a tumor with glandular structure.

The normal course of development of a human being comprises the initial period of growth, a plateau through the years of middle life when maturity is reached and then a gradual decline. Many unjustified or actually fraudulent claims are made that the glands promote rejuvenation. None has been substained and rejuvenation is as far beyond human reach as ever. *See also* ADRENAL GLANDS; ENDOCRINE GLANDS; HORMONES; and under names of separate glands.

GLAUCOMA, a disease of the eyes in which loss of vision is caused by a pressure inside the eyeball. This pressure occurs when optical fluid tends to accumulate there. In one form of glaucoma, this accumulation is caused by improper circulation. Pain results and soon the eyeball is hard and red, and the pupil itself becomes gray and cloudy. Another form of glaucoma, regarded as more serious, results from the accumulation of fluid caused by failure of the drainage system. The internal pressure and loss of vision, however, develop more slowly.

In the earlier stages of glaucoma, visual difficulty occurs at both sides of the area of vision, though the person with glaucoma is able to see in front as well as ever. As the disease develops, however, the area of clear frontal vision gradually becomes narrower until finally the person is completely blind.

In diagnosis of the disease, the

eye specialist employs several mechanical aids. He uses the *ophthalmoscope* to judge whether the internal pressure is sufficient to depress the optic nerve at the rear of the eye. With a *tonometer* he can estimate whether or not the pressure is increasing. The *perimeter* measures the breadth of vision; a progressive decrease in breadth is a sign of glaucoma. These instruments enable a prompt diagnosis which may save the sight.

In all stages of this disease, but especially at the onset, the patient should avoid excitement since the resulting rise in pressure increases the flow of blood into the arteries of the eyes, where the internal accumulation of fluid is already excessive.

In the treatment of glaucoma, eyeglasses are ineffective. Drugs, however, are sometimes successfully used to contract the pupil and also to decrease pressure within the eyeball. Frequently surgery can control glaucoma and actually save the patient's sight. *See also* EYE. *See* MEDIGRAPH page 687.

GLEET, chronic gonorrhea. Modern treatment of gonorrhea with sulfa drugs and with penicillin has made chronic gonorrhea a rather uncommon disease. Indeed few cases are seen now by the physicians who specialize in such conditions. The pain associated with acute gonnorrhea is usually absent, but a transparent discharge occurs regularly, usually upon awakening. This discharge remains highly infectious upon contact with others. *See also* GONORRHEA.

GLIOMA, a tumor of the nervous tissue occurring principally in the brain, spinal cord, peripheral nerves, and the adrenals.

GLOSSITIS, an inflammation of the tip and margin of the tongue, generally caused by a riboflavin deficiency which occurs when the diet consists chiefly of such foods as corn, rice, or potatoes.

GLOSSOPATHY, any disease of the tongue.

GLOSSOPHARYNGEAL NEURALGIA, the result of stimuli to nerves connected with the ninth cranial nerve, which affects the area around the tonsils, back of the tongue, the pharynx, the ear, and the eardrum. This neuralgia is symptomatically similar to *facial neuralgia*. The pain often spreads to the back of the jaw. Patients may not actually complain of pain in the ear but during the attack will point toward the spot where they are feeling the pain. The exact cause of this neuralgia is not known.

GLOTTIS, the opening between the vocal cords which is protected by the *epiglottis*. *See also* EPIGLOTTIS.

GLUCOSE, the chemical term for *dextrose* and for *blood sugar*. The *glucose tolerance test* is used to determine whether or not a diabetic condition exists. For this test a solution of glucose is given intravenously or by mouth and the blood and urine examined to establish the level of the blood glucose at specific

the disease and its causes   Glaucoma is a disease of the eye brought about by an increase in the pressure of the vitreous fluid within the eyeball. This pressure against the retina of the eyeball begins to crush nerves that control side vision and, if unchecked, goes on to destroy nerves controlling frontal vision. The disease affects both sexes equally and occurs in middle and advanced age, often between 40 and 70. Usually it involves both eyes.

The exact cause of glaucoma is unknown, but there are a number of conditions which predispose a patient to the disease—age, heredity, arteriosclerosis, and farsightedness.

symptoms   There are many types of glaucoma. Symptoms vary with the rapidity with which the eyeball pressure rises and the height to which the pressure goes. As shown on the Medi-Graph, early symptoms include a slight fogging of vision and dull pain in the eye. The patient sees colored halos around lights. The pupil may appear somewhat larger than normal, and the eye may appear slightly congested (bloodshot).

These symptoms may occur in attacks that are weeks, months, or even years apart. Between the attacks vision is normal until severe, acute glaucoma develops. This comes on rapidly, with decreasing vision and severe, constant pain all over the head. There may be nausea and vomiting. The eye becomes congested and hard to the touch. The pupil appears steamy and usually remains open and sluggish in its reaction to light. The patient see less and less at the sides of one or both eyes. Glasses have to be changed frequently because of the patient's constantly decreasing vision.

complications   The usual complication of untreated glaucoma is blindness.

prevention (or lessening of impact)   Eye drops and proper medications can prevent acute attacks of glaucoma. These are prescribed by an ophthalmologist (eye specialist), who should be seen as soon as any of the symptoms noted appear. If possible, the patient should avoid tension, insomnia, or sudden shock, because they can precipitate an attack. A patient with any symptom suggesting glaucoma should strenuously avoid taking any medicines or using any eye drops likely to cause widening of the pupils, because this can precipitate an attack. The family physician can give him a list of drugs to avoid.

Glaucoma

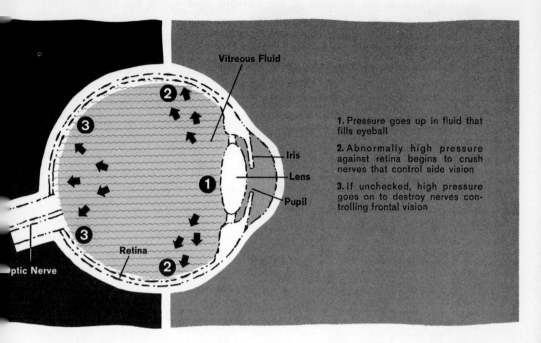

Vitreous Fluid

Iris

Lens

Pupil

Retina

Optic Nerve

1. Pressure goes up in fluid that fills eyeball

2. Abnormally high pressure against retina begins to crush nerves that control side vision

3. If unchecked, high pressure goes on to destroy nerves controlling frontal vision

Glaucoma's Danger Signals

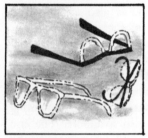

Glasses — even new ones — don't give satisfactory sight

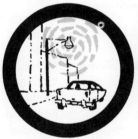

Rainbow colored rings appear around lights

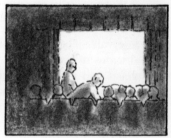

Difficulty with darkened rooms—like movie theatre

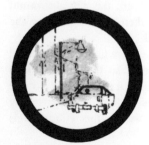

Spells of blurred or foggy eyesight

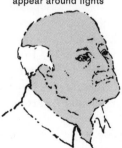

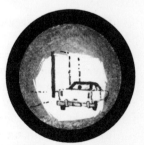

Loss of vision at sides of one or both eyes

687

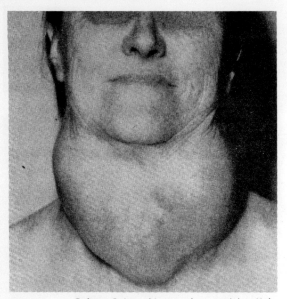

Goiter—Goiter with many large nodules. Multinodular goiter tends to run in families and occurs in middle-aged or elderly persons. These nodules are probably due to iodine deficiency and have been present for many years. The chances of cancer being present in this type of goiter are small, but the patient may want an operation for cosmetic reasons.

intervals. The test is also used in diseases of the liver and the thyroid gland and to determine the absorptive capacity of the gastrointestinal tract.

GOAT FEVER. *See* UNDULANT FEVER.

GOITER, enlargement of the thyroid gland, located in the front of the neck. In *exophthalmic goiter* the gland becomes overactive and is usually but not always enlarged. *Ordinary* or *simple goiter* begins early in adolescence and is directly associated with an inadequate supply of iodine in the diet. Goiter is most common in inland and moun-

tainous areas away from the sea where there is a deficiency of iodine in the soil and water. Simple goiter occurs infrequently in coastal areas, and is five times more common in women than men.

Within the thyroid gland are small vessels which contain a yellow substance called *colloid*. Colloid contains a small amount of iodine, so little that a man weighing 150 pounds has no more than 1/40,000-th of a pound of iodine. Iodine is also present in *thyroxin,* the secretion or hormone of the thyroid gland. The thyroid absorbs the iodine from iodine-containing foods and liquids taken into the body.

As a preventive measure against goiter, small amounts of iodine are sometimes given to young people, particularly those who live in areas where the water and soil are low in iodine. Iodine is also administered to pregnant mothers to prevent undesirable changes in the thyroid gland of the developing embryo. Iodine is often added to table salt, "iodized" salt, and can be added to drinking water. Iodine-containing tablets are also available. The use of iodine should be prescribed by the doctor to assure that the proper amount is given; the actual amount of iodine taken to supplement the diet is small.

In cases in which the thyroid gland becomes so large as to be a deformity and a discomfort to the person, it is ordinarily removed by surgery. However, this condition is rare today.

Exophthalmic goiter is usually more serious than simple goiter. The processes in which the gland is involved through its secretion, thyroxin, are abnormally quickened. A typical symptom of the condition is bulging eyes—the origin of the term "exophthalmic." The disorder occurs most frequently in young adults, especially young women, in urban areas, and is apparently associated with stress on the nervous system. The overactivity of the thyroid gland causes the basic chemical changes throughout the body to accelerate abnormally; the basal metabolism rate rises; the heart beats faster. The person tires easily, his appetite increases, he feels warm, is more nervous than usual and inclined to excitability, he begins to lose weight, his hands may tremble, and he often engages in excessive activity. Substantially these same symptoms can be produced by ingestion of too much extract of the thyroid gland.

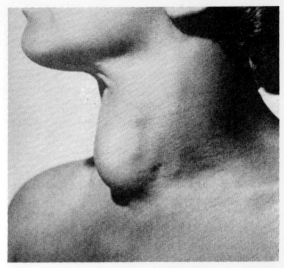

Goiter—A lump in the neck. The huge swelling fills the front and side of the neck. If the growth moves on swallowing the condition is probably nodular goiter, but further examination will have to be done to confirm the diagnosis.

To establish whether or not thyroid activity is excessive, the doctor gives the patient a *basal metabolism test.* Normal basal metabolism ranges from plus 7 to minus 7; in exophthalmic goiter, or *hyperthyroidism,* this measurement may rise as high as plus 15, 30, or even higher. The heart may consequently be forced to work far beyond its capacity. Administration of extra iodine may reduce the heart action and relieve the symptoms, but this is only a partial remedy and should only be prescribed and supervised by a doctor. Physical and mental rest are beneficial to the patient.

For permanent relief part of the thyroid gland is removed surgically.

Enough of the gland is left to perform its normal functions and provide the necessary thyroxin. The amount of the gland to be removed is established by the surgeon at the time of the operation. Sometimes supplemental thyroid material must be given for a time after surgery until the gland and body adjust properly to the loss of part of the thyroid gland.

Other means have also been found for controlling excessive thyroid activity, such as *radioactive iodine*; *thiocyanates,* which lower blood pressure and depress thyroid activity; and *thiouracil,* which controls the major symptoms. Radioactive iodine also assists in diagnosis; since the thyroid gland absorbs iodine entering the body, a test of the amount of radioactivity emanating from the thyroid can be made which guides the doctor in deciding how much radioactive iodine should be given for actual treatment. Radiation from the iodine directly affects the cells of the gland and permanently lowers its activity.

Hyperthyroidism may also result from the growth of a tumor in the gland which may in turn have developed from a simple goiter. Because of the possibility of cancer as well as hyperthyroidism, these tumors are often removed surgically. *See also* EXOPHTHALMIC GOITER. *See* MEDIGRAPH page 769.

GONADS. *See* TESTICLES; OVARIES; REPRODUCTION SYSTEM.

GONORRHEA, a contagious venereal disease, characterized by inflammation of the genital mucous membranes and caused by a microorganism *Neisseria gonorrheae* more commonly known as the *gonococcus* germ. Gonorrhea is the most common venereal disease and occurs throughout the world. Adults are almost always infected by sexual contact with an infected person. An epidemic form occurs in young girls which is spread through nonsexual objects such as clothing or toys.

Symptoms of infection appear in about three days, although they can take as long as three weeks, after exposure. In the male the first symptoms are usually a slight feeling of irritation or burning sensation when urinating because of the inflammation of the urethra. If the person is not treated, a large amount of pus is produced and an increased amount of discharge may be noticed. Complications can ensue which cause damage to other areas of the sex organs, such as the testicles, and to other parts of the body, such as bones, eyes, joints, kidneys, and heart.

In women, gonorrhea affects the urinary passage and may extend to the bladder and kidneys. In the past, treatment of the infection in women was much more difficult than in men, because the organs are less accessible. Formerly a person infected with gonorrhea was incapacitated for weeks or even years, but new methods of treatment with penicillin and other antibiotics, under direction of a physician, can bring about a cure in a few days, provided the infection is brought to the attention of a physician in time. The rapidity and effectiveness of the new drugs had brought about hopes that the disease might eventually be totally eliminated. Unfortunately, new strains of the gonococcus have arisen which are highly resistant to penicillin and other drugs. While new and more effective antibiotics are continually being developed and tested, the complete elimination of gonorrhea from society remains to be accomplished.

Gonorrheal infection of the eyes, although it does occur in adults, is more frequent in newborn infants, who become infected as they pass through the vagina. It is estimated that gonorrheal eye infection is responsible for 10,000 cases of blindness in the United States. Doctors now administer dilute *silver nitrate* solution into the eyes of newborn infants to prevent this infection.

Many urge the use of other drugs such as antibiotics.

In treating gonorrhea with antibiotics, the physician must be particularly careful, since the patient may seem to be cured but still be able to transmit the disease, and the antibiotics, although they may cure the gonorrhea, may cover up, but not cure, an unsuspected case of syphilis, also present. Syphilis requires larger doses of antibiotics. Therefore, if syphilis is also suspected, the physician may use a sulfonamide drug, which will not cover up a developing syphilitic condition. *See also* SYPHILIS; LYMPHOGRANULOMA VENEREUM; GRANULOMA INGUINALE. *See* MEDIGRAPHS pages 995, 1311.

GOUT, a disease in which the primary symptom is a painful inflammation of the joints of the hands or feet, and especially of the big toe. This inflammation arises when *uric acid* in the blood increases, is not destroyed by the body, and accumulates in the blood, where it combines with *sodium* to create *sodium urate*. The sodium urate may eventually be deposited in the cartilage and other tissues. It is not as yet known why the excess of uric acid appears in the blood, why the excess is not destroyed, or why urates are deposited in the tissue.

Gout usually begins with pain in the big toe, occasionally in the ankle, heel, or even instep, and is ordinarily accompanied by chills and fever. The pain resembles that of a violent dislocation. The affected joint becomes so sensitive that any pressure, even that of bedclothes, is unendurable. This disease attacks men, and occasionally women, in their middle thirties as well as in their sixties or later, contrary to popular belief that it is a condition resulting from a diet of rich foods in advanced years. Gout finally becomes chronic.

Among the drugs used in the treatment of gout are *salicylic acid, cortisone, ACTH, Butazolidin, Benemid, anturan* and *colchicine* (a drug used to treat gout since the fifth century). These drugs should be taken only under supervision of a physician, since they can be toxic with many side effects if improperly used. Gout is also relieved by application of *heat* to the painful joint and by protecting it from disturbing external contacts.

Anyone with gout should avoid excesses of diet or exercise. The diet should largely exclude foods containing white crystalline substances known as *purines,* which includes most meats, such as beef, veal, pork, and bacon, and most animal organ foods, such as liver, sweetbreads, kidneys, and brains. Milk, eggs, and cheese, cereals, fruits, green vegetables, cocoa, tea, coffee, sweets, and nuts are relatively low in purines. Alcohol and fats should be avoided. *See* MEDIGRAPHS pages 693, 825.

GRANULOCYTOPENIA.   *See* AGRANULOCYTOSIS.

GRANULOMA INGUINALE, a disease usually regarded as venereal although it is not necessarily transmitted by sexual contact. Its main symptom is deep ulcerations on and

the disease and its causes   Uric acid is one of the many chemicals produced by the body in the course of digestion. Normally it is disposed of, but if there is a disturbance in the protein metabolism of a patient, it collects in his joints and kidneys and results in a condition called gout. The disease tends to run in families, in a wide age group from 20 to 60, affecting mostly men. Attacks can be brought on by excesses in eating or drinking, or by certain acute medical or surgical problems. In such an attack the patient suffers from acute arthritic pain involving any of his joints, particularly those of the large toes.

symptoms   In most cases the first sign of gout is the sudden appearance of pain in one or several joints. These become swollen, red, shiny, and tender to the touch. As the attack subsides, the skin usually peels. During the attack, temperature may be high and there is weakness and headache. The Medi-Graph gives a more detailed picture of the symptoms. Gout may also begin with the sudden appearance of kidney stones. Crystalline deposits (tophi) may be found in the skin—particularly in the ear lobes.

The severity and length of a gout attack depend upon how quickly a diagnosis is made and treatment begun. In the early stages of the disease the joints recover from an acute attack without permanent injury. Months or years elapse between attacks, during which time the patient is quite comfortable. However, as the disease progresses, these intervals become shorter—and chronic, gouty arthritis, resembling rheumatoid arthritis, is likely to develop.

complications   The most serious complication is a slow, progressive kidney involvement which can lead to uremia and death. Younger patients with gout frequently develop high blood pressure and generalized hardening of the arteries. A gout patient can become virtually crippled from the deformation, stiffening, and impaired motion of the involved joints.

prevention (or lessening of impact)   In a family where there is gout, men should routinely be given a blood test for uric acid. A diet may be suggested to delay the onset of gouty symptoms, since there are foods which are thought to predispose to the formation of uric acid. However, it should be noted that while patients are usually given a specific diet to follow, it has not been established that this approach is effective.

A wide range of medication is available which tends to delay the formation of kidney stones and the development of serious joint problems. Patients who are overweight are put on a weight-losing program. Oddly enough, attacks of gout are not unusual during this very program.

692

Gout

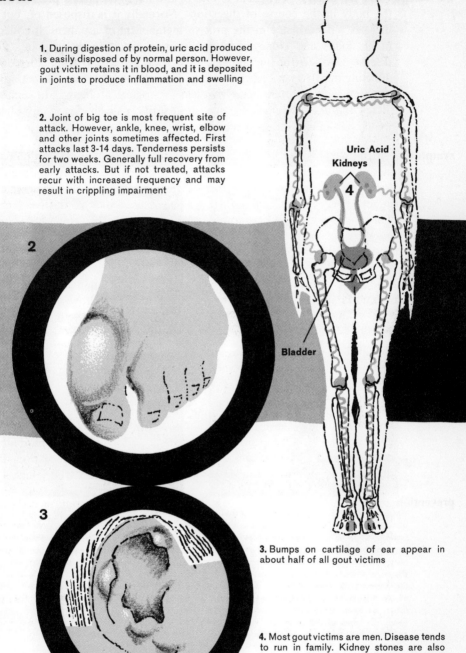

1. During digestion of protein, uric acid produced is easily disposed of by normal person. However, gout victim retains it in blood, and it is deposited in joints to produce inflammation and swelling

2. Joint of big toe is most frequent site of attack. However, ankle, knee, wrist, elbow and other joints sometimes affected. First attacks last 3-14 days. Tenderness persists for two weeks. Generally full recovery from early attacks. But if not treated, attacks recur with increased frequency and may result in crippling impairment

Uric Acid
Kidneys

Bladder

3. Bumps on cartilage of ear appear in about half of all gout victims

4. Most gout victims are men. Disease tends to run in family. Kidney stones are also frequently formed as result of gout attack

693

(A)

(B)

(C)

(D)

(E)

(F)

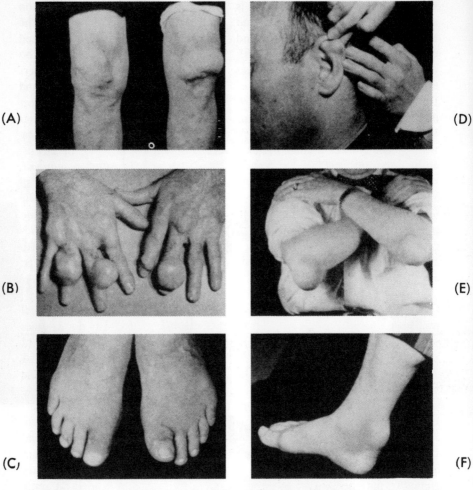

Gout—(A) Gout is a common joint-disabling disease. It affects the extremities and causes redness, swelling and pain. In acute attacks, pain can be excruciating. Lumps or deposits of white material (*tophi*) in the joints indicate presence of gout. Here deposits are shown on the kneecap. (B) Large deposits in the tissue of the fingers causing swelling of the joints. Gout has been present in this patient for 27 years. (C) Tophi of the great toe. Most people get their first attack of gout in the great toe. Gout which begins in some other part of the body eventually involves the great toe. (D) Tophi appear late in the disease, and not all patients with gout develop deposits. This man has a lump in the cartilage of the ear. (E) Deposits on the elbow. The joint is swollen, red and very tender. Pain can be felt simply by touching the area. (F) Tophi of the foot, affecting the heel area and the great toe. In the absence of tophi, gout can be diagnosed by x-ray and laboratory tests.

around the genitals and is thought to be caused by a microorganism. There are usually several thousand cases of granuloma inguinale in the United States and it is associated with uncleanliness.

Following exposure, the disease becomes noticeable one to four weeks later. The first symptom is swelling, usually in the groin, and this swollen area then ruptures and ulcers form. As the ulcers heal, new ulcers continue to appear, and the disease may eventually cover the reproductive organs, lower abdomen and buttocks. These lesions have an unpleasant odor. A person with granuloma inguinale apparently develops little immunity and may have the condition for many years. *Streptomycin* and *terramycin* have both proved successful in treatment of the disease. *See also* CHANCROID; LYMPHOGRANULOMA VENEREUM; GONORRHEA; SYPHILIS. *See* MEDIGRAPH page 1311.

GRAVES' DISEASE, another name for *exophthalmic goiter. See* EXOPHTHALMIC GOITER; GOITER. *See* MEDIGRAPH page 769.

GRIPPE. *See* INFLUENZA.

GUMS, mucous membranes which cover the margin of the jaw and surround the roots of the teeth. Inflammation of the gum, known as *gingivitis,* may be general as in *stomatitis* of the mouth or local as in the area of an infected tooth.

Pyorrhea is the most common and serious purulent infection of the gums. Gums are sensitive and bleed easily, especially when brushed too vigorously, and in certain disorders like *scurvy* they become soft and spongy. The gums are also subject to *tumors* and *alveolar abscesses* which are deep-seated infections. Suppuration of the gum, or ulceration with pus, is called a *gumboil.* Attention by a dental surgeon will prevent permanent scars of the cheek or neck if the infection spreads. After eliminating the infection, the offending tooth or teeth must be treated. *See also* GINGIVITIS; PYORRHEA; TEETH.

GYNECOLOGY, the medical science concerned with the diseases of women, particularly those of the organs related to childbirth. A gynecologist is a specialist in these diseases.

GYNECOMASTIA, (derived form two words meaning women and breasts), a condition of enlargement of the breasts which affects males only. It is usually related to some glandular disturbance. Excessive enlargement may be surgically treated.

H

HABIT SPASM, or *tic*, the habitual and involuntary contraction of a muscle. Habit spasms occur most frequently in the face, perhaps because the facial muscles are remarkably flexible especially when stimulated by emotions. So minute and lively are some of the facial muscles that often their habit spasms are visible only to trained observers. The tiny muscles close to the eye are particularly susceptible to these spasms.

Parents or teachers sometimes mistake a habit spasm for a symptom of *St. Vitus' dance*. The difference between the two, however, is easily defined. Habit spasms are *predictable* and always occur in the same manner; whereas the spasms seen in St. Vitus' dance are *varied* and therefore *unpredictable*.

Habit spasms can be treated effectively only after the cause has been ascertained by expert study. If the cause is physical, the cure may also be physical, via medication or surgery or perhaps merely by the adjustment of eyeglasses. Frequently, however, the cause is emotional. A habit spasm in a child might be traced, for example, to chronic fear of punishment, and the parents might find it desirable to secure psychotherapy for the child. *See* CHOREA; CONVULSION; TIC DOULOUREUX.

HAIR, slender threadlike outgrowths from follicles in the skin.

Structure. The hair root is that part of a hair beneath the surface of the skin. The *sebaceous glands* have their openings in the hair follicles and secrete *sebum* which gives the skin and scalp its oily appearance. The color of the hair is due to the presence of *pigment cells*. Attached to the follicles are tiny muscles which erect the follicle and incidentally the hair. These operate in excitement, when the hair "stands on end," or in chills, when "goose pimples" appear.

Growth. Hair grows at a regular rate in the average person of about an inch in six weeks. Then the follicle rests for a period varying from a few weeks to as much as ten or eleven weeks. The hair of the head, except in baldness, has an almost continuous activity of the follicles, each hair being replaced almost as soon as it reaches its full length.

Several different kinds of hair grow on the body. The hair on the scalp varies considerably, both as to the number of hairs and the length to which they grow. About 125,000 hairs grow on the scalp of the average person. The average length to which a hair will grow on a woman is sixty to seventy centimeters or about twenty-five inches, and it takes about four years to reach that length. Hair that is cylindrical hangs straight from the head and oval hair becomes curly.

The total number of hairs in each eyebrow is around 600 and such hair lasts about 112 days. As people become older the eyebrows tend to curl and grow longer so that they have to be trimmed. The hair of the eyelashes is practically identical with that of the eyebrows except that it is slightly more curved. The average diameter of the hair of the beard increases throughout life, so that these hairs become coarser and more bristling in advanced years. The beard is usually scanty among the more darkly pigmented races. Sexual differences are involved in the distribution of hair on the rest of the body.

Baldness. Alopecia or baldness involves temporary loss of hair due to various causes, or permanent loss of hair due to hereditary causes. *Temporary* falling out of hair may result from an infection or be related to certain diseases like *typhoid, scarlet fever, pneumonia* and other serious infections of the respiratory tract. In such cases, the hair may fall out suddenly, but will be replaced in time without special treatment. Falling hair may be related to excessive activity of the oil glands of the hair.

Hereditary baldness is influenced by sex-limited characteristics. Such baldness is inherited principally through the male as a dominant characteristic, and it is recessive in the female, tending to disappear if it occurs. Not only the baldness but the type of baldness is inherited. Once hereditary baldness appears, little can be done to prevent its development. Possibly the falling of hair in a hereditary case may be delayed somewhat by treatment, but even this is uncertain. Some anthropologists have speculated that the predominating tendency of the human race is toward a complete disappearance of hair from the body and head, and that such a total disappearance is likely to evolve within the next hundred thousand years (assuming man as a species survives that long). Already, the Oriental races, who constitute more than half of all mankind, are largely free of body hair.

Care of the hair. The hair should be washed often enough to keep it clean—usually once a week. For most hair any good toilet soap that will lather freely is satisfactory. After the hair has been washed with soap and water it should be rinsed thoroughly and dried fairly slowly rather than with a hot blower. If the hair is too dry a small amount of oil may be rubbed into it after it has been washed and dried.

All authorities agree that singeing the hair does not accomplish anything for hair health. When the body is in ill health, the hair is likely to react accordingly. Frequently good health and a good state of the skin and hair seem to be related.

The problem of gray or white hair cannot be readily solved. Vitamins or other substances taken internally do not substantially prevent or delay the appearance of gray hair in families in which there is a tendency to early graying. Experts can successfully dye hair. Some people, however, are particularly sensitive to *paraphenylendiamine,* which is an ingredient of many hair dyes, and a careful hairdresser will test the surface of the skin to the reaction of this chemical before using a dye containing it.

Sure methods for growing hair by artificial stimulation are unknown.

Superfluous hair. Hypertrichosis is the scientific name for excessive hairiness. Superfluous hair is not a worry to most men, but it may be a serious problem for a woman.

Expert opinion inclines to the view that the endocrine glands have a definite relationship to excessive growth of hair, particularly on the upper lip and chin of women. Certain forms of overgrowth of glands may be associated with excessive growth of hair. In women this is more likely to occur after they have

passed the menopause. If a young girl has a fine mustache, the matter can be lightly regarded unless the mustache is too dark in color.

For removal of superfluous hair three different methods are known. The safest and the only one generally recommended is the use of the electric needle. This requires patience and endurance both on the part of the woman undergoing the treatment and the doctor. In this process a needle or wire carrying the current is inserted into the hair follicle and a weak current turned on for a brief time. Only from ten to fifteen hairs may be removed in a single session. Since there may be 1200 to 1500 hairs on the upper lip, the time involved is a major consideration. Even with the best operators, from 10 to 50 per cent of the hairs that are removed recur, depending on the efficacy of the electric current in destroying the hair follicles.

Most experts warn against removal of superfluous hair by x-ray. The results are so uncertain and the possibilities of harm so great that this method should not be used except in extreme cases. A dosage of x-ray sufficient to cause the hair to fall out is likely also to produce permanent damage to the skin.

Temporary measures for relief from excess hair are shaving, rubbing with pumice stone, application of depilatory waxes, which harden and are pulled off, taking the hair with them, and other methods. Hydrogen peroxide is sometimes used to bleach the hair so that it is not so visible. *See also* BALDNESS; CRAB

LICE; DEPILATORY; SEBORRHEA; HYPERTRICHOSIS; SKIN. *See* MEDI-GRAPHS pages 1171, 1331.

HAIR REMOVER. *See* DEPILATORY.

HALITOSIS, the scientific name for *bad breath*. The cause may be tooth decay; or an infection of tissue in the mouth, tonsils, or nose; or chronic intestinal disturbances. Certain foods and seasonings, such as garlic, leave a temporary smell on the breath.

Mouthwashes cannot cure halitosis. Professional medical or dental treatment of the basic cause may be required. Teeth should be examined by a dentist every six months. Daily care of the teeth includes regular brushing every morning and evening with a good brush and whatever paste, powder, or solution the person prefers, and the use of dental floss.

When tonsils are infected or the tonsil cavities are filled with food particles, they may produce an unpleasant odor. Tonsils may be cleansed by a doctor and sometimes gargling helps, but surgical removal of tonsils is often the only effective way to combat the problem. Nose infections which may cause halitosis should be treated by a doctor. This may involve special washing.

Some foods, such as garlic, affect the odor of the breath directly from the stomach even when none remains in the mouth or teeth. In this case, flavored oils or mouthwashes may help mask the odor. Substances containing chlorophyll have been tried as antihalitosis agents, but evidence indicates that they do not and cannot prevent mouth odor.

HALLUCINATION, an impression, involving any of the five senses of sight, smell, taste, touch, or hearing, without actual basis in fact. Hallucinations occur frequently in alcoholic delirium, when the victim thinks he sees, for example, rats or snakes. Victims of paranoia often claim to hear voices.

HAND-SCHULLER-CHRISTIAN DISEASE, a rare disease, named for the three medical scientists who first described it, which occurs chiefly in children and young adults. Deposits of cholesterol appear in the bones and subcutaneous tissues with consequent disturbance of the metabolism. Growth and development are retarded and other symptoms usually appear, such as bulging of the eyes, a tendency to develop *diabetes insipidus,* and defects in the formation of the skull.

Direct application of x-ray has been the only effective form of therapy for this condition. Although complete cures have been effected, about a third of the cases terminate fatally.

HANSEN'S DISEASE. *See* LEPROSY.

HARDENING OF THE ARTERIES. *See* ARTERIOSCLEROSIS.

HARELIP, a cleft or clefts in the upper lip, so-called because of its resemblance to a hare's lip. *See also* CLEFT PALATE; LIPS.